BIOTECHNOLOGY
INTELLIGENCE
UNIT

Molecular Imprinting of Polymers

Sergey Piletsky, Ph.D.

Institute of BioScience and Technology
Cranfield University
Silsoe, Bedfordshire, U.K.

Anthony Turner, Ph.D., D.Sc.

Institute of BioScience and Technology
Cranfield University
Silsoe, Bedfordshire, U.K.

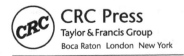

CRC Press
Taylor & Francis Group
Boca Raton London New York

CRC Press is an imprint of the
Taylor & Francis Group, an **informa** business

MOLECULAR IMPRINTING OF POLYMERS

Biotechnology Intelligence Unit

First published 2006 by Landes Bioscience

Published 2018 by CRC Press
Taylor & Francis Group
6000 Broken Sound Parkway NW, Suite 300
Boca Raton, FL 33487-2742

© 2006 by Taylor & Francis Group, LLC
CRC Press is an imprint of Taylor & Francis Group, an Informa business

First issued in paperback 2019

No claim to original U.S. Government works

ISBN 13: 978-0-367-44634-5 (pbk)
ISBN 13: 978-1-58706-219-3 (hbk)

Visit the Taylor & Francis Web site at
http://www.taylorandfrancis.com

and the CRC Press Web site at
http://www.crcpress.com

While the authors, editors and publisher believe that drug selection and dosage and the specifications and usage of equipment and devices, as set forth in this book, are in accord with current recommendations and practice at the time of publication, they make no warranty, expressed or implied, with respect to material described in this book. In view of the ongoing research, equipment development, changes in governmental regulations and the rapid accumulation of information relating to the biomedical sciences, the reader is urged to carefully review and evaluate the information provided herein.

Library of Congress Cataloging-in-Publication Data

Molecular imprinting of polymers / [edited by] Sergey Piletsky, Anthony
   Turner.
      p. ; cm. -- (Biotechnology intelligence unit)
   Includes bibliographical references.
      ISBN 1-58706-219-4
      1. Molecular imprinting. 2. Polymers--Biotechnology.   I. Piletsky,
Sergey. II. Turner, Anthony P. F. III. Series: Biotechnology intelligence
unit (Unnumbered)
      [DNLM: 1. Polymers--chemistry.   QD 382.I43 M718 2006]
   QD382.I43M6517 2006
      660.6'3--dc22

                                    2006008950

CONTENTS

Preface xi

1. **MIP Formats for Analytical Applications** 1
   Natalia Pérez-Moral and Andrew G. Mayes
   Particles 1
   Films 6
   Other Formats 6
   MIP Microstructures 7

2. **Bioimprinting** 12
   Claudio Baggiani and Cristina Giovannoli
   What Bioimprinting Is and How It Works 13
   How to Obtain a Bioimprinted Protein 14
   Properties of Bioimprinted Proteins 17
   Interfacial Bioimprinting 19
   Cross-Linking of Bioimprinted Proteins 21
   Bioimprinted Polysaccharides 22

3. **The Re-Birth of Molecular Imprinting on Silica** 26
   Naonobu Katada and Miki Niwa
   Pioneering Works between 1930s-50s 26
   The Long Winter of the 1960s-1970s 27
   The Re-Birth of Silica Imprinting with Advanced Technologies 30

4. **Chemical Vapor Deposition of Silica Overlayer Using an Organic
   Molecule as Template on Metal Oxide Surface:
   Application to Molecular Sieving Sensor and Adsorbent** 41
   Naonobu Katada and Miki Niwa
   Shape Selective Adsorption 43
   Oxidation Catalysis and Sensing Property 45

5. **Molecularly Imprinted Polymers for Mass Sensitive Sensors:
   From Cells to Viruses and Enzymes** 50
   Franz L. Dickert, Peter A. Lieberzeit and Oliver Hayden
   Principles of Chemical Sensing 51
   Surface Imprinting with Bioanalytes 52

6. **A New Generation of Chemical Sensors Based on MIPs** 64
   Sergey Piletsky and Anthony Turner
   Biosensors 64
   Molecular Imprinting—Introduction 65
   MIP Design 66
   Polymer-Detector Integration 66
   Principal Types of MIP Sensors 67
   MIP Based Affinity Sensors 67

Receptor Sensors 70
Catalytic Sensors Based on MIPs 73
Niche Areas for Application of MIP Sensors 74

7. **Molecularly Imprinted Membranes** **80**
   Mathias Ulbricht
   Membranes and Membrane Technology 81
   Molecularly Imprinted Membranes (MIM) 85

8. **Recognition of Enantiomers Using Molecularly**
   Imprinted Polymers **95**
   Börje Sellergren
   Enantiomers as Model Templates 96
   Use of Enantiomers as Templates to Mimic Natural Binding Sites 100
   Binding Isotherms and Model Fitting 101
   Approaches to Binding Site Design 106
   Combinatorial and Computational Techniques
      to Optimizing MICSPs 106
   MICSPs by Rational Design 107
   MICSPs in Other Formats: Beads, Monoliths and Films 110
   Beads and Nanoparticles 110
   Layers and Films 112
   Superporous Monoliths 115
   Hierarchical Imprinting Techniques 115
   Other Matrices for Imprinting of Enantiomers 116

9. **MIP Catalysts: From Theory to Practice** **122**
   Michael J. Whitcombe
   Transition State Theory 122
   Catalytic MIPs 125
   MIPs as Adjuncts to Synthesis 133

10. **Solid-Phase Extraction on Molecularly Imprinted Polymers:**
    Requirements, Achievements and Future Work **140**
    Lars I. Andersson
    Preparation of Imprinted SPE Sorbents 141
    Development of a Mispe Method 143
    Solid-Phase Extraction Applications 145

11. **Imprinted Polymers in Capillary Electrophoresis**
    and Capillary Electrochromatography **149**
    Alessandra Bossi, Pier Giorgio Righetti and Staffan Nilsson
    The Separation in Capillary Electrophoresis
       and in Capillary Electrochromatography 150
    Column Derivatization Chemistry 153
    The Traditional, Bulk Polymer Approach 154
    Packed Columns 155

Polymer Technology for MIP-CEC 157
Superporous MIP and the Hydrodynamic Pressure 157
MIP Nanoparticles 158
Advantages and Disadvantages of MIP-CEC Separations 158
Applications 159

12. **Molecularly Imprinted Polymers in Drug Screening** 164
    Chris Allender
    The Drug Discovery Process 164
    Molecular Imprinting and Drug Screening 170
    Molecularly Imprinted Receptor Mimics and Drug Screening 179

13. **MIPs in Biotechnology, Perspective and Reality** 182
    David A. Spivak
    Bioactive Pharmaceuticals 182
    Screening Combinatorial Drug Libraries 184
    Bio-(Mimetic)-Sensors 185
    Biocatalysis 186
    Bioimprinting 187
    Bioseparations and Bioassays 188
    Conclusions: Present and Future Role of MIPs in Biotechnology 189

14. **Business Models for the Commercialisation of MIPs** 191
    Peter Leverkus
    Why Commercialise? 191
    Issues in Commercialising Technologies 192
    Challenges and Opportunities for MIPs 194
    From Track Record to Turnover 197
    The Commercial Future for MIPs 198

15. **A General Survey of Patents in the Field of Molecularly
    Imprinted Polymers** 199
    Jeffrey B. McIntyre
    Patents—Generally 199
    Patents/Patent Applications Related to Molecularly
       Imprinted Polymers 200
    Polymers 201
    Methods of Making Polymers 201
    Methods of Using Polymers 203

Index 205

EDITORS

Sergey Piletsky
Institute of BioScience and Technology
Cranfield University
Silsoe, Bedfordshire, U.K.
Email: s.piletsky@cranfield.ac.uk
Chapter 6

Anthony Turner
Institute of BioScience and Technology
Cranfield University
Silsoe, Bedfordshire, U.K.
Email: a.p.f.turner@cranfield.ac.uk
Chapter 6

CONTRIBUTORS

Chris Allender
Welsh School of Pharmacy
Cardiff University
Cardiff, U.K.
Email: allendercj@cf.ac.uk
Chapter 12

Lars I. Andersson
Research DMPK
AstraZeneca R&D Södertälje
Södertälje, Sweden
Email: Lars.i.andersson@astrazeneca.com
Chapter 10

Claudio Baggiani
Dipartimento di Chimica Analitica
Università di Torino
Torino, Italy
Email: claudio.baggiani@unito.it
Chapter 2

Alessandra Bossi
Dipartimento Scientifico e Tecnologico
University of Verona
Verona, Italy
Email: bossi@sci.univr.it
Chapter 11

Franz L. Dickert
Institute of Analytical Chemistry
Vienna University
Vienna, Austria
Email: Franz.Dickert@univie.ac.at
Chapter 5

Cristina Giovannoli
Dipartimento di Chimica Analitica
Università di Torino
Torino, Italy
Chapter 2

Oliver Hayden
Institute of Analytical Chemistry
Vienna University
Vienna, Austria
Chapter 5

Naonobu Katada
Department of Materials Science
Faculty of Engineering
Tottori University
and
Conversion and Control
  by Advanced Chemistry
PRESTO
Japan Science and Technology
  Corporation (JST)
Tottori, Japan
Email: katada@chem.tottori-u.ac.jp
Chapters 3, 4

Peter Leverkus
Department of Technology Transfer
Cranfield Creates
Cranfield University
Cranfield, Bedfordshire, U.K.
Email: p.leverkus@cranfield.ac.uk
Chapter 14

Peter A. Lieberzeit
Institute of Analytical Chemistry
Vienna University
Vienna, Austria
Chapter 5

Andrew G. Mayes
School of Chemical Sciences
  and Pharmacy
University of East Anglia
Norwich, U.K.
Email: andrew.mayes@uea.ac.uk
Chapter 1

Jeffrey B. McIntyre
Oblon, Spivak, McClelland,
  Maier and Neustadt
Alexandria, Virginia, U.S.A.
Email: JMCINTYRE@oblon.com
Chapter 15

Staffan Nilsson
Technical Analytical Chemistry
Center for Chemistry
  and Chemical Engineering
Lund University
Lund, Sweden
Email: staffan.nilsson@teknlk.lth.se
Chapter 11

Miki Niwa
Department of Materials Science
Faculty of Engineering
Tottori University
and
Conversion and Control
  by Advanced Chemistry
PRESTO
Japan Science and Technology
  Corporation (JST)
Tottori, Japan
Chapters 3, 4

Natalia Pérez-Moral
School of Chemical Sciences
  and Pharmacy
University of East Anglia
Norwich, U.K.
Chapter 1

Pier Giorgio Righetti
Dipartimento Scientifico e Tecnologico
University of Verona
Verona, Italy
Email: bossi@sci.univr.it
Chapter 11

Börje Sellergren
INFU
University of Dortmund
Dortmund, Germany
Email: borje@infu.uni-dortmund.de
Chapter 8

David A. Spivak
Department of Chemistry
Louisiana State University
Baton Rouge, Lousiana, U.S.A.
Email: David_Spivak@chem.lsu.edu
Chapter 13

Michael J. Whitcombe
Institute of Food Research
Norwich Research Park, Colney
Norwich, U.K.
Email: Michael.whitcombe@bbsrc.ac.uk
Chapter 9

Mathias Ulbricht
Lehrstuhl für Technische Chemie II
Universität Duisburg-Essen
Essen, Germany
Email: mathias.ulbricht@uni-essen.de
Chapter 7

PREFACE

Molecularly Imprinted Polymers:
A Collective Vision

One of Nature's most important talents is evolutionary development of systems capable of molecular recognition: distinguishing one molecule from another. Molecular recognition is the basis for most biological processes, such as ligand-receptor binding, substrate-enzyme reactions and translation and transcription of the genetic code and is therefore of universal interest. Over the past four decades, researchers have been inspired by Nature to produce biomimetic materials with molecular recognition properties, by design rather than by evolution. A particularly exciting area of biomimetics is *Molecular Imprinting* which can be defined as process of template-induced formation of specific recognition sites (binding or catalytic) in a material where the template directs the positioning and orientation of the material's structural components by a self-assembling mechanism. The material itself could be oligomeric (the typical example is DNA replication process), polymeric (organic MIPs and inorganic imprinted silica gels) or 2-dimensional surface assembly (grafted monolayers: see Scheme 1 below).

The first work on molecular imprinting was published in 1931. Since then this technology has had its "ups" and "downs" with one boom in the sixties (with a major focus on silica imprinting) and a newer period of intensive development which started in 1972 and continues today.

Essentially the current progress is a result of fundamental achievements made by more than a hundred groups working in the areas of non-covalent and reversible covalent imprinting. We believe that the time is now ripe to capture this momentum and publish a new book which will reflect the current situation in this rapidly evolving technology. We are well aware that tens of reviews have been published already on this subject. Very few of them, however, present a critical analysis of the technological aspects of molecular imprinting. We have approached leaders in the field with requests to provide their view and analysis of specific areas of design, characterization and application of these polymers.

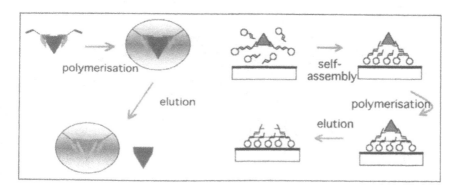

Scheme 1. Three- and two-dimensional imprinting polymerisation (courtesy of VTT, Finland).

The main body of the present book starts with chapters covering polymer design, synthesis and characterization are prepared by well-recognized experts such as Andrew Mayes and Natalia Perez-Moral, Claudio Baggiani, Naonobu Katada and Miki Niwa and Franz Dickert. The key part of the book, dedicated to MIP technology is prepared by MIP pioneers and practitioners who are now at the forefront of the practical application of MIPs: Lars Andersson, Mathias Ulbricht, Borje Sellergren, Michael Whitcombe, Alessandra Bossi, Pier Giorgio Righetti and Staffan Nilsson, Chris Allender, David Spivak, and ourselves. The last but by no means least part of the book is dedicated to often overlooked associated aspects of MIPs such as commercialization strategy and IPR, prepared by Peter Leverkus and Jeffrey McIntyre.

We appreciate very much the enthusiasm of our contributors who kindly volunteered to share their ideas with our readers and spent countless hours in preparing their comprehensive reviews of the field. We are also grateful to the readers of this work who will hopefully find it useful for expanding their knowledge of our favorite area of molecular imprinting. Perhaps some of you will use the accumulated knowledge and collective vision of our contributing authors to help commercialize MIP technology and realise some of the fantastic new products which will make our life more comfortable, richer and safer.

Sincerely,
Sergey and Tony

CHAPTER 1

MIP Formats for Analytical Applications

Natalia Pérez-Moral and Andrew G. Mayes

Abstract

As MIPs make the gradual transition from the academic research laboratory to application areas, it is essential that the MIP is designed, both chemically and structurally, to optimise its performance in that particular application. The optimisation of the chemical design is discussed elsewhere in this volume. In this review, progress in the development of methods for the synthesis of MIPs in controlled and predefined forms is presented. Such methods allow the structural form of the polymer to be selected based on the most desirable properties of the material for the application under consideration. Methods to make MIPs in the form of size-defined spherical particles (at the micro or nano scale), monoliths, films (both thick and thin) and moulded microstructures have all been published in the last few years and are summarised here. It should be noted that the synthetic conditions required to form a specific type of polymer structure are not necessarily compatible with the conditions required for optimal imprinting of the template. All of the methods discussed, however, have been shown to have utility in at least one area of imprinting.

Until recently, most molecularly imprinted polymers have been obtained by bulk polymerisation in the form of a block or monolith and then ground and sieved to generate particles of approximately 10-20 μm before being used. This method, although simple, convenient and reliable, does not allow control of the process and produces highly irregular particles with a loss of up to 80% of the material. Also, some (or most) of the imprinted sites may be located inside the bulk of the polymeric matrix and therefore be inaccessible to some or all of the desired analyte molecules. To improve the design of MIPs for new applications, new formats have been developed.

The format in which the polymer is obtained is very important and will determine to a great extent the application for which the MIP will be suitable. Some applications require specific morphologies and properties, such as micron size beads for more efficient packing into chromatographic columns or SPE cartridges, colloidal particles suspended in solution for binding assays, or films or membranes for coating of sensor devices. In this review, different procedures for producing MIPs in defined formats are considered.

Particles

One of the areas that has attracted considerable interest is the polymerisation of MIPs in the form of spherical particles. Polymeric beads can be obtained by different heterogeneous polymerisation procedures, where the product is a 2-phase system in the form of a fine dispersion of spherical polymer particles in a defined size range. There are methods described in the literature to synthesise polymeric particles in almost any range of sizes, but due to the specific requirements of MIP technology, not all are suitable. Issues like the degree of crosslinking required for receptor formation or the need to maximise the strength of particular types of interactions, means that only a carefully selected subset of the available methods has so far

Molecular Imprinting of Polymers, edited by Sergey Piletsky and Anthony Turner.
©2006 Landes Bioscience.

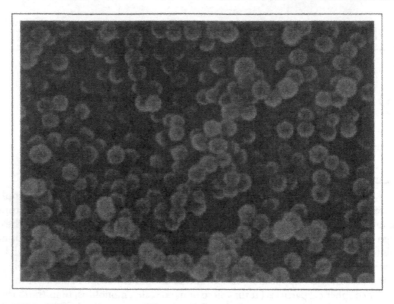

Figure 1. SEM of MIP particles prepared by precipitation polymerisation (15000 x magnification). Reprinted in part with permission from Macromolecules 2000; 33(22):8239-8245 ©2000 American Chemical Society.[6]

proved successful for MIP production, although new systems are continuously being developed. Those that have been successfully applied to date are discussed in more detail below.

Nanoparticles

The first imprinted nanoparticles were reported[1] to recognise metallic Cu(II) at the surface of particles by establishing a complex between a trapped surfactant molecule and an ion template. Similar methods used swelling of particles previously synthesised by emulsion polymerisation to establish a complexation of the metal ion with carboxylic groups from the fuctional particle,[2] or a carboxylic polymeric surfactant bound to the surface of the particles that had a dual role as a ligand to bind metal ions as well as an emulsifier.[3] The final diameter of the particles synthesised to complex metal ions ranged from 0.4 μm to 0.16 mm.

In the submicron scale, MIP nanoparticles for organic templates have been synthesised as organic polymers and on to inorganic silica particles. Ye et al[4] produced imprinted particles with an average diameter of 300 nm by precipitation polymerisation where coagulation is prevented by the rigidity of the crosslinked surfaces (Fig. 1). The polymer grows from a homogeneous solution into insoluble polymeric particles that precipitate once they reach a critical size and are no longer stable in the medium where they grow. This is a simple and fast method that does not need any further steps other than removal of the template before the polymer can be used, but its main limitation is the high dilution of the systems (required to prevent aggregation before the particles have rigidified) that requires higher amounts of solvents and template molecules. The typical ratio of template molecule to functional monomer is from 1:1.3 to 1:5 (in mole). In a new application[5] a UV fluorescent scintillation monomer was incorporated in the composition of the polymer, which allowed the detection of a radiolabelled ligand bound to the imprinted polymer by proximity scintillation counting, without the need for a separation step to remove the unbound ligand. Scintillation proximity assay is an intrinsically inefficient process, however, and further optimisation of scintillant and polymer composition/morphology is required if this application is to become viable as a research tool or an assay technology.

Very small imprinted spherical particles have also been prepared by seeded emulsion polymerisation. Pérez et al[7] synthesised core-shell particles in an oil-in-water system where the

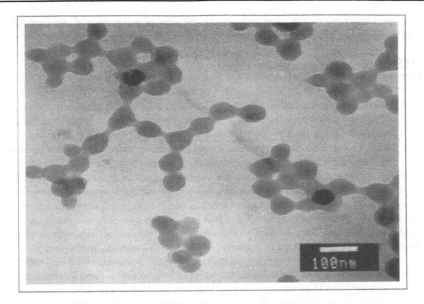

Figure 2. TEM of imprinted core-shell nanoparticles prepared by emulsion polymerisation.

polymerised shell was imprinted with cholesterol using the sacrificial spacer method. The final monodisperse particles had a diameter of 76 nm with a surface area of 82 m^2 g^{-1}. Following the same procedure, imprinted shells were also prepared over superparamagnetic cores with very similar binding properties and with the advantage that they could be sedimented from solution in less than 30 seconds in a magnetic field. This approach was also developed to prepare surface-imprinted particles in the shell of core-shell nanoparticles.[8] In this case, in the second stage of the polymerisation the shell was imprinted with a molecule that can work both as a template and a surfactant, placing itself at the interface of the particle and the aqueous medium, and therefore creating all the binding sites at the surface. The hydrophilicity at the surface of the particle was also regulated with the incorporation of a polymerisable surfactant that formed a hydrophobic surface covered by long chained sulphate groups that, if required, could be hydrolysed to create a hydrophilic surface in the particles covered with short chained alcohols. The position of the imprinted sites at the surface of the polymeric beads was proved by their ability to flocculate when they were in the presence of a multiligand template, like PEG-bis-cholesterol. A range of agglutination-type assays can be envisaged based on this approach. The imprinting of core-shell particles has also been successfully tested for production of receptors by noncovalent imprinting using hydrogen-bonding and ion-pair interactions[9] in aqueous emulsion systems. In this procedure, since the particles are only imprinted in the outer shell, the imprinted sites should have better accessibility for molecules such as template-tagged enzymes that would be used in competitive assay formats. The core-shell structure also allows extra properties such as magnetism or fluorescence to be incorporated into the core, giving many additional opportunities for assay development[9,10] (see Fig. 2).

Miniemulsion polymerisation is another method used to prepare imprinted nanospheres.[11,12] Using this technique a relatively polydisperse distribution of particles with diameters between 50-300 nm were imprinted and characterised. These nanoparticles were subsequently used to prepare a selective membrane by coating the MIP onto the surface of a membrane disc.

In silica particles, Markowitz et al developed a template-directed imprinting procedure in the surface of the silica by using a transition-state analogue acting as both the template and the head group of a surfactant molecule in a synthesis carried out by microemulsion polymerisation.[13] Also, in a more general approach, they prepared imprinted small sized silica particles where, since no grinding process was used, only imprinted sites at the surface of the particles were accessible. The effect of different functional silanes[14] on this process was studied.

Microparticles

Sometimes particles with a larger size are required. Depending on whether the particles are synthesised in an aqueous or organic medium, imprinted micron-sized beaded polymers can be prepared by a two-step procedure or by suspension, dispersion or precipitation polymerisation.

The difference between dispersion and precipitation polymerisation is based on the solubility of the monomer in the growing polymer and the loci of polymerisation. The first example of the imprinting technology applied to micron sized globular particles was reported by Sellergren et al in 1994[15] where the influence of the solvent, template and monomer concentration on the morphology of the imprinted particles and their chromatographic evaluation was studied. Precipitation polymerization, on the other hand, has also be adjusted to prepare particles in the nano or micro domain, producing imprinted beads with better imprinting characteristics.[16]

As one of the best known methods for making micron size polymer beads, suspension polymerisation has also been applied to the synthesis of imprinted polymers. It is used to produce particles within the range of 3 micron -20 mm with a certain distribution of sizes. The monomer is insoluble in the polymerisation medium (usually aqueous) and is suspended in the form of small droplets before it is polymerised with the help of a stirrer and a suitable stabiliser. This approach was tested by various authors,[17-19] but so far it has not been further developed as a convenient procedure, probably due to the low specificity in the imprinting effect of the particles.

A few years ago, a new method that employed a liquid fluorocarbon as the continuous suspending phase was developed for use with imprinting methodology.[20] Fluorocarbons are inert solvents that allow the establishment of the interactions needed for the recognition of the template molecules without interfering with them. They are also immiscible with most monomers and solvents used in imprinting technology. Therefore, with the aid of a suitable surfactant, this method can produce imprinted polymeric beads in the range of 5-50 µm that show some of the best performances achieved to date for beaded polymers in rebinding experiments, both in organic and aqueous solvents.[21-23] Take up of this methodology for routine application has been slow, however, possibly due to a misconception that it is a complex procedure requiring reoptimisation for each new system (Fig. 3).

Aqueous 2-step swelling is another method that produces particles from 2 micron to more than 50 micron with a good control over the particle size. It was first employed to prepare imprinted polymers by Hosoya[24] and has subsequently been used by many other groups.[25,26] The procedure consists of the consecutive swelling of a small monodisperse polymeric seed with activating solvents and monomers until they reach the desired size, before the swollen particles are polymerised. Many templates have been imprinted by this method. The polymers generally show good rebinding properties, despite the aqueous dispersing phase present during polymerisation (Fig. 4).

Zimmerman et al[27,28] have recently reported a new way of polymerizing dendrimers with a covalently attached template (porphyrin) in the core of the monomers that ultimately crosslink by their end-groups. This approach produces nearly homogeneous sites and a complete removal of template after hydrolysis. It also offers the ability to make particles with one receptor cavity each, thus coming closer to mimicking natural protein receptors such as enzymes and antibodies

Another interesting method that also produced imprinted micron-sized beaded polymers is cationic aerosol polymerisation.[29] The beads obtained were polydisperse in terms of size with an average diameter of 31µm and showed only moderate levels of rebinding for noncovalent interactions (14-16%). It has the advantage that the polymerisation is continuous and very rapid, but certain common functionalities may interfere with the cationic polymerisation, thus limiting its applicability. This probably explains why the procedure has not been investigated further.

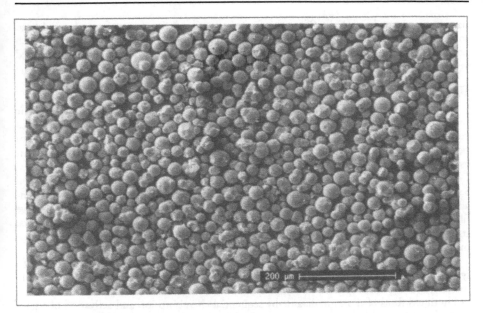

Figure 3. SEM of imprinted particles synthesised by suspension polymerisation (fluorocarbon solvent).

Finally, imprinted polymers in the form of particles can also be produced by immobilising the template in pores of a preformed silica bead and filling the pores with the imprinting mixture before polymerising. In the last step, the silica support is dissolved, leaving behind a polymer structure in a beaded format with the receptors situated on the surface of the polymer.[30] This surface localisation of the receptors has many interesting and useful advantages, though the method of preparation is quite complex. Also, in a similar way, imprinted polymers

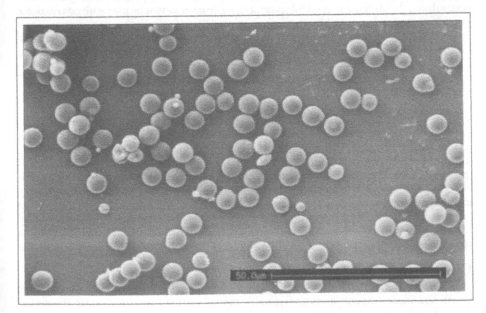

Figure 4. SEM of particles synthesised by aqueous 2-step swelling method.

have been prepared simply by filling the pores or coating the surfaces of a preformed bead made of silica or polymer.[31-34] This offers a simple route to beaded polymers, but the approach has probably been superseded by more direct synthetic methods that avoid the cost and wasted volume of the original bead.

Films

Another major area of interest concerning the formats and the applications of MIPs is the production of films or membranes. In the last years, a variety of approaches have been tested to control the synthesis of MIP in the format of films. Some of these include sandwiching, in-situ polymerisation, deposition on membranes, phase inversion precipitation, spin coating, solvent evaporation or grafting from or to a polymer or surface.

Briefly, sandwiching methods consist of trapping the necessary amount of solution between a surface that has been previously treated (e.g., with a methacryloyl silane) and a smooth non-adhesive surface such as a metallised film. After polymerisation, the layers are separated to leave films of 2-10 μm thick adhering to the silanised surface.[35-38] Although this method works, reproducibility can be a problem, as can film instability due to shrinkage and stresses introduced during polymerisation or subsequent evaporation of porogenic solvent.

Another method for preparing a MIP film coating an electrode was demonstrated by modifying a quartz crystal microbalance (QCM) electrode with a vinyl-terminated self assembly monolayer, and photo- or electro-polymerising the film in situ at the electrode.[39-43] Synthesis of imprinted films of titanium dioxide by sequential chemisorption and activation of a gold coated quartz crystal microbalance electrode has also been demonstrated.[44-46] Also, imprinted films on layers have been synthesised by polycondensation of urethanes.[47-49]

Composite membranes can be prepared by deposition of MIP layers onto the surface of a polymeric PVDF microfiltration membrane that has been precoated with a photoinitiator[50-52] or from an aqueous solution on polypropylene membranes.[53] Coating of imprinted nanoparticles between two membranes of polyamide that cover and support the film has also been reported.[12]

Phase Inversion Precipitation is another technique that can also be used to synthesise imprinted membranes. It requires spreading a liquid phase of the cast solution containing the imprinting mixture on a glass plate and coagulating the imprinted polymer membrane with a poor solvent.[54-56] As it involves soluble polymers, however, it cannot be used with conventional imprinting approaches in highly cross-linked polymers.

An alternative method for the preparation of imprinted membranes is based on a solubilised prepolymer that establishes the interactions between template and polymer while the polymer is adopting its final conformation.[57,58]

Other methods also employed to prepare films of MIPs include evaporation of solvent[59,60] polymerisation on a glass slide,[55,61,62] soft lithography[63] and spin coating.[64-66]

Finally, one of the most promising methods is the grafting of polymers "to" or "from" a support. Grafting imprinted polymers from a support can be achieved by firstly immobilising initiators on a surface and subsequently polymerising imprinted polymers from that point of attachment.[67-69,53,70] However, gelation and polymerisation in solution can occur and these sometimes are difficult to avoid. This problem has been solved by using initiators where one of the radicals formed by their decomposition is unable to initiate polymerisation but is capable of recombining and therefore terminating the growing polymers.[71,72] There is currently a lot of research activity in this general area, due to the technological importance of controlled surface architecture and surface properties, so it is likely that better understanding and control of such methods will emerge in the near future, though not all the initiation methods developed will be applicable to imprinting.

Other Formats

Hydrogels are insoluble crosslinked polymer network structures that have the ability to absorb significant amounts of water. Typically, normal hydrogels are very lightly crosslinked (0.1-3% mole per mole of monomer) and therefore not very appropriate for conventional imprinting technology, but so far a few groups have managed to revise the imprinting approach

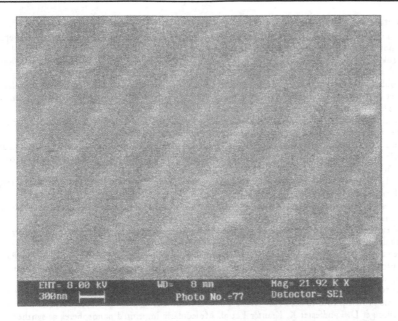

Figure 5. S.E.M. image of a diffraction grating moulded using a typical EDMA/MAA imprinting mixture. The mould was a gold-coated photoresist diffraction grating on a glass backing (rigid). The substrate was glass, pretreated with methacryloxypropyl trimethoxysilane (rigid). Mould release is facilitated if either the substrate or the mould is flexible, but for small amplitude structures such as this rigid moulds and substrates can also be separated easily

and still obtain specific recognition with lower percentage of crosslinking,[73] hence making it possible to combine this type of recognition with hydrogels.[74,75] Some attempts include the preparation of materials for stimuli-sensitive recognition,[76-80] their use as drug delivery devices[75,81] or using a prepolymer that binds the template molecule before being crosslinked into a MIP hydrogel.[74]

Biffis et al[82] tested a new approach by preparing highly crosslinked microgels (50-90%) by radical solution polymerisation in a range of solvents, but the imprinted polymers obtained exhibited low selectivities to date. This approach is interesting, however, since it generates polymer particles with similar sizes and general properties to proteins, so it truly represents an approach towards "soluble" MIPs that have truly "antibody-like" properties.

More formats also applied to MIP technology include: in situ polymerisation of MIP into stainless steel columns or silica capillaries[83-87] molecular imprinting in liquid crystalline polymers,[88] and surface imprinting using bifunctional molecules (emulsifier+functional host), obtaining a polymer in block that needs to be ground into particles of 30 μm.[89]

MIP Microstructures

With rapid progress in the field of microfabricated analytical systems, it seems likely that MIPs will find their way into such devices. This will require MIPs to be constructed on and in devices in the form of patterned structures, monoliths and surface coatings, using synthetic methods compatible with the manufacture of such devices. To date, there has been relatively little work in this area. Yan and Kapua[90] used silicone elastomer moulds to produce "micro-monoliths", though this approach is limited by solvent swelling of the elastomer mould. Pérez-Moral and Mayes[91] have circumvented this problem by using moulds made from aluminised polyester that had been embossed to produce a surface relief pattern. Using this approach features with dimensions below 100 nm can be reproduced, giving access to many types of surface structures (see Fig. 5).

References

1. Kido H, Miyajima T, Tsukagoshi K et al. Metal-ion complexation behavior of resins prepared by a novel template polymerization technique. Anal Sci 1992; 8(6):749-53.

2. Tsukagoshi K, Yu K, Maeda M et al. Metal ion-selective adsorbent prepared by surface-imprinting polymerization. Bull Chem Soc Jpn 1993; 66:114-20.

3. Koide Y, Senba H, Shosenji H et al. Selective adsorption of metal ions to surface-template resins prepared by emulsion polymerization using 10-(p- vinylphenyl)decanoic acid. Bull Chem Soc Jpn 1996; 69(1):125-30.

4. Ye L, Cormack PAG, Mosbach K. Molecularly imprinted monodisperse microspheres for competitive radioassay. Analytical Communications 1999; 36(2):35-38.

5. Ye L, Mosbach K. Polymers recognizing biomolecules based on a combination of molecular imprinting and proximity scintillation: A new sensor concept. J Amer Chem Soc 2001; 123(12):2901-02.

6. Ye L, Weiss R, Mosbach K. Synthesis and characterization of molecularly imprinted microspheres. Macromolecules 2000; 33(22):8239-45.

7. Perez N, Whitcombe MJ, Vulfson EN. Molecularly imprinted nanoparticles prepared by coreshell emulsion polymerization. J Appl Poly Sci 2000; 77(8):1851-59.

8. Pérez N, Whitcombe MJ, Vulfson EN. Surface imprinting of cholesterol on submicrometer coreshell emulsion particles. Macromolecules 2001; 34(4):830-36.

9. Pérez-Moral N, Mayes AG. Molecular imprinting of polymeric coreshell nanoparticles. Paper presented at: Molecularly Imprinted Materials-Sensors and other Devices; MRS Symposium Proceedings. 2002.

10. Carter SR, Rimmer S. Molecular recognition of caffeine by shell molecular imprinted coreshell particles in aqueous media. Adv Mater 2002; 14:667-70.

11. Vaihinger D, Landfester K, Krauter I et al. Molecularly imprinted nanospheres as synthetic affinity receptors obtained by miniemulsion polymerisation. Macromol Chem Phys 2002; 203:1965-73.

12. Lehmam M, Brunner H, Tovar GEM. Selective separations and hydrodynamic studies: A new approach using molecualrly imprinted nanosphere composite membranes. Desalination 2002; 149:315-21.

13. Markowitz MA, Kust PR, Deng G et al. Catalytic silica particles via template-directed molecular imprinting. Langmuir 2000; 16(4):1759-65.

14. Markowitz MA, Deng G, Gaber BP. Effects of added organosilanes on the formation and adsorption properties of silicates surface-imprinted with an organophosphonate. Langmuir 2000; 16(15):6148-55.

15. Sellergren B. Imprinted dispersion polymers - a new class of easily accessible affinity stationary phases. J Chromatogr A 1994; 673:133-41.

16. Ye L, Mosbach K. Molecularly imprinted microspheres as antibody binding mimics. Reactive & Functional Polymers 2001; 48:149-57.

17. Flores A, Cunliffe D, Whitcombe MJ et al. Imprinted polymers prepared by aqueous suspension polymerization. J Appl Poly Sci 2000; 77:1841-50.

18. Byström S, Börje A, Åkermark B. Selective reduction of steroid 3- and 17-Ketones using LiAlH$_4$ activated template polymers. J Am Chem Soc 1993; 115:2081-83.

19. Damen J, Neckers DC. Memory of synthesized vinyl polymers for their origins. J Organ Chem 1980; 45:1382-87.

20. Mayes A, Mosbach K. Molecularly imprinted beaded polymers: Suspension polymerisation using a perfluorocarbon liquid as the dispersing phase. Anal Chem 1996; 68:3769-3774..

21. Pérez-Moral N, Mayes AG. A comparative study of imprinted polymer particles prepared by different polynerisation methods. Analytica Chimica Acta 2004; 504:15-21.

22. Ansell R, Mosbach K. Molecularly imprinted polymers by suspension polymerisation in perfluorocarbon liquids, with emphasis on the influence of the porogenic solvent. J Chromatogr A 1997; 787:55-66.

23. Ansell R, Mosbach K. Magnetic Molecularly Imprinted Polymer Beads for Drug Radioligand Binding Assay. Analyst 1998; 123(7):1611-16.

24. Hosoya K, Yoshikazo K, Tanaka N et al. Uniform-size macroporous polymer-based stationary phase for hplc prepared through molecular imprinting technique. Chem Lett 1994; 1437-38.

25. Haginaka J, Sanbe H. Uniform-sized molecularly imprinted polymers for beta-estradiol. Chem Lett 1998; 1089-90.

26. Haginaka J, Sakai Y, Narimatsu S. Uniform-size molecularly imprinted polymer material for propanolol. Recognition of Propranolol and its Metabolites. Anal Sci 1998; 14(4):823-26.

27. Mertz E, Zimmerman SC. Cross-linked dendrimer hosts containing reporter groups for amine guests. J Am Chem Soc 2003; 125(12):3424-25.

28. Zimmerman SC, Wendland MS, Rakow NA et al. Synthetic hosts by monomolecular imprinting inside dendrimers. Nature 2002; 418:399-403.
29. Vorderbruggen MA, Wu K, Breneman CM. Use of cationic aerosol photopolymerization to form silicone microbeads in the presence of molecular templates. Chem Mater 1996; 8:1106-11.
30. Yilmaz E, Haupt K, Mosbach K. The use of immobilized templates - a new approach in molecular imprinting. Angew Chem Int Ed Engl 2000; 39:2115-18.
31. Wulff G, Oberkobusch D, Minarik M. Enzyme-analogue built polymers 18. Chiral cavities in polymer layers coated on wide-pore silica. Reactive Polymers 1985; 3:261-75.
32. Plunkett SD, Arnold FH. Molecularly imprinted polymers on silica - selective supports for high-performance ligand-exchange chromatography. J Chromatogr A 1995; 708:19-29.
33. Glad M, Reinholdsson P, Mosbach K. Molecularly imprinted composite polymers based on trimethylolpropane trimethacrylate (TRIM) Particles for efficient enantiomeric separations. Reactive Polymers 1995; 25:47-54.
34. Vidyasankar S, Ru M, Arnold FH. Molecularly imprinted ligand-exchange adsorbents for the chiral separation of underivatized aminoacids. J Chromatogr A 1997; 775:51-63.
35. Kugimiya A, Takeuchi T. Molecularly imprinted polymer-coated quartz crystal microbalance for detection of biological hormone. Electroanalysis 1999; 11:1158-60.
36. Hedborg E, Winquist F, Lundström I et al. Some studies of molecularly-imprinted polymer membranes in combination with field-effect devices. Sensors and Actuators A-Physical 1993; 37(8):796-99.
37. Jakusch M, Janotta M, Mizaikoff B et al. Molecularly imprinted polymers and infrared evanescent wave spectroscopy. A chemical sensors approach. Anal Chem 1999; 71(20):4786-91.
38. Haupt K, Noworyta K, Kutner W. Imprinted polymer-based enantioselective acoustic sensor using a quartz crystal microbalance. Analytical Communications 1999; 36(11-12):391-93.
39. Cao L, Zhou XC, Li SFY. Enantioselective sensor based on microgravimetric quartz crystal microbalance with molecularly imprinted polymer film. Analyst 2001; 126:184-88.
40. Malitesta C, Losito I, Zambonin PG. Molecularly imprinted electrosynthesized polymers: New materials for biomimetic sensors. Anal Chem 1999; 71(7):1366-70.
41. Panasyuk TL, Mirsky VM, Piletsky SA et al. Electropolymerized molecularly imprinted polymers as receptor layers in a capacitive chemical sensors. Anal Chem 1999; 71:4609-13.
42. Deore B, D ZDCZ, Nagaoka T. Potential-induced enantioselective uptake of amino acid into molecularly imprinted overoxidized polypyrrole. Anal Chem 2000; 72:3989-94.
43. Peng H, Liang CD, Zhou AH et al. Development of a new atropine sulfate bulk acoustic wave sensor based on a molecularly imprinted electrosynthesized copolymer of aniline with o-phenylenediamine. Analytica Chimica Acta 2000; 423:221-28.
44. Lahav M, Kharitonov AB, Willner I. Imprinting of chiral molecular recognition sites in thin TiO2 films associated with field-effecttransistors: Novel functionalized devices for chiroselective and chirospecific analyses. Chemistry-A European Journal 2001; 7:3992-97.
45. Lee S, Ichinose I, Kunitake T. Molecular imprinting of azobenzene carboxylic acid on a TiO2 ultrathin film by the surface sol-gel process. Langmuir 1998; 14(10):2857-63.
46. Lahav M, Kharitonov AB, Katz O et al. Tailored chemosensors for chloroaromatic acids using molecular imprinted TiO2 thin films on ion-sensitive field-effect transistors. Anal Chem 2001; 73:720-23.
47. Dickert FL, Tortschanoff M, Bulst WE et al. Molecularly imprinted sensor layers for the detection of polycyclic aromatic hydrocarbons in water. Anal Chem 1999; 71(20):4559-63.
48. Dickert FL, Besenbock H, Tortschanoff M. Molecular imprinting through van der Waals interactions: Fluorescence detection of PAHs in water. Adv Mater 1998; 10(2):149-52.
49. Dickert FL, Lieberzeit P, Torstschanoff M. Sens Actuator B 2000; 65:186-89.
50. Kochkodan V, Weigel W, Ulbricht M. Desalination 2002; 149:323-28.
51. Kochkodan V, Weigel W, Ulbricht M. Thin layer molecularly imprinted microfiltration membranes by photofunctionalization using a coated alpha-cleavage photoinitiator. Analyst 2001; 126(6):803-09.
52. Hilal N, Kochkodan V. Surface modified microfiltration membranes with molecularly recognising properties. J Memb Sci 2003; 213(1-2):97-113.
53. Piletsky SA, Matuschewski H, Schedler U et al. Surface functionalization of porous polypropylene membranes with molecularly imprinted polymers by photograft copolymerization in water. Macromolecules 2000; 33:3092-98.
54. Wang HY, Kobayashi T, Fukaya T et al. Molecular imprint membranes prepared by the phase inversion precipitation technique 2. Influence of coagulation temperature in the phase inversion process on the encoding in polymeric membranes. Langmuir 1997; 13:5396-400.
55. MathewKrotz J, Shea K. Imprinted polymer membranes for the selective transport of targeted neutral molecules. J Am Chem Soc 1996; 118(34):8154-55.

56. Wang H, Kobayashi T, Fujii N. Molecular imprint membranes prepared by the phase inversion precipitation technique. Langmuir 1996; 12(20):4850-56.
57. Yoshikawa M, Izumi J, Kitao T et al. Molecularly imprinted polymeric membranes containing DIDE derivatives for optical resolution of amino acids. Macromolecules 1996; 29:8197-203.
58. Yoshikawa M, Izumi JI, Kitao T. Alternative molecular imprinting,a facile way to introduce chiral recognition sites. Reactive and Functional Polymers 1999; (42):93-102.
59. Yoshikawa M, Izumi J, Ooi T et al. Carboxylated polysulfone membranes having a chiral recognition site induced by an alternative molecular imprint technique. Polym Bull 1998; 40(4-5):517-24.
60. Yoshikawa M, Ooi T, Izumi JI. Alternative molecularly imprinted membranes from a derivative of natural polymer cellulose acetate. J Appl Poly Sci 1999; 72:493-99.
61. Duffy DJ, Das K, Hsu SL et al. Binding efficiency and transport properties of molecularly imprinted polymer thin films. J Am Chem Soc 2002; 124:8290-96.
62. Marx S, Liron Z. Molecular imprinting in thin films of organic-inorganic hybrid sol-gel and acrylic polymers. Chem Mater 2001; 13:3624-30.
63. Yan M, Kapua A. Polymer Preprints 2000; 41:264-65.
64. Percival CJ, Stanley S, Braithwaite A et al. Molecular imprinted polymer coated QCM for the detection of nandrolone. Analyst 2002; 127:1024-26.
65. Sneshkoff N, Crabb K, BelBruno JJ. An improved molecularly imprinted polymer film for recognition of amino acids. J Appl Poly Sci 2002; 86:3611-15.
66. Liang CD, Peng H, Bao XY et al. Study of a molecular imprinting polymer coated BAW bio-mimic sensor and its application to the determination of caffeine in human serum and urine. Analyst 1999; 124(12):1781-85.
67. Sulitzky C, Ruckert B, Hall AJ et al. Grafting of molecularly imprinted polymer films on silica supports containing surface-bound free radical initiators. Macromol 2002; 35:79-91.
68. Wang H, Kobayashi T, Fujii N. Surface molecular imprinting on photosensitive dithiocarbamoylpolyacrylonitrile membranes using photograft polymerization. J Chem Technol Biotechnol 1997; 70(4):355-62.
69. Quaglia M, Lorenzi ED, Sulitzky C et al. Surface initiated molecularly imprinted polymer films: A new approach in chiral capillary electrochromatography. Analyst 2001; 126:495-1498.
70. Titirici MM, Hall AJ, BS, B. Hierarchically imprinted stationary phases: Mesoporous polymer beads containing surface-confined binding sites for adenine. Chem Mater 2002; 14:21-23.
71. Ruckert B, Hall A, Sellergren B. Molecularly imprinted composite materials via iniferter-modified supports. J Mater Chem 2002; 12:2275-80.
72. Sellergren B, Ruckert B, Hall AJ. Layer-by-layer grafting of molecularly imprinted polymers via iniferter modified supports. Adv Mater 2002; 14:1204-08.
73. Byrne ME, Park K, Peppas NA. Molecular imprinting within hydrogels. Adv Drug Delivery Rev 2002; 54:149-61.
74. Wizeman WJ, Kofinas P. Molecularly imprinted polymer hydrogels displaying isomerically resolved glucose binding. Biomaterials 2001; 22:1485-91.
75. Hiratani H, Alvarez-Lorenzo C. Timolol uptake and release by imprinted soft contact lenses made of N,N-diethylacrylamide and methacrylic acid. J Control Release 2002; 83(2):223-30.
76. Enoki T, Tanaka K, Watanabe T et al. Frustrations in polymer conformation in gels and their minimization through molecular imprinting. Physical Review Letters 2000; 85:5000-03.
77. Alvarez-Lorenzo C, Guney O, Oya T et al. Polymer gels that memorize elements of molecular conformation. Macromolecules 2000; 33(23):8693-97.
78. Alvarez-Lorenzo C, Guney O, Oya T et al. Reversible adsorption of calcium ions by imprinted temperature sensitive gels. J Chem Physics 2001; 114(6):2812-16.
79. Hiratani H, Alvarez-Lorenzo C, Chuang J et al. Effect of reversible cross-linker, N,N'-Bis(acryloyl)cystamine, on Calcium Ion Adsorption by imprinted gels. Langmuir 2001; 17(14):4431-36.
80. Kanekiyo Y, Sano M, Iguchi R et al .Novel nucleotide-responsive hydrogels designed from copolymers of boronic acid and cationic units and their applications as a QCM resonator system to nucleotide sensing. Journal Of Polymer Science Part A-Polymer Chemistry 2000; 38:1302-10.
81. Peppas NA, Keys KB, TorresLugo M et al. Poly(ethylene glycol)-containing hydrogels in drug delivery. J Control Release 1999; 62:81-87.
82. Biffis A, Graham NB, Siedlaczek G et al. The synthesis characterization and molecular recognition properties of imprinted microgels. Macromolecular Chemistry And Physics 2001; 202:163-71.
83. Schweitz L, Spegel P, Nilsson S. Approaches to molecular imprinting based selectivity in capillary electrochromatography. ELECTROPHORESIS 2001; 22(19):4053-63.
84. Svec F, Frechet JMJ. Continuous rods of macroporous polymer as high-performance liquid-chromatography separation media. Anal Chem 1992; 64(7):820-22.

85. Matsui J, Kato T, Takeuchi T et al. Molecular recognition in continuous polymer rods prepared by a molecular imprinting. Technique Anal Chem 1993; 65:2223-24.
86. Brüggemann O, Freitag R, Whitcombe M et al. Comparison of polymer coatings of capillary electrophoresis with respect to their applicability to molecular imprinting and electrochromatography. J Chromatogr A 1997; 781:43-53.
87. Tan Z, Remcho V. Molecular imprint polymers as highly selective stationary phases for open tubular liquid chromatography and capillary electrochromatography. Electrophoresis 1998; 19(12):2055-60.
88. Marty JD, Tizra M, Mauzac M et al. New molecular imprinting materials: Liquid crystalline networks. Macromolecules 1999; 32:8674-77.
89. Araki K, Goto M, Furusaki S. Enantioselective polymer prepared by surface imprinting technique using a bifunctional molecule. Analytica Chimica Acta 2002; 469:173-81.
90. Yan M, Kapua A. Fabrication of molecularly imprinted polymer microstructures. Analytica Chimica Acta 2001; 435:163-67.
91. Pérez-Moral N, Mayes AG. Novel MIP formats. Bioseparation 2002; 10:287-99.

CHAPTER 2

Bioimprinting

Claudio Baggiani and Cristina Giovannoli

Abstract

Besides mainstream, molecular imprinting based on man-made synthetic polymers or silica-imprinted materials, proteins too can be considered as building blocks to prepare artificial molecular recognition systems. The technique of bioimprinting is based on reversible changes in the three dimensional structure of a protein induced by noncovalent interactions with a ligand in mild denaturing conditions such as lyophilization or precipitation with a polar solvent. After these changes, a protein shows altered binding properties, with a reversal of enantioselectivity, enhancement of enzyme activity or de novo binding features. The principles of bioimprinting, nature of the protein and of the template, experimental techniques (lyophilization or solvent precipitation) and some progress, such as interfacial bioimprinting, stabilization by cross-linking and polysaccharide-based bioimprinting are discussed referring to examples reported in literature for enzymes and binding proteins.

Introduction

Besides mainstream, molecular imprinting based on man-made fully synthetic polymers or silica-imprinted materials, over the last fifteen years several papers have been dedicated to studying and describing the approach to bioimprinting, relying on the use of proteins (or less frequently polysaccharides) to obtain artificial molecular recognition systems.

As biopolymers, proteins have interesting molecular recognition properties. Their highly organized molecular architecture comes from ordered folding of the amino acid sequence, and consists in a flexible but well defined three-dimensional structure, generally provided with clefts and cavities, chirally active and provided with a large array of functional groups which are able to establish interactions with other biopolymers, low mass ligands and several kinds of surfaces by means of an ion pair, hydrogen bond or hydrophobic noncovalent interactions. These properties make proteins very attractive building blocks to prepare molecularly imprinted matrices which are potentially useful for selective recognition of ligands and for stereo / chemoselective catalysis in biotransformations.

The first published attempt to use a biopolymer to obtain an imprinted artificial receptor is due to the pioneering work of Pauling on the instructional theory of immunological response. This theory, later proven incorrect, relied on the concept of antibody proteins as a well-defined biopolymer with a unique amino acid sequence and multiple variable conformations complementary to different antigens.[1] In accordance with Pauling's idea, a nonspecific γ-globulin could be "imprinted" with an "antigen" under denaturing conditions. Thus, after exhaustive dialysis, the protein should retain molecular recognition properties toward the molecule used as an "antigen". Experiments performed by precipitation of polyclonal γ-globulins with *Pneumococcus* polysaccharide Type III seemed to show a certain degree of selective recognition.[2,3] Apart from the questionability of the experimental results obtained, the idea of

Molecular Imprinting of Polymers, edited by Sergey Piletsky and Anthony Turner.
©2006 Landes Bioscience.

artificial antibodies was shifted towards silica-based materials,[4] and protein-based imprinting was not further studied.

In 1988, after more than four decades of silence, bioimprinting of proteins was proposed again by Russell and Klibanov, that focused their attention on the modified protease activity of subtilisine, lyophilized in the presence of N-acetyl-L-amino acids as templates.[5] For the pecision's sake, it should be mentioned that five years before, Sinkai and coworkers had briefly described the molecular recognition properties of starch towards methylene blue, which was cross-linked with s-trichlorotriazine in the presence of the same dye used as a template.[6]

What Bioimprinting Is and How It Works

It is well known that a progressive reduction of water content in a water-solvent mixed medium generally reduces enzyme activity as an effect of the progressive denaturation of the protein tertiary structure. On the other hand, when the dissolving medium is represented by a nearly anhydrous solvent, many enzymes retain their tertiary structures and catalytic properties. The reason for this apparently anomalous behaviour has been identified as the stiffening of the protein structure. This is due to the nearly complete desolvation of the amino acid substituents. When the protein is dissolved in water, its tertiary structure is characterized by a marked conformational flexibility that makes denaturation easier, while a non aqueous solvent causes a significant reduction of this mobility without loss of tertiary structure.[7-9]

To avoid irreversible denaturation, lyophilization is the main technique to bring a protein from an aqueous environment to an organic one. Nevertheless, there is much experimental evidence of structural modification of proteins as a direct effect of the lyophilization process. Thus, to avoid unwanted and potentially irreversible modification that could cause loss of protein activity, it is a good laboratory practice to add some substances to the solution to be lyophilized; the so called "lyoprotectants", that prevent a dangerous denaturation maintaining a very thin shell of water molecules around the protein structure.[10-12]

In several cases, it has been observed that a protein which is lyophilized in the presence of a molecule able to act as a template and dispersed again in a nonaqueous solvent showed molecular recognition properties towards the template. This effect, called "bioimprinting" has been verified for a broad variety of proteins (see Table 1), showing clear evidence of newly formed catalytic or binding sites. These structures are stabie in anhydrous conditions where the protein architecture is in a frozen conformational state, whereas an aqueous environment causes the disappearance of these structures as an effect of the conformational relaxation due to the increased motility of the protein.

The bioimprinting effect can be better interpreted as the ultimate consequence of reversible changes in the structure of a protein induced by a noncovalent interaction with a ligand. In water, these changes are transient and cannot be observed, because of the conformational flexibility of the protein backbone that causes a rapid disappearance of them. Contrarily, when protein molecules are dispersed in a nonaqueous solvent, a change in the binding site structure induced by a ligand can be preserved because of the acquired conformational stiffness of the protein backbone. Thus, each change in the protein structure can be "frozen" and retained unchanged after the removal of the ligand that acts as an effective template. When the protein possesses enzymatic properties and the noncovalent interaction involves the binding site, its catalytic activity could be increased or changed towards unnatural substrates. Obviously, if the protein is transferred back into water, its tertiary structure relaxes and the newly formed binding properties are lost again.

Experimental evidence of reversible changes in the structure of bioimprinted proteins have been given from Mishra and coworkers.[20] Using L-malic acid as a template, the secondary structure of imprinted and nonimprinted bovine serum albumin, chymotrypsinogen and lysozyme was quantitatively examined using Fourier-transform infrared spectroscopy (FTIR). A marked difference in β-sheet, α-helix and disordered structure contents (see Table 2) between nonimprinted and imprinted structures was observed for all the proteins considered

Table 1. A list of bioimprinted proteins

Protein	Template	Activity	References
α-chymotrypsin	N-acetyl-D-tryptophane	catalysis	13,15,27
α-chymotrypsin	N-acetyl-L-phenylalanine	catalysis	23
β-lactoglobulin	N-isopropyl-4-nitrobenzylamine	catalysis	24
bovine hemoglobin	L-malic acid	ligand binding	11
bovine serum albumin	L-malic acid	ligand binding	11,20
bovine serum albumin	4-hydroxybenzoic acid, L-tartaric acid	ligand binding	14,31
bovine serum albumin	N-methyl-N-(4-nitrophenyl)-δ-aminovaleric acid	catalysis	19
bovine serum albumin	N-isopropyl-4-nitrobenzylamine	catalysis	24,31
chicken ovalbumin	L-malic acid	ligand binding	11
chicken ovalbumin	N,S-bis(2,4-dinitrophenyl) glutathione	catalysis	28
chymotrypsinogen	L-malic acid	ligand binding	20
epoxide hydrolase	(S)-1,2-epoxyoctane	catalysis	31
lipase F-AP	(R)-(-)-2-octanol	catalysis	36
lipase OF	(R)-1-phenylethanol	catalysis	18
lipase TL	17β-estradiol	catalysis	33
liver alcohol dehydrogenase	NADP+	catalysis	16
lysozime	L-malic acid	ligand binding	20
myoglobin	4-hydroxymethylpyridine (and other templates, less efficient)	catalysis	30
papaine	N-isopropyl-4-nitrobenzylamine	catalysis	24
subtilisin	N-acetyl-L-amino acids	catalysis	5,27,29
subtilisin	tymidine	catalysis	21
subtilisin	17β-estradiol-3-sulphate, 17β-estradiol	catalysis	33
thermolysin	paclitaxel-2'-adipic acid, paclitaxel	catalysis	33

when suspended in ethylacetate, whereas there were no differences when imprinted proteins were dissolved in water again. Interestingly, imprinted proteins suspended in ethylacetate showed secondary structures more similar to native proteins than nonimprinted ones, while imprinted proteins suspended in water showed secondary structures more similar to lyophilized, nonimprinted proteins. The authors interpreted these results as a consequence of the presence of L-malic binding sites formed by bioimprinting during the lyophilization process, stable in organic solvents but transient in a water environment.

How to Obtain a Bioimprinted Protein

As reported in Figure 1, protein bioimprinting consists of several consecutive steps: template binding, protein denaturation, template removal and rebinding. These involve both the template and protein. Each of these steps should be carefully planned to obtain a positive result, and consideration can be made on the basis of what is reported in literature.

The Template

It is possible to observe from the literature data (see tab. 3.1), that bioimprinting has been performed with a panel of very different templates. Amino acid derivatives,[5,13,15,23,27,29] carboxylic acids,[11,14,19,20,24,31] and amphiphilic substances[17,22,25,26,34,35] are the most preferred, but also more exotic substances such as glutathione,[28] 17β-estradiol[33] or paclitaxel[33] have been considered. Some considerations need to be made on these templates. First of all, the template

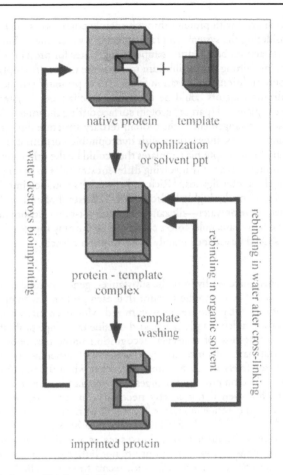

Figure 1. Simplified scheme of bioimprinting process.

Table 2. Changes in the secondary structure of three proteins after lyophilization with and without presence of L-malic acid as a template. Data taken from ref. 20.

Protein		% α-helix	% β-Sheet	% Others*
bovine serum	native	34 ± 1	15 ± 1	51 ± 2
albumin	not imprinted	30 ± 1	25 ± 1	45 ± 1
	imprinted	25 ± 1	16 ± 1	59 ± 2
chimotrypsinogen	native	6 ± 1	42 ± 1	52 ± 1
	not imprinted	2 ± 1	62 ± 1	36 ± 1
	imprinted	11 ± 2	41 ± 1	48 ± 3
lysozime	native	34 ± 2	18 ± 2	48 ± 3
	not imprinted	24 ± 1	45 ± 1	31 ± 1
	imprinted	17 ± 2	34 ± 2	49 ± 4

*Including β-turns, random coils and extended chains

described seems to interact with proteins through mainly polar forces, such as hydrogen bond and ion pair. Considering the system template / protein / water, there should be competition for noncovalent interactions between the template and water for protein. Also, with an excess of template, useful for shifting the equilibrium towards the protein / template complex, it can be observed that only additional stabilization factors make protein / template interactions feasible. These stabilization factors could be identified in changes of system entropy due to desolvation of the template and (part of) protein surface during the interaction, but also due to the denaturation and rearrangement of the protein tertiary structure during the lyophilization process. For the same reasons, interactions with hydrophobic portions of the template should not be ruled out, and for hydrophobic templates they could be the driving force for a successful interaction with a protein. In a study involving different strategies to bioimprint subtilisin and thermolysin with hydrophobic ligands,[33] Rich and coworkers obtained imprinted proteins able to catalyze the acylation of the highly hydrophobic 17β-estradiol and paclitaxel using water soluble template derivative or water—dioxane and water—t-butyl alcohol mixtures to dissolve the templates. In the latter case, polar forces could not be the only source of protein—template interaction, but it should be ascribed mainly to hydrophobic forces.

The Protein

As regards proteins, these are hydrophilic substances, generally soluble in water and aqueous buffers. It should be taken into the account that each protein has an optimal pH range in which its binding or catalytic properties are maximized. Moreover, many proteins have a stable tertiary structure only in a defined pH range, and outside this range profound and sometimes irreversible changes causes loss of molecular recognition properties. Some proteins, such as bovine serum albumin, have a distinct tertiary structure with different binding properties, and these conformations are freely interconverting each other when the pH changes.[37] Nevertheless, bioimprinting is based on profound changes in the tertiary structure, thus acidic (or basic) buffers could be useful, even if not strictly necessary. In fact, even if many examples of bioimprintings have been described in water[16,19,28,31,32] or near neutral buffer solutions, such as phosphate[5,15,21,23,25,27,30,33-36] and TRIS buffers,[17,22,26] other successful bioimprintings have been reported from more denaturing conditions, such as acidified water as a dissolving medium.[11,14,20,24] In many cases protein solutions are not buffered, and pure water, that can be also adjusted with concentrated chlorhydric acid, seems to work well. Anyway, it should be taken into account that pure water (i.e., nearly neutral, not buffered) assumes a pH value that could be largely conditioned by the amounts of protein and template dissolved. Thus, after the addition of the template, the pH of the protein solution could change, and bioimprinting will be performed in an environment quite far from the assumed neutrality.

For several systems, the acidity and ionic strength of the protein solution seems to be related to bioimprinting efficiency. As reported by Kwon and coworkers,[29] subtilisine Carlsberg bioimprinted with N-acetyl-L-phenylalanine showed an increasing catalytic activity for the transesterification of N-acetyl-L-phenylalanine ethyl ester when the pH of the protein solution gradually changed from acidic to slightly basic, and the amount of potassium salts (especially chloride and nitrate) increased. It should be stressed anyway that increased enzyme activity, as an effect of ionic strength is not uncommon and is also described for not-imprinted enzymes operating in organic solvents.[38] The same pH effect was also reported for a nonenzymatic protein.[19] Oya and coworkers described the bioimprinting of bovine serum albumin with substituted benzoic acids to create an artificial receptor, and with N-methyl-N-(4-nitrobenzyl)-4-aminovaleric acid as transition state analog to create an artificial dehydrofluorinase. All the bioimprinted systems showed binding capacity and enzyme activity proportional to the initial pH of the protein solution. On the basis of the experimental results and considering the template acidity, the authors concluded that the positive effect of pH and ionic strength on the bioimprinting efficacy was due to the ionic nature of the newly created binding sites.

Lyophilization or Precipitation?

As seen previously, to obtain a bioimprinted protein it is important to partially denaturise its tertiary structure in presence of a template molecule. The lyophilization technique assures that such denaturation is far from complete, and that the protein architecture is approximately preserved, introducing only minor alterations regarding preexisting or newly formed binding sites.[39] Lyophilization is simple, suitable for all the proteins and fully compatible with a wide range of buffers and templates. Moreover the use of volatile buffers, such as ammonium formiate or acetate, lets us obtain the lyophilized protein free from potentially interfering salts. Apart from its advantages, lyophilization also has some drawbacks, such as the need for a dedicated apparatus and the difficulty of completely evaporating the buffers from very viscous solutions as concentrated proteins are. Moreover, lyophilization does not let us remove salts and other very polar substances, posing consequent problems for the use of bioimprinted proteins in organic solvents.

Beside lyophilization, some authors have considered precipitation with organic solvents as an alternative technique in protein bioimprinting.[13,15,23,27,32] To precipitate a protein from an aqueous solution with an organic solvent it is necessary to use a substance provided with moderate denaturing properties towards proteins, mixable with water in all proportions, easily removable by vacuum drying, and without chemical reactivity towards proteins.[40,41] Moreover, it would be useful if protein solubility in water-solvent mixtures decreased very rapidly when the amount of solvent increases. The possible choice is restricted between some lower alcohols (methanol, ethanol, 1-propanol), cyclic ethers (1,4-dioxane, tetrahydrofurane), acetonitrile and acetone, even if all the authors reported the use of 1-propanol, ignoring other possible solvents.

From the experimental data reported in literature it is quite difficult to judge what method is better, because it is not possible to find data which compares the enzyme activity (or the binding properties) of a bioimprinted protein directly with the same template by lyophilization or solvent precipitation. Anyway, it should be taken into account that the first method for protein denaturation is a milder technique than the second. In fact, proteins subjected to lyophilization are rarely irreversibly denatured with a loss of binding properties, while in many cases solvent precipitation may cause the complete loss of molecular recognition properties. Obviously, it is a matter of discussion if a complete protein denaturation should be detrimental for a successful bioimprinting or not.

Properties of Bioimprinted Proteins

Bioimprinted proteins retain many of the properties typical of the native proteins. The primary sequence and other related features, such as disulfide bonds, are not involved in the imprinting process that acts exclusively on the noncovalent architecture of the protein. In fact, as seen previously, extensive modifications of the secondary and tertiary structures are involved, and the formation of binding sites by imprinting is the effect of the protein structure alteration due to the reshaping of intra-protein noncovalent interactions, such as hydrogen bond, saline bridges or hydrophobic interactions between the amino acid side chains. Thus, it is plausible that a bioimprinted protein could retain most of its properties related to the primary structure without changes (such as molecular mass), while properties influenced by secondary and tertiary structures, such as isoelectric point or hydrodynamic volume could be changed more or less significantly.

On the contrary, bioimprinting has a profound effect on the binding properties. It should be taken into account that the bioimprinting can involve both the formation of new binding sites and the modification of previously existent structures. In the first case, the function of the protein drastically changes, assuming de novo binding properties, while in the latter, the nature of the protein does not change, except for the behaviour of the modified binding site.

The formation of binding sites with enhanced properties can be well exemplified by the bioimprinting of β-lactoglobulin and papaine with N-isopropyl-4-nitrobenzylamine, a transition state analog for the dehydrofluorination of 4-fluoro-4-(4-nitrophenyl)-butan-2-one to

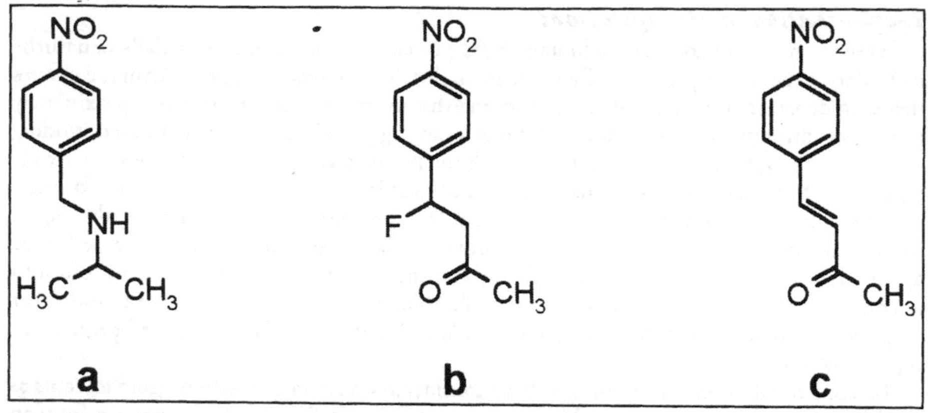

Figure 2. Bioimprinting of b-lactoglobulin and papaine witn the transition state analog N-isopropyl-4-nitrobenzylamine (a). Modified proteins show enzyme-like activity, catalyzing the dehydrofluorination of 4-fluoro-4-(4-nitrophenyl)-butan-2-one (b) to 4-(4-nitrophenyl)-3-buten-2-one.

4-(4-nitrophenyl)-3-buten-2-one (see Fig. 2).[24] The imprinted proteins show a catalytic behavior which is not stated for the native form. The β-elimination of fluorine was catalyzed in acetonitrile with rate constants of 0.036 min^{-1} for β-lactoglobulin and 0.013 min^{-1} for papain. It should be considered that catalytic activity was also experimentally observed for the non imprinted proteins, but in this case values (0.011 min^{-1} for β-lactoglobulin and 0.0049 min^{-1} for papaine) compare unfavorably with those of imprinted proteins, that increase 3.3 times for β-lactoglobulin and 2.7 times for papaine.

At present there could be matter for discussion if bioimprinting (involving the formation of new binding sites) can only be made on proteins with latent binding sites, in which new binding properties are obtained by modification of a preexistent and suitable tertiary structure, or the denaturation of the protein structure in the presence of a template is so deep that a binding site is formed anyway, without regard for the nature of the preexistent tertiary structure. Nowadays an answer based on experimental data remains difficult, because of the limited number of bioimprinted proteins reported in literature.

Bovine serum albumin bioimprinted with L-malic acid is an example of protein modification in which multiple binding sites were formed.[11] In this case, imprinting with an excess of template (about 1 mole of albumin against 670 moles of L-malic acid) produced a bioimprinted protein with a large number of binding sites. Interestingly, the number of these binding sites changed when the solvent in which rebinding was measured was changed (see Table 3), with a marked inverse proportion between the number of L-malic acid molecules bounded and the solvent ability to form hydrogen bonds. The authors interpreted this as a clear indication that the noncovalent interaction between the ligand and the binding site was based on hydrogen bonds, but it could also be considered as an indication of binding site heterogeneity. Also the binding selectivity was considered in the same study. It was observed that the net amount of ligand bound to the bioimprinted protein was strongly influenced by the structure of the ligand itself (see Table 4). In fact, bicarboxylic acids provided with 4 carbon atoms and no hindering substituents, such as L-malic (the template), succinic, mercaptosuccinic, N-acetylaspartic, tartaric, fumaric or maleic acid showed good recognition by the binding sites, while cyclic bicarboxylic or substituted acids, such as monomethylsuccininc, phenylsuccininc, phtalic or 1,2-cyclohexandicarboxylic acid showed poor recognition. It can be interpreted as the effect of shape selective binding sites in which noncovalent interaction with a ligand is based principally on multiple hydrogen bonds.

Table 3. *Effect of organic solvent hydrogen bonding parameter on rebinding of L-malic acid to bioimprinted bovine serum albumin. Data taken from ref. 11.*

Solvent	Molar Equivalent Amount of L-Malic Acid Bound
tetrahydrofurane	0.9 ± 1
pyridine	3.1 ± 1.6
N,N-dimethylformamide	3.2 ± 1.7
1,4-dioxane	4.8 ± 1.2
diisobutylketone	6.5 ± 1.7
acetone	10.6 ± 2.5
t-butylmethylether	11.0 ± 1.3
2-ethoxyethyl acetate	11.1 ± 1.8
2-butanone	14.5 ± 1.4
isobutylethylketone	14.8 ± 0.6
pentylethylketone	15.0 ± 1.7
butyl acetate	17.6 ± 2.4
hexyl acetate	21.3 ± 1.4
ethyl acetate	24.2 ± 1.8

Interfacial Bioimprinting

A peculiar kind of bioimprinting introduced for the first time by Mingarro and coworkers is defined as "surfacial activation" or more appropriately "interfacial bioimprinting".[17] It involves a protein and a surface-active molecule able to act as a template (see Fig. 3). The bioimprinting effect is due to protein activation by the presence of an amphiphilic interface constituted by an structured layer of surface-active molecules, ordered in micelles, liposomes or Langmuir-Blodgett surfaces.

The amphiphilic interface does not provide lyoprotection and solubilization of the protein only, but is responsible for the bioimprinting effect or directly inducing the formation of conformationally rigid binding sites onto the protein surface, or improving the interaction between binding site and hydrophobic template.[22] In fact, crystallographic studies have shown that lipases have the catalytic site partially blocked by a helical loop, that makes it unaccessible to many substrates, and that surface-active agents and organic solvents can open the catalytical site exposing it to the substrate molecules.[42]

It should be mentioned that, in these terms, not all the bioimprinted proteins obtained in the presence of surface-active agents can be classified as produced by interfacial bioimprinting. In fact, in literature several examples are reported of bioimprinted proteins obtained in presence of surface-active agents acting as solubilizing agents only, but not directly involved in the bioimprinting process.[18,25]

This technique is particularly efficient to enhance the catalytic properties of enzymes acting on hydrophobic substances in nonaqueous media, such as lipases.[22,26,34,35] An interesting application that demonstrates the potentialities of bioimprinting has been reported for the synthesis of industrial flavours starting from oleic acid and geraniol, rac-citronellol, geranylgeraniol or (-)-menthol.[26] This technique not only enhanced the catalytic reaction rate for the esterification, but also widened the reactivity spectrum of substrates suitable for catalysis of fatty acids either not esterificable or nearly so from non imprinted lipases.

It should be mentioned that interfacial bioimprinting of lipases has been enhanced using air-water amphiphilic surfaces produced by foaming a buffered solution of lipase in the presence of a surface active agent such as tween 20.[35]

Table 4. Binding selectivity of bovine serum albumin bioimprinted with L-malic acid. Selectivty is calculated as the ratio between the molar equivalent amounts of bicarboxylic acid and L-malic acid bound. Data taken from ref. 11.

Ligand	Structure	Net Amount of Ligand Bound (Mol Eqv)	Binding Selectivity
L-malic acid (template)		24.2 ± 1.8	1.00
maleic acid		35.6 ± 1.1	1.47
meso-tartaric acid		32.6 ± 1.2	1.35
L-tartaric acid		29.5 ± 1.4	1.22
N-acetyl-L-aspartic acid		23.8 ± 2.0	0.98
phtalic acid		19.4 ± 1.8	0.80
fumaric acid		16.9 ± 1.5	0.69
mercaptosuccininc acid		15.3 ± 1.7	0.63
succininc acid		11.0 ± 1.5	0.45
cis-cyclohexandicarboxylic acid		7.4 ± 1.1	0.31
phenylsuccinic acid		7.0 ± 1.3	0.29

Table continued on next page

Table 4. Continued

Ligand	Structure	Net Amount of Ligand Bound (Mol Eqv)	Binding Selectivity
trans-cyclohexandicarboxylic acid		6.8 ± 1.3	0.28
methylsuccinate		1.1 ± 1.6	0.05

Cross-Linking of Bioimprinted Proteins

One of the main drawbacks of protein bioimprinting consists of the unsuitability of these modified proteins in aqueous environments. In fact, the bioimprinting mechanism is based on the structural modification of the protein architecture, and its stabilization is due to the stiffening of the tertiary structure in the absence of polar and hydrogen bond inducing solvents. It has been shown that limited but increasing amounts of water irreversibly destroy the binding properties of bioimprinted proteins.[5,16,21,34] Moreover, not only water, but also other solvents are able to reduce or destroy these binding properties. A clear relation between solvent polarity and catalytic activity of bioimprinted lipase AK was observed when catalysis was measured in different solvents ranging from the apolar hexane to polar methanol.[35] Such instability of imprinted binding sites poses severe limitations to the use of bioimprinted proteins such as artificial receptors in aqueous environments.

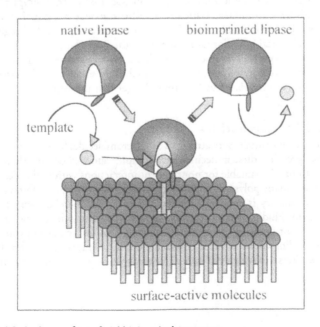

Figure 3. Simplified scheme of interfacial bioimprinting process.

To overcome this problem, the use of cross-linking agents has been proposed in order to preserve the binding properties of the bioimprinted protein, able to "freeze" the altered tertiary structure introducing additional covalent bonds between functionalities which are present on the protein surface (and sometimes between distinct protein molecules). Such agents act by reacting with functional groups present on the native protein surface or introduced artificially. Protein covalent cross-linking techniques are well known and crystallized enzymes stabilized by glutaraldehyde cross-linking through so-called "CLEC technology" (CLEC: cross-linked enzyme crystal) are widely used as catalysts for biotechnological and fine chemistry applications.[43]

Subtilisin and α-chimotrypsin were vinylated by acylation with itaconic anhydride before being bioimprinted with N-acetyl-D-tryptophane by precipitation with 1-propanol.[27] The precipitated proteins were cross-linked with etrhylenglycole dimethacrylate in cyclohexane, and their catalytic activity towards the unnatural substrate N-acetyl-D-tryptophane ethyl ester was measured in phosphate buffer. The reaction rate acceleration compared to a noncatalyzed system for the hydrolysis reaction was found to be enhanced by almost two orders of magnitude (and the same order of magnitude was observed for the backward reaction, measured in cyclohexane). These results indicated that cross-linking procedure stabilized the structure of bioimprinted protein in such a manner as to preserve its template-induced catalytic properties even in a highly polar medium such as a phosphate buffer.

The itaconic anhydride method was also shown to be efficient in the stabilization of epoxide hydrolase from *Rhodotorula glutinis*, bioimprinted to enhance its enantioselectivity towards the hydrolysis of several 1,2-epoxyalkanes from R to S isomers.[32] The modified enzyme activity of the cross-linked protein was found essentially preserved when measured in buffer, and cross-linking increased the protein stability by at least 7 times compared to the native enzyme. It should be noted that—as an effect of the large inter-protein cross-linking—the itaconic anhydride-mediated cross-linking produces mostly insoluble agglomerates of proteins. Moreover, this is not a serious drawback, because insoluble but active enzymes find advantageous applications in biotechnological processes, due to the ease of biocatalyst recycling and product-biocatalyst separation.

Direct post-imprinting modification of a protein was used in an attempt to generate an artificial glutathione peroxidase. Chicken ovalbumin was bioimprinted with N,S-bis-(dinitrophenyl)glutathione, and the modified protein was cross-linked with glutaraldehyde and subjected to a chemical mutation procedure with the insertion of a selenium atom in the newly formed catalytic center. The resulting modified protein showed a markedly enhanced glutathione peroxidase activity of about 800 U/μmol, only seven times less than the native rabbit liver glutathione peroxidase but 800 times bigger that the best mimic known not obtained by bioimprinting.[28]

Bioimprinted Polysaccharides

Polysaccharides are potentially very attractive biomacromolecules for the bioimprinting technique. In fact, like proteins, these molecules have complex and well defined three dimensional architecture, functionalities suitable for noncovalent interactions with molecules able to act as templates. Moreover, many polysaccharides, such as cellulose, dextran or starch are very cheap materials, whose chemistry is very well known. Despite this, there are very few reports of bioimprinting on this kind of macromolecule. In fact, apart from the use of cyclodextrins as building blocks,[44-47] or putative functional monomers[48] in molecular imprinting, there are only three papers dealing with the use of polysaccharides in bioimprinting. After the early work of Sinkai and coworkers,[6] in which the molecular recognition properties of starch cross-linked with s-trichlorotriazine in presence of the same dye used as a template towards methylene blue is briefly described, a more elaborate work on amylose was reported by Wulff and coworkers.[49] In those papers, several inclusion complexes were prepared by cross-linking with s-trichlorotriazine or epichloridryne, and the binding selectivity behaviour of the modified polysaccharide was studied.

More recently,[50] Kanekiyo and coworkers have been reporting the preparation of cross-linked amylose able to selectively bind the environmental significant bisphenol A and other alkylphenols. In this case the approach is different, because starch is functionalized with acryloyl chloride to provide it with cross-linkable additional functions. After that, the polysaccharide is cross-linked with N,N-bismethylenacrylamide in presence of a saturated solution of template. The binding capacity, the effect of the amount of cross-linking agent introduced and the binding selectivity of the modified amylose were measured and the presence of a bioimprinting effect was demonstrated.

Considering that polysaccharides are not less complex, more difficult to find or manipulate than proteins, what is the cause of such a substantial absence of a large body of experimental work on bioimprinting involving these biomacromolecules? A precise answer is not forthcoming, but it is plausible that the absence in nature of catalytic systems based on polysaccharides has largely reduced the interest in bioimprinting–directed studies. In fact, in contrast with protein-based systems, all the examples of bioimprinted polysaccharides describe the rebinding of templates, and not de novo catalytic properties. As a consequence, the potential practical applications are less evident.

Conclusions

Taking into account the whole body of papers on bioimprinting published from 1988 to today, it is clear that the most of the efforts have been dedicated to demonstrating the feasibility of bioimprinting, and that several features of this technology are not well known today or have not been explored yet.

As a significant example, the templates considered are low mass substances, rarely with molecular mass greater than 1000 D, and no bioimprinting of a protein using an oligopeptide, oligonucleotide or oligosaccharide as a template has been described. There are no physical obstacles to bioimprinting with high molar mass templates (provided that they are soluble in water). In fact, in analogy with what happens in nature with anti-macromolecule antibodies or DNA-binding protein, it is not necessary that a bioimprinted protein recognizes all the template structure. It is sufficient that a limited part of the protein (i.e., the binding site) and a limited part of the biopolymer (i.e., the epitope) will be able to interact because molecular recognition happens successfully. On this route, a successful bioimprinting of proteins which uses nucleic acid sequences, oligosaccharides with a physiological role, or whole cells could open unexpected possibilities in molecular biology, medicine and, generally speaking, biotechnology. It should be noted that while molecular imprinting of nucleic acid remains elusive today, surface imprinting of bacteria using a lithographic approach has been clearly shown.[51]

Year after year new literature on bioimprinting accumulates, new proteins are used and practical applications are described. The growth rate of this particular kind of molecular imprinting cannot be compared with the very rapidly growth of papers describing molecularly imprinted polymers (see Fig. 4), but it has found its niches of interest, especially in the field of biotechnology, where modified proteins and new enzymes with unprecedented properties are welcomed. Even if it is difficult for the authors of this review to make predictions on what the future holds, it would be quite strange if bioimprinting techniques do not find their right place at the side of the other imprinting techniques.

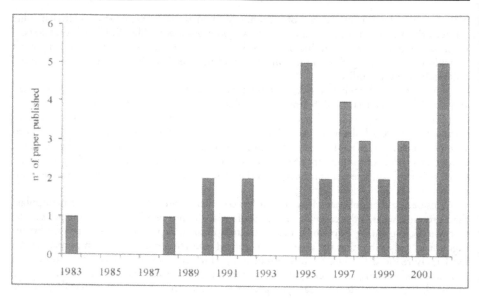

Figure 4. Papers related to bioimprinting published between 1988 and 2002. Data taken from refs. 52,53.

References

1. Pauling L. A theory of the structure and process of formation of antibodies. J Am Chem Soc 1940; 62:2643-2657.
2. Pauling L, Campbell DH. The production of antibodies in vitro. Science 1942; 95:440-441.
3. Pauling L, Campbell DH. The manufacture of antibodies in vitro. J Exptl Med 1942; 76:211-220.
4. Dickey FH. The preparation of specific adsorbents. Proc Natl Acad Sci USA 1949; 35:227-229.
5. Russell AJ, Klibanov AM. Inhibitor-induced enzyme activation in organic solvents. J Biol Chem 1988; 263:11624-11626.
6. Shinkai S, Yamada M, Sone T et al. Template synthesis from starch as an approach to tailor-made "cyclodextrins". Tetrahedron Lett 1983; 24:3501-3504.
7. Klibanov AM. Improving enzymes by using them in organic solvents. Nature 2001; 409:241-246.
8. Braco L. Biocatalysis and biorecognition in nonaqueous media. Some perspectives in analytical biochemistry. Mikrochim Acta 1995; 120:231-242.
9. Krishna SH. Developments and trends in enzyme catalysis in nonconventional media. Biotechnol Adv 2002; 20:239-266.
10. Engbersen JFJ, Broos J, Verboom W et al. Effects of crown ethers and small amounts of cosolvent on the activity and enantioselectivity of α-chymotripsin in organic solvents. Pure Appl Chem 1996; 68:2171-2178.
11. Dabulis K, Klibanov AM. Molecular imprinting of proteins and other macromolecules resulting in new adsorbents. Biotechnol Bioeng 1992; 39:176-185.
12. Klibanov AM. Improving enzymes by using them in organic solvents. Nature 2001; 409:241-246.
13. Ståhl M, Månsson M, Mosbach K. The synthesis of a D-amino acid ester in an organic media with α-chymotrypsin modified by a bio-imprinting procedure. Biotech Lett 1990; 12:161-168.
14. Braco L, Dabulis K, Klibanov AM. Production of abiotic receptors by molecular imprinting of proteins. Proc Natl Acad Sci USA 1990; 82:274-277.
15. Ståhl M, Jeppson-Wistand U, Månsson M et al. Induced stereoselectivity and substrate specificity of bioimprinted α-chymotrypsin in anhydrous organic media. J Am Chem Soc 1991; 113:9366-9368.
16. Johansson A, Mosbach K, Månsson M. Horse liver alcohol dehydrogenase can accept NADP+ as coenzyme in high concentration of acetonitrile. Eur J Biochem 1995; 227:551-555.
17. Mingarro I, Abad C, Braco L. Interfacial activation-based molecular bioimprinting of lipolytic enzymes. Proc Natl Acad Sci USA 1995; 92:3308-3312.
18. Okahata Y, Hatano A, Ijiro K. Enhancing enantioselectivity of a lipid-coated lipase via imprinting methods for esterification in organic solvents. Tetrahedron Asymm 1995; 6:1311-1322.
19. Ohya Y, Miyaoka J, Ouchi T. Recruitment of enzyme activity in albumin by molecular imprinting. Macromol Rapid Comm 1996; 17:871-874.

20. Mishra P, Griebenov K, Klibanov AM. Structural basis for the molecular memory of imprinted proteins in anydrous media. Biotechnol Bioeng 1996; 52:609-614.
21. Rich JO, Dordick JS. Controlling subtilisin activity and selectivity in organic media by imprinting with nucleophylic substrates. J Am Chem Soc 1997; 119:3245-3252.
22. Gonzales-Navarro H, Braco L. Improving lipase activity in solvent-free media by interfacial activation-based molecular bioimprinting. J Mol Catal B 1997; 3:111-119.
23. Lion-Dagan M, Willner I. Nitrospiropyran-modified α-chymotrypsin, photostimulated biocatalyst in an organic solvent: Effects of bioimprinting. J Photochem Photobiol 1997; 108:247-252.
24. Slade CJ, Vulfson EN. Induction of catalytic activity in proteins by lyophilization in the presence of a transition state analogues. Biotechnol Bioeng 1998; 59:211-215.
25. Kamiya N, Goto M. Preparation of surfactant-coated lipases utilizing the molecular imprinting technique. J Ferm Bioeng 1998; 85:237-239.
26. Gonzales-Navarro H, Braco L. Lipase-enhanced activity in flavour ester reactions by trapping enzyme conformers in the presence of interfaces. Biotechnol Bioeng 1998; 59:122-127.
27. Peissker F, Fischer L. Crosslinking of imprinted proteases to maintain a tailor-made substrate selectivity in aqueous solutions. Bioorg Med Chem 1999; 7:2231-2237.
28. Liu J, Luo G, Gao S et al. Generation of a gluthatione peroxidase-like mimic using bioimprinting and chemical mutation. Chem Comm 1999; 199-200.
29. Kwon OH, Imanishi Y, Ito Y. Enhancement of catalytic activity of chemically modified subtilisin Carlsberg in benzene by adjustment of lyophylization conditions. Bull Chem Soc Jpn 2000; 73:1277-1282.
30. Ozawa S, Klibanov AM. Myoglobin-catalyzed epoxidation of styrene in organic solvents accelerated by bioimprinting. Biotechnol Lett 2000; 22:1269-1272.
31. Slade CJ. Molecular (or bio-)imprinting of bovine serum albumin. J Mol Catal B 2000; 9:97-105.
32. Kronenburg NAE, de Bont JAM, Fischer L. Improvement of enantioselectivity by immobilized imprinting of epoxide hydrolase from Rhodotorula glutinis. J Mol Catal B 2001; 16:121-129.
33. Rich JO, Mozhaev VV, Dordick JS et al. Molecular imprinting of enzymes with water-insoluble ligands for nonaqueous biocatalysis. J Am Chem Soc 2002; 124:5254-5255.
34. Yilmaz E. Improving the application of microbial lipase by bioimprinting at substrate-interfaces. World J Microbiol Biotechnol 2002; 18:37-40.
35. Yilmaz E. Bio-imprinting of microbial lipase at air-water interface. World J Microbiol Biotechnol 2002; 18:141-145.
36. Furukawa S, Ono T, Ijima H et al. Effect of imprinting sol–gel immobilized lipase with chiral template substrates in esterification of (R)-(+)- and (S)-(-)-glycidol. J Mol Catal A 2002; 17:23-28.
37. Carter DC, Ho JX. Structure of serum albumin. Adv Protein Chem 1994; 45:153-203.
38. Bedell BA, Mozhaev VV, Clark DS et al. Testing for diffusion limitations in salt-activated enzyme catalysts operating in organic solvents. Biotechnol Bioeng 1998; 58:654–657.
39. Pohl T. Concentration of proteins and removal of solutes. Methods Enzymol 1990; 182:68-82.
40. Schein CH. Solubility as a function of protein structure and solvent components. Biotechnology 1990; 8:308-317.
41. Houen G. The solubility of proteins in organic solvents. Acta Chem Scand 1996; 50:68-70.
42. Cajal Y, Svedsen A, Girona V et al. Interfacial control of lid opining in thermomyces lanuginonsa lipase. Biochemistry 2000; 39:413-423.
43. Margolin AL. Novel crystalline catalysts. Trends Biotechnol 1996; 4:223-230.
44. Asanuma H, Kakazu M, Shibata M et al. Molecularly imprinted polymer of β-cyclodextrin for the efficient recognition of cholesterol. Chem Commun 1997; 1971-1972.
45. Asanuma H, Kajiya K, Hishiya T et al. Molecularly imprinting of cyclodextrin in water for the recognition of peptides. Chem Lett 1999; 665-666.
46. Hishiya T, Shibata M, Kakazu M et al. Molecularly imprinted cyclodextrins as selective receptors for steroids. Macromolecules 1999; 32:2265-2269.
47. Asanuma H, Akiyama T, Kajiya K et al. Molecular imprinting of cyclodextrin in water for the recognition of nanometer-scaled guests. Anal Chim Acta 2001; 435:25-33.
48. Piletsky SA, Andersson SA, Nicholls IA. Combined hydrophobic and electrostatic interaction-based recognition in molecularly imprinted polymers. Macromolecules 1999; 32:633-636.
49. Kubik S, Höller O, Steinert A et al. Inclusion compounds of derivatized amyloses. Macromol Symp 1995; 99:93-102.
50. Kanekiyo Y, Naganawa R, Tao H. Molecular imprinting of bisphenol A and alkylphenols using amylose as a host matrix. Chem Commun 2002; 2698-2699.
51. Aherne A, Alexander C, Payne MJ et al. Bacteria-mediated lithography of polymer surfaces. J Am Chem Soc 1996; 118:8771-8772.
52. ISI's Web of Science. http://www.isinet.com/isi/
53. Society for Molecular Imprinting Database. http://www.smi.tu-berlin.de/SMIbase.htm

CHAPTER 3

The Re-Birth of Molecular Imprinting on Silica

Naonobu Katada and Miki Niwa

Abstract

Molecular imprinting was first attempted between the 1930s-50s on silica surfaces, but later studies were carried out mainly on organic polymers. However, with advances in technology for the inorganic synthesis of siliceous materials, molecular imprinting on silica has, since the late of 1980s, again become a focus of attention and is now applied to sensor, adsorbent and catalyst preparation. This is a short review on the history and recent topics of molecular imprinting on silica and related materials.

Pioneering Works between 1930s-50s

The active centre of an enzyme selectively interacts with a specific reactant molecule like the combination of a lock and a key, as explained by Fischer in 19th century.[1] Such a reaction centre in an antibody molecule is considered to be formed in the presence of a template molecule, as explained by Pauling in 1940.[2] The concept of molecular imprinting to synthesize a reaction field can be found in this explanation.

Prior to this explanation in 1930s, the first attempt at molecular imprinting on a solid was carried out by Poljakov. A silica gel was prepared in the presence of aromatic hydrocarbons as the templates and, after drying, a relatively high adsorption capacity was observed when the adsorbed molecule was smaller than the template molecule used.[3] Because the original paper was written in Russian, this first work is frequently ignored by the scientists.

Further literature appeared in 1940s-50s. Dickey utilized the methyl orange molecule as the template to form a silica gel and after the removal of the template, the adsorption capacity for methyl orange was several times higher than that for ethyl orange.[4] The dependence of selectivity on the preparation method was investigated in the other studies.[5,6] During this period, the first enantiometric separation using silica gel was reported. Curti and Colombo prepared a silica gel in the presence of (S)-10-camphorsulfonic acid as the template. Selective adsorption of the S-isomer from a racemic 10-camphorsulfonic acid solution was observed on the thus prepared silica gel.[7,8] Later, the stereo selective adsorption of alkaloid molecule was also reported.[9]

These studies are the pioneering works of molecular imprinting to construct an adsorption cavity on a solid surface. All of these works utilized organic molecules as the templates, because various molecular shapes and sizes can be selected from a large range of organic compounds. In addition, all of these studies utilized silica as the substrate. This is presumably because silica is a thermally and chemically stable metal oxide in which the chemical bond between silicon and oxygen has a strongly covalent character. It is easily synthesized from such a precursor as sodium silicate. The microstructure is expected to be controlled easily by the template and the

Molecular Imprinting of Polymers, edited by Sergey Piletsky and Anthony Turner.
©2006 Landes Bioscience.

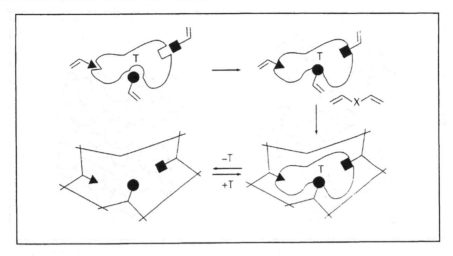

Figure 1. Fundamental concept of molecular imprinting on organic polymer, where T is the template molecule organizing three kinds of functional monomers into a controlled arrangement. Reproduced from ref. 12 with permission. ©1994 Elsevier Science B. V.

controlled structure is expected to be kept even after the removal of the template on the basis of its covalent nature. However, silica has limitations. Among metal oxides, silica is known to possess a substantially inactive surface. Usually, adsorption on silica is weak and the silica surface has few functions. As shown below, introduction of an additional metal element or functional group is required to construct a reaction field suitable for various practical purposes such as electrochemical sensing and catalysis.

The Long Winter of the 1960s-1970s

Molecular Imprinting on Organic Polymers
After the first development of molecular imprinting, attention moved in the 1970s to the use of organic polymers as solid substrates[10] following the significant development of polymer science in industry. The progress of molecular imprinting method during this period was not only due to the utilization of a new substrate; a new strategy was also clearly established. Today, molecular imprinting involves not only the formation of a controlled cavity as Dickey envisaged, but also the precise arrangement of functional groups induced by the template molecule, as shown in Figure 1. This principle was introduced when synthetic polymers were adopted as the substrate.

There are many excellent reviews on molecular imprinting on organic polymers.[11-16] Their application to sensors, chromatographic adsorbents and catalysts in the chemical and biochemical fields rapidly developed after this period.[17-24]

Ordered Porous Silicas and Related Materials Using Templates or Structural Directing Agents
This section summarizes advance in the synthesis of silicates and related metal oxides with ordered porous structures. It is not a type of molecular imprinting, but the final purpose of these studies is to obtain a reaction field with a well defined shape in a similar way to the aim of molecular imprinting. Moreover, the techniques utilized in the porous silica synthesis are closely related to the molecular imprinting method.

Among the ordered porous silicates, zeolite is a quite important group, because the reaction field in the zeolite has been utilized practically for the shape selective adsorption or catalytic

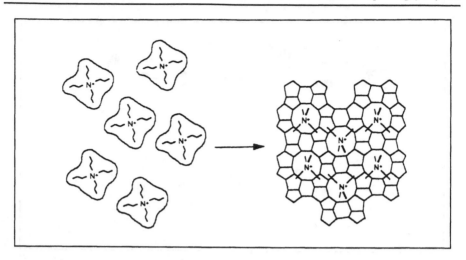

Figure 2. Schematic drawing of formation of zeolite crystallite from primary units consisting of silicon compounds and organoammonium cations. Reproduced from ref. 28 with permission. ©1996 Elsevier Science B. V.

reactions in industry. It is one of the biggest applications of nanotechnology, although the word nanotechnology was not used when the practical application of zeolite started.

Zeolite is a class of crystal aluminosilicates with micropores, whose diameter is close or smaller than 1 nm. It was first found as a natural mineral and later has been hydrothermally synthesized in a mixed solution of metal (silicon and aluminum) sources and a basic compound such as sodium hydroxide. In 1960s, a novel synthetic technique using an organoammonium salt as a fraction of the basic compound was established by a group of Mobil Research and Development. Among the thus synthesized group of zeolites, ZSM-5 type was rapidly applied to a wide variation of chemical industry as a catalyst and therefore this synthetic technique is quite important. The ZSM-5 zeolite with a small concentration of aluminum generally shows high catalytic activities for various acid-catalyzed reactions due to the strong Brønsted acidity. In addition, the shape selectivity in the catalytic reaction was clearly demonstrated by this zeolite.[25] The molecular sieving effects by the zeolites had been observed and utilized for gas separation and oil refinery catalysis before the appearance of the ZSM-5 type. However, the ZSM-5 zeolite has an excellent characteristic, because it catalyzes an important shape selective reaction, namely the synthesis of *para*-substituted aromatic compounds. For example, *para*-xylene, which has been in huge demand as a raw material of plastics, is selectively produced by methylation or disproportionation of toluene in the micropore of ZSM-5 zeolite prior to the *ortho*- and *meta*-isomers. This reaction is, still now, one of a few industrialized reactions which produce only desired products, while other isomers are not formed. With a post modification technique, namely the chemical vapor deposition (CVD) of silicon alkoxide on the external surface, the shape selectivity can be increased close to 100%, where almost no undesired isomers are produced.[26-27] This fact must encourage researchers in the field of molecular imprinting. By using a silicate framework, if suitable microstructure and chemical nature are obtained, almost 100% selectivity can be realized in catalysis.

Here we note that the synthesis of zeolite using such an organic species as alkylammonium cation is closely related to molecular imprinting on silica. The organic compound was called a "template" in the early studies, because it was believed that the shape of molecule affected on the structure of micropore, as represented in Figure 2.[28] It has however been clarified that the microporous structure formed is correlated not only with the shape but also with the chemical property, e.g., hydrophobicity, of the organic species.[29] At present, the added organic

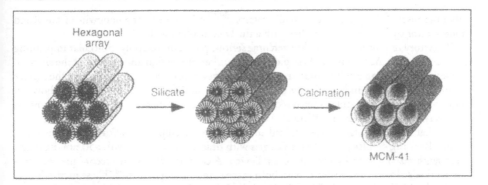

Figure 3. Speculated mechanism of formation of MCM-41 mesoporous silica. Hexagonal arrays of cylindrical mecelles with the polar groups of the surfactants (light gray) to the outside. Silicate species (dark gray) then occupy the spaces between the cylinders. The final calcination steps burns off the organic material, leaving hollow cylinders of inorganic material. Reproduced from ref. 31 with permission. ©1992 Nature Publishing Group.

compound is therefore called "SDA (structure-directing agent)", but there are several examples of zeolite synthesis in which the added organic molecule must play a role of the template. For example, in the synthesis of UTD-1 type zeolite, bis-(pentamethyl-cyclopentadienyl)-cobalt (III) hydroxide probably plays a role of the template to form a large micropore.[30] The reader can refer to some excellent reviews dealing with recent advances in zeolite synthesis.[28]

We should mention here another important advance in a related field. In the 1990s, a class of novel silicate, mesoporous silica, was synthesized. The research group of Kresge et al (Mobil Research and Development) synthesized a silicate MCM-41 in the presence of a surfactant liquid crystal, i.e., ammonium salt with a long chain of alkyl group. The obtained silicate possessed an ordered structure in which the pore diameter was several nanometers. The linear pores were arranged in hexagonal arrays, as controlled by a cluster of the surfactant (liquid crystal) molecules (Fig. 3). The pore size was controllable from 2 to 10 nm by selecting the length of the alkyl chain of the template surfactant.[31] Independently of this study, Inagaki and Kuroda et al synthesized a similar mesoporous silica FSM-16 from a layered silicate material using the surfactant as the template.[32] These are the first group of silicates with controlled pore sizes in a mesoporous region (diameter 2 to 50 nm). Many researchers followed these studies to synthesize a series of mesoporous silicas and related materials.[33] Some layered silicates[34] synthesized before these studies may be classified into the same group of the mesoporous silicates, although the researchers did not recognize this at the time.

Catalytic cracking is one of the most important chemical industries and has been catalyzed by the zeolites. It produces gasoline fraction of hydrocarbons from crude oil. Recently, demand has emerged for a new catalyst which catalyzes the reaction of heavier hydrocarbons. In the early 1990s, mesoporous silica with a small concentration of aluminum was predicted to be a good catalyst for the cracking of heavy hydrocarbons, because it has a composition similar to that of the conventional cracking catalyst (some types of zeolite) and the pore size is far larger than that of the zeolites. The cracking properties of zeolites results from the Brønsted acidity; the acid site (H^+) is generated by the substitution of a silicon atom (Si^{4+}) by an aluminum atom (Al^{3+}).[25] However, as clarified recently, the acidic property of zeolite cracking catalyst depends critically on the microstructure but not on the composition.[35,36] In other words, the origin of high cracking activity on the zeolite is a specific microstructure relating to the specific bond angle and length. The wall of mesoporous silica is substantially amorphous and hence different from that of zeolite. It is difficult to generate strong Brønsted acidity by incorporating aluminum on the wall of mesoporous silica and no application of the mesoporous silica to the cracking process has been achieved. Attempts are now being made to apply mesoporous silica for other purposes,[37,38] e.g., as a Lewis acidic catalyst,[39,40] microvessel for a nanowire of metal and microreactor to form a polymer fibre with a finely controlled width.[42]

This story tells us how we might overcome serious problems to apply molecular imprinting for practical uses. According to these pioneering studies, the design and control of the shape of the reaction cavity on a solid surface is possible. However, the chemical property of the surface should be controlled independently of the structure modification. As mentioned above, in order to apply the molecular-imprinted silica in practice, the creation of a function group is necessary, but in many cases difficult.

Further large templates were utilized to synthesize macroporous silicas and other metal oxides. By using emulsion droplets, silica gels with ordered pore arrays with >50 nm diameters were synthesized[43-45] and several studies followed. A combination of this technique with zeolite synthesis also created a silicate with both macro- and microporosity.[46] These methods may not be classified as "molecular" imprinting, but are in a closely related field.

We should also mention a different approach by Feng and Bein. They attached the zeolite particles on a solid surface.[47] The target of this study must be considered the same as the goal of molecular imprinting, to give a shape selective reactivity on a solid surface.

Sol-Gel Techniques for Synthesis of Siloxane Network

With the development of the science of and synthetic methods for ordered porous silicates, sol-gel technology, to synthesis amorphous, porous metal oxides, has developed since the 1980s.[48,49] At the time of Dickey, the silica gel was simply synthesized by the hydrolysis of sodium silicate.[4] However, nowadays, various organosilicon precursors can be used and various conditions can be selected. The kinetics and the resulting microstructure have been analyzed[50] and the optimization of procedures and conditions for the synthesis of intentionally designed porous structure is now possible. Control of the mean pore size and its distribution in amorphous silica is a well established technique even without using template material.[51] This accelerates the application of molecular imprinting on silica as shown later.

The Re-Birth of Silica Imprinting with Advanced Technologies

Design and Construction of Silica-Organic Hybrid Surface

The development of molecular imprinting on silica recommenced in the 1980s. It developed not only to design structure, but also to combine it with surface function.

At first we will review advances in silicon sources for the molecular imprinting. Stradub and Piletsky et al selected vapor of alkylchlorosilane. They modified a transition metal oxide surface originally possessing electrochemical functions. This target is also new and such a suitable application was not found in the period of Poljakov[3] and Dickey.[4] As shown in Figure 4, a template molecule, e.g., phenylalanine, was adsorbed on the electrode surface, e.g., indium tin oxide (ITO). The uncovered surface was subsequently modified with the silane deposited from the gas phase, followed by removal of the template. Finally, the uncovered space whose shape was controlled by the template molecule was expected to be formed to show shape-selective sensing ability. Phenylalanine showed a relatively large current change on the ITO covered by silane in the presence of phenylalanine template, while tryptophane showed a small change on the same ITO, and both reactants showed small responses on the ITO covered by silane without using the template.[52] However, the differences among these responses were approximately 2 to 3 times, not high.

Modification of an electrode surface was also carried out by Makote and Collinson. They introduced an advanced technique of the sol-gel process. Silicon sources, tetramethoxysilane, phenyltrimethoxysilane and methyltrimethoxysilane were mixed and the template, dopamine, and some necessary organic compounds were then added. The coverage of the surface by the organic-silica hybrid layer suppressed the response to various molecules in cyclic voltammetry. The modified electrode showed almost no response (close to 0%) to chemical species with a

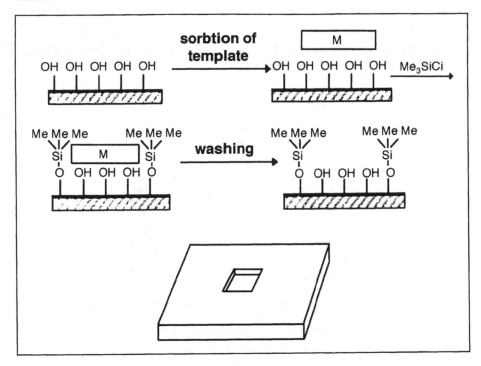

Figure 4. Process of modification on silica surface adopted by Starodub and Piletsky et al. Reproduced from ref. 52 with the permission. ©1993 Elsevier Science B. V.

large molecular size, while dopamine itself retained quite a high response (67% of the unmodified electrode).[53] In other words, the selectivity as a sensor was very clear. This is presumably owing to the advanced method of silicate synthesis.[54] Enantioselective adsorption was also reported by the application of the organic-inorganic hybrid sol-gel method.[55,56]

A simpler introduction of the molecular imprinting technique found on organic polymers to the silica surface was also carried out. The surface of silica can be coated with polymer synthesized by the molecular imprinting method. For example, Burow and Minoura coated the surface of silica beads with a thin layer of polymer synthesized in the presence of an enzyme as the template.[57] After the removal of template by washing, the surface showed a strong adsorption for the template itself. Application in a sensor has been reported. The organic polymer layers synthesized in the presence templates were loaded on a quartz microbalance surface and the selective detection of specific molecules was reported.[58,59]

Another application of the molecular imprinting technique developed with organic polymers applied to silica is the use of the polymerization of silicon alkoxide with a large organic group. Wulff et al constructed a silica gel surface with aminosilane groups as shown in Figure 5. The amino groups were fixed at a controlled distance on the silica gel. Carboxylic compounds with two carboxylic groups with different distances were tested as the adsorbates and selective adsorption and separation in liquid chromatography were observed.[13,60] The surface modification of silica or other metal oxide with silane coupling reagent is a traditional method in manufacturing adsorbents for gas and liquid chromatography.[21] Therefore, this technique is considered to be a combination of silane modification and the molecular imprinting.

Principally the same strategy, but using more sophisticated approaches have been reported recently using the polymerization of alkoxysilanes.[61-63] Among them, Katz and Davis recently constructed an adsorption site with three binding points at precisely controlled positions in a

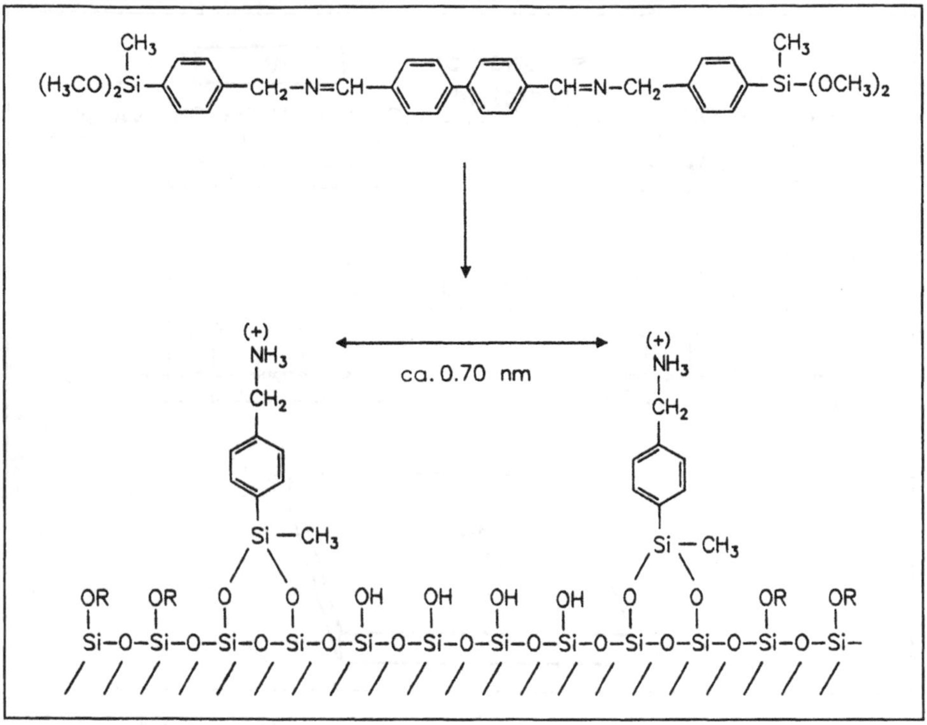

Figure 5. Preparation of silica gel with two amino groups on the surface with a controlled distance proposed by Wulff. Reproduced from ref. 13 with permission. ©1995 Wiley-VCH Verlag GmbH & Co. KGaA.

cavity, as shown in Figure 6. This material was applied to a base-catalyzed reaction and showed a shape selectivity, although its magnitude was not reported. In addition, the microporosity formed by the molecular imprinting could be observed by the physical adsorption of argon.[62] This is the first case where the reaction cavity was directly observed by physical measurement. The key technique to realize this attempt was the organic synthesis of the specific template molecule.

Also recently, enantioselective activity for catalytic hydrolysis of amide was observed on silica particles modified with organosilane compound in the presence of the template.[64]

Purely Inorganic Surface

Another important attempt is the construction of a reaction field purely consisting of inorganic oxides on an inorganic oxide surface, because the inorganic oxide has advantages in thermal and chemical stability compared to the organic materials. The pioneering works by Poljakov[3] and Dickey[4] sought this goal. From the late 1980s, this field again gathered interest. One possible reason is the advances in silicate synthesis discussed above.

More than 30 years after Dickey,[4] in the late 1980s, Morihara et al presented new results on molecular imprinting on a purely inorganic substrate. This is the first attempt to create a chemically active site by metal loading with a controlled position on the silica surface and the first application of molecular imprinting on the purely inorganic surface to the catalysis. Aluminum cation was precipitated on a silica gel, followed by adsorption of the template molecule. The resulting solid was treated in an acidic solution, as it was expected that the silicon, aluminum and oxygen atoms on the surface were arranged to form a reaction cavity in which an acid site (aluminum cation) was generated at a controlled position after the removal of the

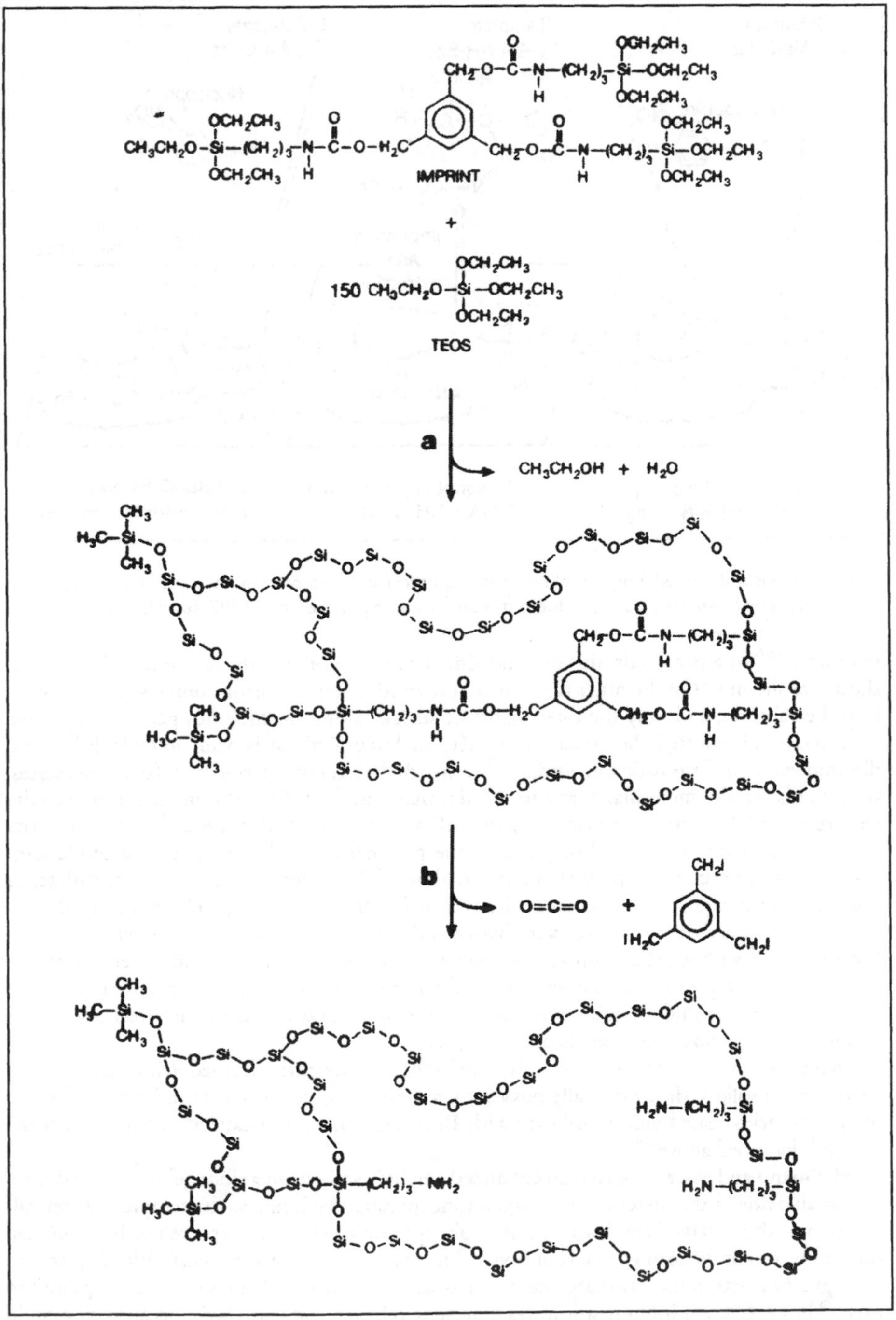

Figure 6. Formation of a cavity with three binding points on silica proposed by Katz and Davis. Reproduced from ref. 62 with permission. ©2000 Nature Publishing Group.

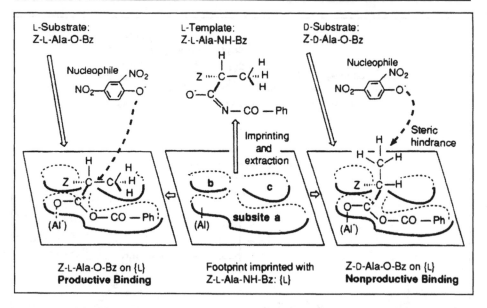

Figure 7. Models of formed footprint of L-template (center) and adsorption of the L- (left) and D-reactants (right) drawn by Morihara et al. Reproduced from ref. 71 with permission. ©1992 Royal Chemical Society.

template.[65,66] In other words, this method aimed to form not only the reaction cavity but also the active site in it. On the other hand, it is noteworthy that no silicon source was introduced into the solution, and only the movements of surface atoms on the silica gel were expected. Morihara et al reported the enhanced activity of butanolysis of benzoic anhydride[65,67] and dinitrophenolysis of aromatic anhydrides[68-70] in which the reaction intermediates (transition states) were similar in the molecular shape to the templates utilized. In addition, enantioselectivity was reported for the catalytic reaction of a substituted alanine anhydride on the aluminum-containing silica gel prepared in the presence of a substituted alanineamide template, whose molecular shape was similar to that of the expected reaction intermediate, as postulated in Figure 7.[71-72] The selectivity was unfortunately not large. Difference in the apparent catalytic activity for one reactant between the imprinted catalyst and the reference catalyst (modified without the template) was generally within several fold and difference in the activity on one imprinted catalyst between different reactants were also within several times the rate. However, this study is quite important because of its priority. Kaiser and Andersson tried to apply this principle to liquid chromatography.[73]

In place of the effort to create an active site in the reaction cavity formed, Morihara et al also tried to use a solid surface originally possessing a catalytic function. They modified the surface of clay, an acid-treated aluminosilicate with Brønsted acidity and catalytic activity, with the method described above.[74]

Heilmann and Maier reported an enhanced catalytic activity on a silica gel synthesized from silicon alkoxide in the presence of an organophosphonate molecule as the template. After calcination of the obtained solid, an acid site (phosphoric species) was expected to be generated on the bottom of the formed reaction cavity. The reaction tested was transesterification and an analogue of reaction intermediate was selected as the template. Shape selectivity appeared to exist,[75] but a different interpretation was represented by Ahmad and Davis, because they could not reproduce the effects of molecular imprinting.[76] Maier et al claimed[77] that impurity in the reactants induced the autocatalytic reaction which affected the selectivity and that this was the major reason for the observation by Ahmad and Davis.[76] However, at least in ref. 77, Maier et al themselves also have not reproduced the original selectivity shown in ref. 75. Subsequent

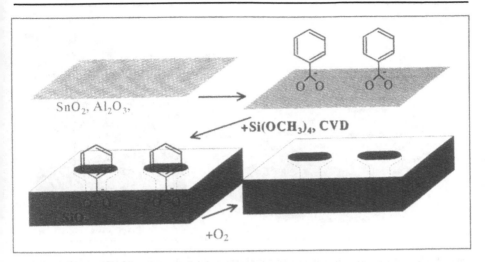

Figure 8. Schematic drawing of CVD of silica overlayer in the presence of template carboxylate anion on weakly basic metal oxide proposed by Katada and Niwa et al.

studies by Maier et al showed that the adsorption property on the modified silica was strongly affected by the modification of the chemical property, while the molecular imprinting effect was not clear.

Katada and Niwa et al utilized metal oxide with a high surface area and possessing catalytic function as the substrate, in order to form a shape selective catalyst. In addition, they introduced the CVD method of silicon alkoxide, which had first been developed to improve the zeolite catalysis[26] and then applied to prepare a model compound of an amorphous mixed oxide catalyst[79-84] and to enhance the thermal stability of the oxide surface.[85] On such weakly basic metal oxides as alumina and tin oxide, three kinds of aldehydes with different molecular sizes were adsorbed as the templates. Subsequently vapor of silicon alkoxide was admitted onto the surface to form a silica overlayer with cavities whose shape and size were controlled by the template molecule. The silica overlayer readily covered the surface almost completely, as shown in Figure 8. After the removal of template, the modified surface showed the function which was originally observed on the unmodified surface, but only molecules smaller than the template could reach the surface.[86] Thus a shape selectivity was generated in chemisorption of such molecules as aldehyde and alcohol[87,88] and catalytic oxidation of aldehyde, alcohol and alkane. The selectivity found is the first in oxidation catalysis on solids and also this is the first case where isomers were distinguished on a metal oxide catalyst other than with the zeolites. Also it was the first case where it was applied to a semiconductor chemical sensor.[89-91] The characteristic result of this study was that the catalytic selectivity was high and changed according to the varied molecular size of the template. Further details are given elsewhere.[92]

Later, Tada and Iwasawa et al followed this study. Alumina was covered by silica with the CVD technique in the presence of an analogue molecule of the desired reaction intermediate.[93] In this case, the unmodified alumina had no activity for the reaction tested, hydrolysis of ester. It needs Brønsted acidity, and the deposition of silica overlayer on alumina has been known to generate Brønsted acidity.[81,83,84] The acidic property of silica-alumina interface strongly depends on the microstructure.[35,94,95] and therefore the control of catalytic activity is generally difficult. Although it is still unclear why a suitable property was generated on the thus formed interface, the reactant shape selectivity was observed. Esters with molecular sizes smaller than the template were hydrolyzed on the thus modified alumina at relatively high reaction rates.[93]

This research group extended this technique to construct a catalytic site with a noble metal. An organophosphoric complex of rhodium was utilized as the template and after the CVD of

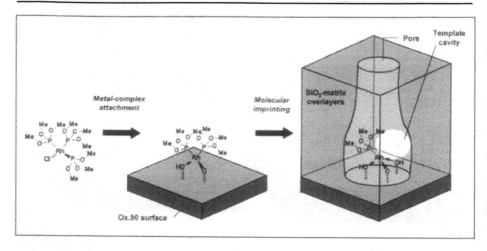

Figure 9. Model of formation of rhodium monomer in the cavity of silica overlayer deposited on the alumina surface proposed by Tada and Iwasawa et al. Reproduced from ref. 97 with permission. ©2003 Elsevier Science B. V.

silica, a fraction of the organophosphoric group of the template was eliminated under a specific set of conditions. Finally, a reaction cavity was formed with a metal complex on its bottom,[96] as shown in Figure 9. The hydrogenation of alkene with a relatively small molecular size was significantly enhanced by the attached rhodium complex.[97] Although the effect of not only the structure but also the chemical nature of the reactant would influence the activity, the high selectivity is characteristic of this study.

As stated in the previous section, the modification of a quartz microbalance surface was reported with some organic polymers. In place of the organic polymers, Kunitake et al coated the quartz surface with a titania layer with controlled cavities. They treated the quartz surface with a mixed solution of titanium alkoxide (as a polymer precursor) and an amino acid (template). The resulting quartz microbalance sensors adsorbed the analogue molecules of the templates in relatively high capacities.[98-100] These titania-coated silicas must have a large potential as novel functional materials, because titania-silica has various functions such as photocatalysis as well as chemical and thermal stability.

Conclusion

Following a long period when the interests of researchers moved to other fields, molecular imprinting of silica is now gathering attention. Techniques are being developed under the influence of advances in the technology of silicate synthesis. The field of application is also being extended with the development of sensor technology and bioscience. High performance has been exhibited for specific sensing and as catalysts, and shape selectivity has been observed in limited areas. However, all of the selectivities already observed are categorized as reactant shape selectivity, in which only raw materials fitting to the reaction cavity can be reacted. The molecular imprinting method has failed to achieve more valuable selectivity, namely the transition state or product shape selectivity in which only a specific product is formed among possible products. For such a difficult target, it is further required to develop the synthetic technique and combination of cavity shape and function. Quantum chemical calculation will help the advance; in some cases establishment of a model of the reaction field has been started,[97] and theoretical study of the siloxane network formation will be continued.[101]

References

1. Lichtenthaler FW. 100 years "Schlüssel-Schloss-Prinzip": What made Emil Fischer use this analogy? Angew Chem Int Ed Engl 1994; 33:2364-2373.
2. Pauling L. A theory of the structure and process of formation of antibodies. J Am Chem Soc 1940; 62:2643-2657.
3. Poljakov MW. Adsorbzionnie svojstva silikagelja i ego struktura. Russian J Phys Chem 1931; 2:799-805.
4. Dickey FH. Specific adsorption. J Phys Chem 1955; 59:695-707.
5. Bernard SA. The preparation of specific adsorbents. J Am Chem Soc 1952; 74:4946-4947.
6. Haldeman RG, Emmett PH. Specific adsorption of alkyl orange dyes on silica gel. J Phys Chem 1955; 59:1039-1043.
7. Curti R, Colombo U. E fortunato clerici:cromatografia con adsorbenti specifici. Gazzeta Chimica Italiana 1952; 82:491-502.
8. Curti R, Colombo U. Chromatography of stereoisomers with "tailor made" compounds. J Am Chem Soc 1952; 74:3961.
9. Beckett AH, Anderson P. A method for the determination of the configuration of organic molecules using 'stereo-selective adsorbents'. Nature 1957; 179:1074-1075.
10. Wulff G, Sarhan A. The use of polymers with enzyme-analogues structures for the resolution of racemates. Angew Chem Int Ed Engl 1972; 84:364-365.
11. Wulff G. Molecular recognition in polymers prepared by imprinting templates. ACS Symp Ser 1986; 308:186-230.
12. Shea KJ. Molecular imprinting of synthetic network polymers:the de novo synthesis of macromolecular biding and catalytic sites. Trends Polym Sci 1994; 5:166-173.
13. Wulff G. Molecular imprinting in cross-linked materials with the aid of molecular templates-a way towards artificial antibodies. Angew Chem Int Ed Engl 1995; 34:1812-1832.
14. Steinke J, Sherrington DC, Dunkin IR. Imprinting of synthetic polymers using molecular templates. Adv Polym Sci 1995; 123:81-125.
15. Sellergren B. Noncovalent molecular imprinting:antibody-like molecular recognition in polymeric network materials. Trends Anal Chem 1997; 16(6):310-320.
16. Hentze H-P, Antionietti M. Template synthesis of porous organic polymers. Curr Opinion Solid State Mater Sci 2001; 5:343-353.
17. Kempe M, Mosbach K. Molecular imprinting used for chiral separations. J Chromatogr A 1995; 694:3-13.
18. Ramström O, Ansell RJ. Molecular imprinting technology:challenges and prospects for the future. Chirality 1998; 10:195-209.
19. Haupt K, Mosbach K. Molecularly imprinted polymers and their use in biometic sensors. Chem Rev 2000; 100(7):2495-2504.
20. Martín-Esteban M. Molecularly imprinted polymers:new molecular recognition materials for selective solid-phase extraction of organic compounds. Fresenius J Anal Chem 2001; 370:795-802.
21. Buchmeiser MR. New synthetic ways for the preparation of high-performance liquid chromatography supports. J Chromatography A 2001; 918:233-266.
22. Piletsky SA, Turner PF. Electrochemical sensors based on molecularly imprinted polymers. Electroanal 2002; 14(5):317-323.
23. Peppas NA, Huang Y. Polymers and gels as molecular recognition agents. Pharmaceutical Res 2002; 19(5):578-587.
24. Byrne ME, Park K, Peppas NA. Molecular imprinting within hydrogels. Adv Drug Delivery Rev 2002; 54:149-161.
25. Breck DW. Zeolite molecular sieves: structure, chemistry and use. New York: John Wiley & Sons, 1974.
26. Niwa M, Kawashima Y, Hibino T et al. Mechanism of chemical vapour deposition of silicon alkoxide on mordenites. J Chem Soc, Faraday Trans, 1 1988; 84(1):4327-4336.
27. Halgeri AB, Das J. Recent advances in selectivity of zeolites for para-disubstituted aromatics. Catal Today 2002; 73(1-2):65-73.
28. Zones SI, Davis ME. Zeolite materials:recent discoveries and future prospects. Curr Opinion Solid State Mater Sci 1996; 1:107-117.
29. Kubota Y, Helmkamp MM, Zones SI et al. Properties of organic cations that lead to the structure-direction of high-silica molecular sieves. Microporous Mater 1996; 6:213-229.
30. Freyhardt CC, Tsapatsis M, Lobo RF et al. A high-silica zeolite with a 14-tetrahedral-atom pore opening. Nature 1996; 381:295-298.

31. Kresge CT, Leonowicz ME, Roth WJ et al. Ordered mesoporous molecular sieves synthesized by a liquid-crystal template mechanism. Nature 1992; 359:710-712.

32. Inagaki S, Fukushima Y, Kuroda K. Synthesis of highly ordered mesoporous materials from a layered polysilicate. J Chem Soc, Chem Commun 1993; 680-682.

33. Biz S, Occelli ML. Synthesis and characterization of mesoporous materials. Catal Rev-Sci Eng 1998; 40(3):329-407.

34. For example, Sakata K, Kunitake T. Siloxane polymer films with varied microstructures. Chem Lett 1989; 2159-2162.

35. Katada N, Igi H, Kim J-H et al. Determination of the acidic properties of zeolite by theoretical analysis of temperature-programmed desorption of ammonia based on adsorption equilibrium. J Phys Chem, B 1997; 101(31):5969-5977.

36. Katada N, Kageyama Y, Niwa M. Acidic property of Y- and mordenite-type zeolites with high aluminum concentration under dry conditions. J Phys Chem, B 2000; 104(31):7561-7564.

37. Sayari A. Catalysis by crystalline mesoporous molecular sieves. Chem Mater 1996; 8(8):1840-1852.

38. Corma A. From microporous to mesoporous molecular sieve materials and their use in catalysis. Chem Rev 1997; 97(6):2373-2419.

39. Tanaka Y, Sawamura N, Iwamoto M. Highly effective acetalization of aldehydes and ketones with methanol on siliceous mesoporous material. Tetrahedron Lett 1998; 39(51):9457-9460.

40. Katada N, Fujinaga H, Nakamura Y et al. Catalytic activity of mesoporous silica for synthesis of methyl N-phenyl carbamate from dimethyl carbonate and aniline. Catal Lett 2002; 80(1-2):47-51.

41. Fukuoka A, Sakamoto Y, Guan S et al. Novel templating synthesis of necklace-shaped mono- and bimetallic nanowires in hybrid organic-inorganic mesoporous material. J Am Chem Soc 2001; 123(14):3373-3374.

42. Kageyama K, Tamazawa J, Aida T. Extrusion polymerization catalyzed synthesis of crystalline linear polyethylene nanofibers within a mesoporous silica. Science 1999; 285:2113-21158.

43. Imhof A, Pine DJ. Ordered macroporous materials by emulsion templating. Nature 1997; 389(6654):948-951.

44. Velev OD, Jede TA, Lobo RF et al. Porous silica via colloidal crystallization. Nature 1997; 389(6650):447-448.

45. Chia S, Urano J, Tamanoi F. Patterned hexagonal arrays of living cells in sol-gel silica films. J Am Chem Soc 2000; 122(27):6488-6489.

46. Schmidt I, Madsen C, Jacobsen CJH. Confined space synthesis. A novel route to nanosized zeolites. Inorg Chem 2000; 39(11):2279-2283.

47. Feng A, Bein T. Growth of oriented molecular sieve crystals on organophosphate films. Nature 1994; 368:834-836.

48. Brinker CJ, Schere GW. Sol-Gel science. San Diego: Academic Press, 1990.

49. Attia YA. Sol-Gel Processing and applications. New York: Prenum Press, 1994.

50. Sefcík J, McCormick AV. Kinetic and thermodynamic issues in the early stages of sol-gel processes using silicon alkoxides. Catal Today 1997; 35:205-223.

51. Lin YS, Kumakiri I, Nair BN et al. Microporous inorganic membranes. Separation Purification Methods 2002; 31(2):229-379.

52. Starodub NF, Piletsky SA, Lavryk NV et al. Template sensors for low weight organic molecules based on SiO₂ surfaces. Sens Actuators, B 1993; 13-14:708-710.

53. Makote R, Collinson MM. Template recognition in inorganic-organic hybrid films prepared by the sol-gel process. Chem Mater 1998; 10(9):2440-2445.

54. Collinson MM. Sol-gel strategies for the preparation of selective materials for chemical analysis. Critical Rev Anal Chem 1999; 29(4):289-311.

55. Pinel C, Loisil P, Gallezot P. Preparation and utilization of molecularly imprinted silicas. Adv Mater 1997; 9(7):582-585.

56. Marx S, Liron Z. Molecular imprinting in thin films of organic-inorganic hybrid sol-gel and acrylic polymers. Chem Mater 2001; 13(10):3624-3630.

57. Burow M, Minoura N. Molecular imprinting:synthesis of polymer particles with antibody-like binding characteristics for glucose oxidase. Biochem Biophys Res Commun 1999; 227(2):419-422.

58. Kugimiya A, Takeuchi T. Molecularly imprinted polymer-coated quartz crystal microbalance for detection of biological hormone. Electroanal 1999; 11(15):1158-1160.

59. Hirayama K, Sakai Y, Kameoka K et al. Preparation of a sensor device with specific recognition sites for acetaldehyde by molecular imprinting technique. Sens Actuators, B 2002; 86:20-25.

60. Wulff G, Heide B, Helfmeier G. Enzyme-analog built polymers 20:molecular recognition through the exact placement of functional groups on rigid matrixes via a template approach. J Am Chem Soc 1986; 108(5):1089-1091.

61. Boury B, Corriu RJP, Strat VL et al. Generation of porosity in a hybrid organic-inorganic xerogel by chemical treatment. New J Chem 1999; 23:531-538.
62. Katz A, Davis ME. Molecular imprinting of bulk, microporous silica. Nature 2000; 403:286-289.
63. Ki CD, Oh C, Oh S-G et al. The use of a thermally reversible bond for molecular imprinting of silica spheres. J Am Chem Soc 2002; 124(50):14838-14839.
64. Markowitz MA, Kust PR, Deng G et al. Catalytic silica particles via template-directed molecular imprinting. Langmuir 2000; 16(4):1759-1765.
65. Morihara K, Kurihara S, Suzuki J. Footprint catalysis I:a new method for designing „tailor-made" catalysts with substrate specificity:silica (alumina) catalysts for butanolysis of benzoic anhydride. Bull Chem Soc Jpn 1988; 61(11):3991-3998.
66. Morihara K, Doi S, Takiguchi M et al. Footprint catalysis VII:reinvestigation of the imprinting procedures for molecular footprint catalytic cavities:the effects of imprinting procedure temperature on the catalytic characteristics. Bull Chem Soc Jpn 1993; 66(10):2977-2982.
67. Morihara K, Nishihata E, Kojima M. Footprint catalysis II:molecular recognition of footprint catalytic sites. Bull Chem Soc Jpn 1988; 61(11):3999-4003.
68. Morihara K, Tanaka E, Takeuchi Y et al. Footprint catalysis III:inducible alteration of substrate specificities of silica (alumina) gel catalysts for 2,4-dinitrophenolysis of toluic anhydrides by footprint imprinting. Bull Chem Soc Jpn 1989; 62(2):499-505.
69. Shimada T, Nakanishi K, Morihara K. Footprint catalysis IV:structural effects of templates on catalytic behavior of imprinted footprint cavities. Bull Chem Soc Jpn 1992; 65(4):954-958.
70. Shimada T, Kurazono R, Morihara K. Footprint catalysis V:substituent effects of template molecules on the catalytic behavior of imprinted molecular footprint cavities. Bull Chem Soc Jpn 1993; 66(3):836-840.
71. Morihara K, Kurokawa M, Kamata Y et al. Enzyme-like enantioselective catalysis over chiral ,molecular footprint' cavities on a silica (alumina) gel surface. J Chem Soc, Chem Commun 1992; 358-360.
72. Matsuishi T, Shimada T, Morihara K. Footprint catalysis IX:molecular footprint catalytic cavities imprinted with chiral hydantoins; enantioselective hydantoinase mimics. Bull Chem Soc Jpn 1994; 67(3):748-756.
73. Kaiser GG, Andersson JT. Sorbents for liquid chromatography based on the footprint principle:an exploratory study. Fresenius J Anal Chem 1992; 342:834-838.
74. Morihara K, Iijima T, Usui H. Footprint catalysis VIII:molecular imprinting for footprint cavities on an active clay surface. Bull Chem Soc Jpn 1993; 66(10):3047-3052.
75. Heilmann J, Maier WF. Selective catalysis on silicon dioxide with substrate-specific cavities. Angew Chem Int Ed Eng 1994; 33(4):471-473.
76. Ahmad WR, Davis ME. Transesterification on „imprinted" silica. Catal Lett 1996; 40(1-2):109-114.
77. Maier WF, BenMustapha W. Transesterification on imprinted silica-reply. Catal Lett 1997; 46(1-2):137-140.
78. Hunnius M, Rufinska A, Maier WF. Selective surface adsorption versus imprinting in amorphous microporous silicas. Micro- Mesoporous Mater 1999; 29:389-403.
79. Niwa M, Hibino T, Murata H et al. A silica monolayer on alumina and evidence of lack of acidity of silanol attached to alumina, J Chem Soc, Chem Commun 1989; (5):289-290.
80. Xu B-Q, Yamaguchi T, Tanabe K. Dehydrogenation of alkylamines on acid-base hybrid catalyst. Chem Lett 1989; 149-152.
81. Sato S, Toita M, Sodesawa T et al. Catalytic and acidic properties of silica-alumina prepared by chemical vapour deposition. Appl Catal 1990; 60:73-84.
82. Sarrazin P, Kasztelan S, Zanier-Szydlowski N et al. Interaction of oxomolybdenum species with γ_c-Al_2O_3 and γ_c-Al_2O_3 modified by silicon 1:the SiO_2/γ_c-Al_2O_3 system. J Phys Chem 1993; 97(22):5947-5953.
83. Sheng T-C, Gay ID. Measurement of surface acidity by ^{31}P NMR of adsorbed trimethylphosphine: application to vapor deposited SiO_2 on Al_2O_3 monolayer catalysts. J Catal 1994; 145:10-15.
84. Katada N, Niwa M. Silica monolayer solid-acid catalyst prepared by CVD. Adv Mater, Chem Vap Deposition 1996; 2(4):125-134.
85. Katada N, Ishiguro H, Muto K et al. Heat-resisting acid catalyst:thermal stability and acidity of thin silica layer on alumina calcined at 1493 K. Adv Mater, Chem Vap Deposition 1995; 1(2):54-60.
86. Kodakari N, Katada N, Niwa M. Molecular sieving silica overlayer on tin oxide prepared using an organic template. J Chem Soc, Chem Commun 1995; 623-624.
87. Kodakari N, Katada N, Niwa M. Silica overlayer prepared using an organic template on tin oxide and its molecular sieving property. Adv Mater, Chem Vap Deposition 1997; 3(1):59-66.
88. Kodakari N, Tomita K, Iwata K et al. Molecular sieving silica overlayer on g-alumina:the structure and acidity controlled by the template molecule. Langmuir 1998; 14(16):4623-4629.

89. Kodakari N, Sakamoto T, Shinkawa K et al. Molecular-sieving gas sensor prepared by chemical vapor deposition of silica on tin oxide using an organic template. Bull Chem Soc Jpn 1998; 71(2):513-519.
90. Tanimura T, Katada N, Niwa M. Molecular shape recognition by tin oxide chemical sensor coated with silica overlayer precisely designed using organic molecule as template. Langmuir 2000; 16(8):3858-3865.
91. Katada N, Niwa M. Silica-tin oxide sensor with molecular recognition ability. Sens Update 2001; 9:225-254.
92. Katada N, Niwa M. Chemical vapor deposition of silica overlayer using an organic molecule as template on metal oxide surface:application to molecular sieving sensor and adsorbent. this book.
93. Suzuki A, Tada M, Sasaki T et al. Design of catalytic sites at oxide surfaces by metal-complex attaching and molecular imprinting techniques. J Mol Catal, A: Chemical 2002; 182-183:125-136.
94. Niwa M, Katada N, Murakami Y. Thin silica layer on alumina:evidence of the acidity in the monolayer. J Phys Chem 1990; 94(16); 6441-6445.
95. Katada N, Toyama T, Niwa M. Mechanism of growth of silica monolayer and generation of acidity by chemical vapor deposition of tetramethoxysilane on alumina. J Phys Chem 1994; 98(31):7647-7652.
96. Tada M, Sasaki T, Iwasawa Y. Performance and kinetic behavior of a new SiO$_2$-attached molecular-imprinting Rh-dimer catalyst in size- and shape-selective hydrogenation of alkenes. J Catal 2002; 211:496-510.
97. Tada M, Iwasawa Y. Design of molecular-imprinting metal-complex catalysts. J Mol Catal, A: Chemical 2003; 199:115-137.
98. Lee S-W, Ichinose I, Kunitake T. Molecular imprinting of protected amino acids in ultrathin multilayers of TiO$_2$ gel. Chem Lett 1998:1193-1194.
99. Lee S-W, Ichinose I, Kunitake T. Molecular imprinting of azobenzene carboxylic acid on a TiO$_2$ ultrathin film by the surface sol-gel process. Langmuir 1998; 14(10):2857-2863.
100. Ichinose I, Kikuchi T, Lee S-W et al. Imprinting and selective binding of di- and tri-peptides in ultrathin TiO$_2$-gel films in aqueous solutions. Chem Lett 2002:104-105.
101. Srebnik S, Lev O. Theoretical investigation of imprinted crosslinked silicates. J Sol-Gel Sci Tech 2003; 26:107-113.

CHAPTER 4

Chemical Vapor Deposition of Silica Overlayer Using an Organic Molecule as Template on Metal Oxide Surface:
Application to Molecular Sieving Sensor and Adsorbent

Naonobu Katada and Miki Niwa

Abstract

Recent progress is reviewed on the studies carried out to design a reaction field on surfaces consisting purely of metal oxides. Chemical vapor deposition (CVD) of silicon alkoxide, using a molecule as a template, formed a silica overlayer on a weakly basic metal oxide surface with molecular sieving properties of adsorption, catalysis and chemical sensing. The observed shape selectivity was consistent with the molecular shape and size and was high in comparison with that obtained by liquid phase preparation attempts to molecularly imprint metal oxides.

Introduction

Molecular imprinting is a method to design and construct a reaction field on a solid surface in atomic dimensions. Most of the studies in the field of molecular imprinting have been done using organic molecules as templates to form organic polymers with reaction cavities on the surfaces. There have been many attempts using organic modifiers to construct reaction fields on inorganic solids.[1] However, in comparison with organic materials, metal oxides possess advantages in thermal and mechanical stability, and various functions such as catalysis, semi-conducting property and sensing ability. There have been many proposals to design a reaction field on a metal oxide. In order to construct a porous structure inside a bulk of metal oxide, numerous attempts have been made to create micro- and mesoporous[3,4] oxides using organic molecules as templates.

Only a few studies, however, have been carried out to design a reaction field on a surface consisting purely of metal oxides. Dickey proposed a concept for the design of a specific adsorption site using a molecule as the template. The adsorption capacity of a particular molecule on the silica gel was preferably increased when the silica gel was prepared under the presence of the organic molecule.[5] In this study, for example, the adsorption capacity of methyl orange was higher than that of ethyl orange on the silica gel prepared in the presence of methyl orange. The presence of the methyl orange during the preparation of silica gel was expected to form a cavity whose shape was controlled by the molecular shape of methyl orange template. However, the selectivity was not clearly demonstrated, although some studies followed continued this work.[6] Morihara et al proposed a 'footprint catalyst' based on the surface design using an organic molecule as the template.[7] A silica-alumina gel was exposed to a dibenzamide (or similar

Molecular Imprinting of Polymers, edited by Sergey Piletsky and Anthony Turner.

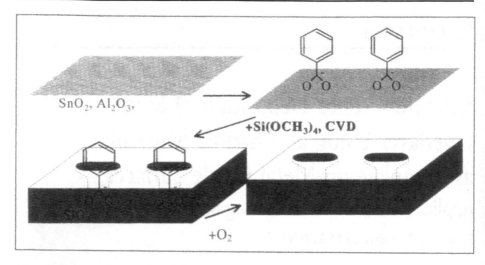

Figure 1. Concept of preparation of silica overlayer with cavities controlled by organic template.

molecules) solution, and the surface dehydration was carried out to fix the surface structure. After the removal of template, the thus obtained silica-alumina catalyst showed high catalytic activity selectively for butanolysis of benzoic anhydride, in which the reaction intermediate was speculated to fit with the reaction field. Recently, Heilmann and Maier used organic phosphonates as the templates to control the microstructure of silica gel.[8] However, as Maier et al stated, the observed selectivity in adsorption ability was generally low in these studies and not only the shape of the reaction field but also the chemical nature affected the specific adsorption property.[9] All of these studies utilized the hydrolysis of silicon alkoxide into silica in a solution to construct a reaction field on the surface. The hydrolysis of silicon alkoxide usually forms a highly porous silica gel. It is speculated that the thus formed silica wall possesses many terminal silanols and defects in atomic dimension. It is supposed that a high selectivity requires a structure of silica in which silicon and oxygen atoms are packed in a high density without defects. In other words, a network of siloxane (Si-O-Si) should be well developed to realize the design of a reaction field using silica and the template.

We have developed a method of chemical vapor deposition (CVD) of silicon alkoxide to design the structure of external surface of zeolite. The structure of silica layer was well controlled to a scale of several angstroms to finely tune the shape selectivity of zeolite.[10] This method has been applied to a practical use for shape selective synthesis of *para*-xylene from toluene and methanol in several countries.[11] Subsequently the CVD method was applied to the surfaces of such metal oxides as alumina, titania and zirconia, i.e., weakly basic metal oxides.[12-14] CVD of tetramethoxysilane [$Si(OCH_3)_4$] resulted in a monolayer of silica almost completely covering the surface.[15] The microstructure of a silica monolayer on alumina consists of a two dimensional network of siloxane[16] with a high concentration of $Si(OSi)_3(OAl)_1$ species and a quite low concentration of silanols[18] under selected preparation conditions. On the other hand, we found the strong chemisorption of aldehyde on these basic oxides formed a stable carboxylate anion.[19] By combining these two studies, we started to apply this method to prepare a silica overlayer with the cavity designed using a template molecule, as shown in Figure 1.[20] We named the resulting material a "molecular-sieving silica overlayer", because it sieves molecules before they reach the substrate surface. This method can add shape selectivity to a surface that possesses an original function such as catalysis.

In order to realize this procedure, the following parameters are required:

    1. The density of adsorbed template can be controlled.

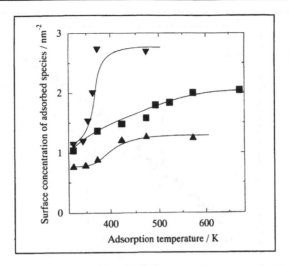

Figure 2. Chemisorption capacities of butanal (▼), benzaldehyde (■) and 1-naphthaldehyde (▲) on tin oxide.

   2. The adsorbed template is stable under the conditions of the subsequent CVD. Moreover, the adsorbed molecules do not form the domain by self-condensation. For these two requirements, the bond between the template and substrate surface should be a strong chemical bond.

   3. The deposited silica distributes homogeneously on all the surfaces of oxide particles. For this, the mass-transfer limitation should be avoided during the CVD.

   4. The bonding between silica and the template can be avoided. The silicon alkoxide is preferentially deposited in a high density on the surface uncovered by the template. For these requirements, the interaction between the silica and the oxide surface should also be strong.

As detailed,[21] the proposed system satisfies these requirements. The thus prepared SiO_2/MO_x has many potential applications for separation, adsorption and catalysis, i.e., all the functions that the substrate material originally had.

Shape Selective Adsorption

   Figure 2 shows the adsorption capacities of butanal, benzaldehyde and 1-naphthaldehyde on a tin oxide surface, divided by the surface area.[22] The adsorption capacity generally increased with increasing adsorption temperature. This suggests that the adsorption of these molecules under these conditions is classified as chemisorption, which can be controlled by kinetics; therefore the adsorption amount is enhanced by increasing the temperature. The mechanism of chemisorption of aldehyde has been studied;[19] it is considered that the corresponding carboxylate anion was formed from the aldehyde on such basic metal oxides as alumina and tin oxide. The maximum concentration of adsorbed species was observed above 400, 600 and 450 K to be ca. 2.8, 2.0 and 1.3 molecules nm^{-2} for butanal, benzaldehyde and 1-naphthaldehyde, respectively. These maximum concentrations are in agreement with the simulated values for the surface saturated with the carboxylate anions. Therefore, it is estimated that the surface was completely covered by the carboxylate anions at the high temperatures above 400, 600 and 450 K for butanal, benzaldehyde and 1-naphthaldehyde, respectively. Such a high coverage has to be avoided for preparation of SiO_2/MO_x with molecular recognition ability. Therefore low adsorption temperatures were selected for these aldehydes.

   It was found that the CVD of tetramethoxysilane selectively formed a monolayer of silica, in which all the silicon atoms possessed 1 : 1 bonding to the aluminum cations on the alumina surface.[15] Later, this was also observed commonly on such basic oxides as titania and zirconia.[24]

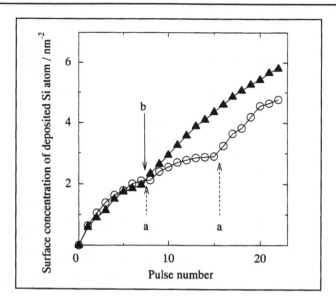

Figure 3. Example of deposition behavior of silica by pulse of tetramethoxysilane. In the experiment shown by O, water was injected at (a). In the another experiment shown by ▲, aqueous solution of acetic acid was injected at (b).

The formation of a silica monolayer is based on the nature of silica and the metal oxide support; different properties of these metal oxides bring about strong interactions between them and forms the monolayer of deposited oxide. The mechanism of the CVD of silicon alkoxide on the basic metal oxide surface has been detailed elesewhere.[16]

By combining these two backgrounds, the CVD of tetramethoxysilane after the adsorption of benzaldehyde was tested at 423 K. The deposition of tetramethoxysilane was immediately saturated by several injections and the introduction of water vapor made it possible to continue further deposition, as shown in Figure 3 (O). Finally the template was removed by calcination in oxygen.

Thus the SiO_2/SnO_2 sample was prepared using an aldehyde molecule as the template. Although it is generally difficult to find an experimental method which can evaluate the shape of the adsorption site apart from the chemical nature,[9] we could utilize the chemisorption of aldehydes themselves. As stated above, the adsorption of aldehyde occurs on the surface of uncovered basic metal oxide to cover the surface completely at a high temperature. In contrast, it does not occur on the silica surface.[25] The adsorption capacities of three kinds of aldehydes on the thus prepared SiO_2/SnO_2 sample were displayed in Figure 4 (A) as the relative values divided by the capacities on SnO_2. The utilized template was benzaldehyde. The deposition of silica decreased the amount of adsorbed material in all the cases. The adsorption capacity for 1-naphthaldehyde, the molecule larger than the template, was relatively low on the SiO_2/SnO_2 sample (A). This is possibly due to the shape selectivity generated by the controlled cavity size. However, the selectivity was low; a considerable adsorption of 1-naphthaldehyde was observed on the sample (A), showing that there were considerable amount of adsorption sites whose size was larger than the template molecule.

In order to improve the selectivity, we tested some additional reagents to accelerate the formation of siloxane bond from the silicon alkoxides. By adding acetic acid during the CVD, the deposition of tetramethoxysilane was enhanced, as shown in Figure 5 (▲). The adsorption of 1-naphthaldehyde was almost completely suppressed on the SiO_2/SnO_2 sample prepared using the benzaldehyde template under the presence of acetic acid, as shown in Figure 7 (C).

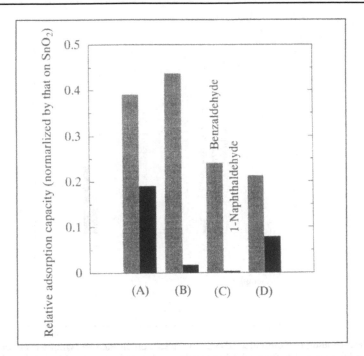

Figure 4. Relative adsorption capacities (adsorption capacity on the modified sample / adsorption capacity on the unmodified tin oxide) of benzaldehyde (gray bar) and 1-naphthaldehyde (black bar) on SiO_2/SnO_2 prepared using benzaldehyde as the template under the co-presence of water (A), trifluoroacetic acid + water (B), acetic acid + water (C) and ammonia + water (D).

Trifluoroacetic acid also showed high selectivity (B), whereas ammonia showed no positive effect (D). In summary, the presence of a volatile acid during the CVD of silicon alkoxide seems to improve the shape selectivity. Although the mechanism has not been clarified, the importance of the preparation conditions for silica layers should be noted.

The deposition of silica without the template suppressed the adsorption capacities for all the used aldehydes, as shown in Figure 5. On the SiO_2/SnO_2 sample prepared using butanal as the template, only butanal itself showed a high adsorption capacity, while the larger molecules, i.e., benzaldehyde and 1-naphthaldehyde, showed quite low adsorption capacities. On the SiO_2/SnO_2 sample prepared using benzaldehyde as the template, butanal and benzaldehyde, namely the molecules smaller than the template and the template itself, showed high adsorption capacities, while the larger molecule, i.e., 1-naphthaldehyde, showed almost no adsorption capacities. When 1-naphthaldehyde was used as the template, all the used aldehydes were adsorbed in high capacities. Thus, the shape selectivity was performed in the chemisorption of aldehyde; a molecule whose size is smaller or the same as the template molecule can be penetrate into the surface cavity, while a larger molecule is not adsorbed.[26,27] We have reported similar selective adsorption on SiO_2/Al_2O_3 prepared by this method and the analysis by solid state NMR (nuclear magnetic resonance) was adopted in this case.[28]

Oxidation Catalysis and Sensing Property

Tin oxide has an activity as an oxidation catalyst. Figure 6 shows that the unmodified tin oxide possessed an activity for complete oxidation of alkane into carbon dioxide; under the utilized conditions, the conversion of C_6 alkane isomers was 50 to 85% on the unmodified tin oxide. CVD of silica did not affect the reaction of *n*-hexane, i.e., the linear molecule. The high

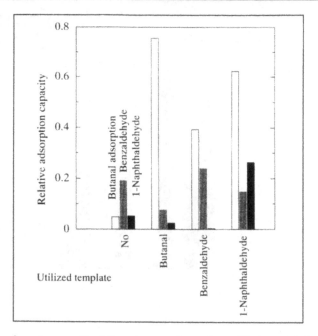

Figure 5. Relative adsorption capacities (adsorption capacity on the modified sample/adsorption capacity on the unmodified tin oxide) of butanal (white bar), benzaldehyde (gray bar) and 1-naphthaldehyde (black bar) on SiO$_2$/SnO$_2$ prepared using various aldehydes under the co-presence of acetic acid and water.

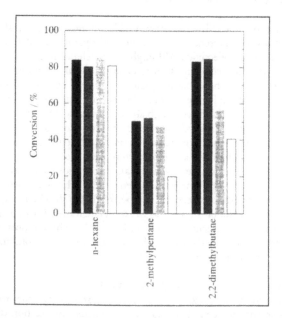

Figure 6. Conversion of C$_6$ alkane on SnO$_2$ (black bar), and SiO$_2$/SnO$_2$ prepared using 1-naphthaldehyde (dark gray bar), benzaldehyde (light gray bar) and butanal (white bar) as template.

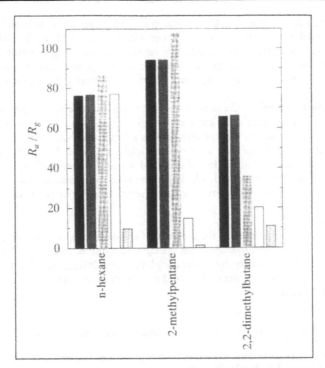

Figure 7. Sensitivity to C_6 alkane on SnO_2 (black bar), and SiO_2/SnO_2 prepared using 1-naphthaldehyde (dark gray bar), benzaldehyde (light gray bar) and butanal (white bar) as template, and without template (cross-hatched bar).

conversion, close to 80%, was maintained on the SiO_2/SnO_2 samples prepared using various aldehydes as the templates. However, the isomer with one methyl branch, namely 2-methylpentane, showed relatively low conversion on the SiO_2/SnO_2 sample prepared under the presence of butanal template. This suggests that the branched molecule cannot penetrate into the surface cavity whose shape was controlled by the template aldehyde with a linear alkyl group. In the case of the isomer with two methyl branches (2,2-dimethylbutane), the SiO_2/SnO_2 sample prepared using the benzaldehyde template also showed the low conversion as well as the sample prepared using the butanal template. The SiO_2/SnO_2 sample prepared using the 1-naphthaldehyde template showed high activities for all the isomers. The thus observed selectivity is consitent with the molecular size, as explained in detail elsewhere.[22] The selectivity was also observed for the C_8 alkane isomers. This is the first report of clear reactant shape selectivity on an inorganic solid catalyst other than zeolites.[22] Recently Suzuki and Shido et al reported the selectivity in acid-catalyzed hydrolysis of esters on SiO_2/Al_2O_3 prepared by CVD under the presence of template molecule.[29]

Tin oxide also possesses an ability as a chemical sensor. Because the catalytic oxidation proceeds on the tin oxide surface as above, the concentration of surface oxygen is changed by contact with organic vapor, resulting in a change of electric resistance.[30] Figure 7 shows the sensitivities of the SiO_2/SnO_2 samples to the C_6 alkane isomers. The unmodified tin oxide showed high sensitivities to all the isomers. In contrast, the SiO_2/SnO_2 prepared using no template showed low sensitivities to all the isomers. Probably all the surface was covered by silica, which has no oxidation activity. The high sensitivity to n-hexane was maintained on the SiO_2/SnO_2 samples prepared using various aldehydes as the templates. The isomer with one methyl branch showed a low sensitivity on the SiO_2/SnO_2 sample prepared under the presence of butanal template. The SiO_2/SnO_2 samples prepared using the butanal and benzaldehyde templates showed low sensitivities to the isomer with two methyl branches. The SiO_2/SnO_2 sample prepared using the 1-naphthaldehyde template showed high sensitivities for all the isomers. Thus, the sensitivity changed according to the change in oxidation activity, and shape selectivity due to the cavity size is suggested. Selective recognition for alcohols and aldehydes was also found.[31]

It is proposed to combine the sensors which possess characteristic responses to a specific compound in order to establish a 'chemical imaging system' or 'electronic nose'.[32] For this purpose, a set of many sensor devices with various selectivities should be developed, and furthermore a method to design such a set systematically is needed. There are a number of researches dealing with the modification of chemical sensor,[21] but control of the chemical reaction on the solid surface has been difficult. The present series of chemical sensors with adjustable molecular shape recognition properties are presumed to have major potential.

Conclusion

The CVD of silicon alkoxide in the presence of aldehyde template on a weakly basic metal oxide surface forms an silica overlayer with selective adsorption, catalytic and sensing properties. Precise control of the cavity size by the template molecule is suggested by the high selectivity. The formation of a silicate network should be important to realize the design of a reaction field as shown in Figure 1.

References

1. Haupt K. Imprinted polymers-Tailor-made mimics of antibodies and receptors. Chem Commun 2003; (2):171-178.
2. Freyhardt CC, Tsapatsis M, Lobo RF et al. A high-silica zeolite with a 14-tetrahedral-atom pore opening. Nature 1996; 381(23):295-298.
3. Kresge CT, Leonowicz ME, Roth WJ et al. Ordered mesoporous molecular sieves synthesized by a liquid-crystal template mechanism. Nature 1992; 359:710-712.
4. Inagaki S, Fukushima Y, Kuroda K. Synthesis of highly ordered mesoporous materials from a layered polysilicate. J Chem Soc, Chem Commun 1993:680-682.
5. Dickey FH. Specific adsorption. J Phys Chem 1955; 59:695-707.
6. Bernhard SA. The preparation of specific adsorbants. J Am Chem Soc 1952; 74:4946-4947.
7. Morihara K, Kurihara S, Suzuki J. Foot print catalysis. I. A new method for designing "tailor-made" catalysts with substrate specificity:silica (alumina) catalysts for butanolysis of benzoic anhydride. Bull Chem Soc Jpn 1988; 61(11):3991-3998.
8. Heilmann J, Maier WF. Selective catalysis on silicon dioxide with substrate-specific cavities. Angew Chem Int Ed Engl 1994; 33(4):471-473.
9. Hunnius M, Rufinska A, Maier WF. Selective surface adsorption versus imprinting in amorphous microporous silicas. Micro- Mesoporous Mater 1999; 29:389-403.
10. Niwa M, Kato S, Hattori T et al. Fine control of pore-opening size of zeolite ZSM-5 by chemical vapor deposition of silicon methoxide. J Phys Chem 1986; 90:6233-6237.
11. Halgeri AB, Das J. Recent advances in selectivation of zeolites for para-disubstituted aromatics. Catal Today 2002; 73(1-2):65-73.
12 Jin T, Okuhara T, White JM. Ultra-high vacuum preparation and characterization of ultra-thin layers of SiO_2 on ZrO_2 and TiO_2 by chemical vapour deposition of Si(OEt)$_4$. J Chem Soc, Chem Commun 1987; 248-249.
13. Niwa M, Hibino T, Murata H et al. A silica monolayer on alumina and evidence of lack of acidity of silanol attached to alumina. J Chem Soc, Chem Commun 1989; (5):289-290.
14. Sato S, Toita M, Sodesawa T et al. Catalytic and acidic properties of silica-alumina prepared by chemical vapor deposition. Appl Catal 1990; 62:73-84.
15. Niwa M, Katada N, Murakami Y. Thin silica layer on alumina:evidence of the acidity in the monolayer. J Phys Chem 1990; 94(16):6441-6445.
16. Katada N, Toyama T, Niwa M. Mechanism of growth of silica monolayer and generation of acidity by chemical vapor deposition of tetramethoxysilane on alumina. J Phys Chem 1994; 98(31):7647-7652.
17. Katada N, Niwa M. Microstructure of silica monolayer solid acid catalyst determined by 29Si NMR spectroscopy. Res Chem Intermed 1998; 24(5):481-494.

18. Katada N, Fujii T, Iwata K et al. Concentration of hydroxyl groups on silica monolayer solid acid catalyst. J Catal 1999; 186:478-480.
19. Niwa M, Inagaki S, Murakami Y. Alumina:sites and mechanism for benzaldehyde and ammonia reaction. J Phys Chem 1985; 89(12):2550-2555.
20. Kodakari N, Katada N, Niwa M. Molecular sieving silica overlayer on tin oxide prepared using an organic template. J Chem Soc, Chem Commun 1995:623-624.
21. Katada N, Niwa M. Silica-tin oxide sensor with molecular recognition ability. Sensors Update 2001; 9:225-254.
22. Tanimura T, Katada N, Niwa M. Molecular shape recognition by tin oxide chemical sensor coated with silica overlayer precisely designed using organic molecule as template. Langmuir 2000; 16(8):3858-3865.
23. Kodakari N, Katada N, Niwa M. Silica overlayer prepared using an organic template on tin oxide and its molecular sieving property. Adv Mater, Chem Vap Deposition 1997; 3(1):59-66.
24. Niwa M, Katada N, Murakami Y. Generation of acid sites by SiO_2 deposition on groups IVB metal oxides. J Catal 1992; 134:340-348.
25. Niwa M, Suzuki K, Kishida M et al. Benzaldehyde-ammonia titration method for discrimination between surfaces of metal oxide catalysts. Appl Catal 1991; 67:297-305.
26. Akazawa S, Shimogai M, Magata K et al. Preparation of molecular sieving silica layer by chemical vapor deposition with acetic acid as a condensation reagent. In: Preprint of 89th Catalysis Society of Japan Meeting A. Tokyo: Catalysis Society of Japan, 2002:1P06.
27. Katada N, Akazawa S, Niwa M. Improvement of selectivity in specific adsorption by addition of acetic acid during chemical vapor deposition of silicon alkoxide to form a silica overlayer with molecular sieving property. Adv Mater, Chem Vap Deposition, in press.
28. Kodakari N, Tomita K, Iwata K et al. Molecular sieving silica overlayer on g-alumina:the structure and acidity controlled by the template molecule. Langmuir 1998; 14(16):4623-4629.
29. Suzuki A, Tada M, Sasaki T et al. Design of catalytic sites at oxide surfaces by metal-complex attaching and molecular imprinting techniques. J Mol Catal, A: Chemical 2002; 182-183:125-136.
30. Yamazoe N, Miura N. Some basic aspects of semiconductor gas sensors. Chem Sensor Tech 1992; 4:19-42.
31. Kodakari N, Sakamoto T, Shinkawa K et al. Molecular-sieving gas sensor prepared by chemical vapor deposition of silica on tin oxide using an organic template. Bull Chem Soc Jpn 1998; 71(2):513-519.
32. Göpel W. Nanosensors and molecular recognition. Micoelectr Eng 1996; 32:75-110.

CHAPTER 5

Molecularly Imprinted Polymers for Mass Sensitive Sensors:
From Cells to Viruses and Enzymes

Franz L. Dickert, Peter A. Lieberzeit and Oliver Hayden

Abstract

Artificial recognition layers for bioanalytes (cells, bacteria, viruses, proteins etc.) combine biological selectivity with the long-term stability of tailored polymers. They can be produced by surface imprinting procedures where the analyte-to-be is used as template and pressed into a prepolymerized reaction mixture of a highly cross-linked polymer during curing of the material. The cells removed from the surface leave behind adapted cavities that are ideally shaped for reincorporation, as they are formed by self-organization processes of the prepolymer around the cell walls. As these biological samples consist of high molecular weight substances or their assemblies, no bulk imprinting routines can be used as a result of unfavorable layer height and diffusion behavior into the layer. Combining such a layer with a befitting transducer yields sensor devices being highly suitable for the fast, reversible and straightforward on-line detection of these analytes.

Introduction

Deeper chemical insight into the processes occurring in living organisms and the application of these results in gene technology has triggered off extraordinary scientific progress in a variety of fields such as pharmacy, healthcare, food technology and many more. On the other hand, infections caused by contaminated water and food but also in hospitals, where especially multi-resistant microorganisms occur, still impose one of the most fundamental threats to man. During the last few years this was complemented by the danger of terrorist attacks making use of e.g., biological warfare agents such as anthrax spores. Therefore, developing methods for the fast and straightforward detection of biogenous species is an urgent necessity. Of course, there is a variety of well-developed analytical routines, such as breeding on culture plates or PCR for bacteria, fungi and viruses or modern chromatography, electrophoresis[1] and soft-ionisation techniques for proteins but also entire microorganisms. All these methods, however, have in common that they are usually time consuming (e.g., breeding procedures in a Petri dish last for several days before a result is obtained) or require high-end apparatus as well as extensively trained personnel. Huge effort has thus to be done to miniaturize classical appliances or to develop (bio-) chemical sensor systems for bioanalyte detection.

Molecular Imprinting of Polymers, edited by Sergey Piletsky and Anthony Turner.
©2006 Landes Bioscience.

Principles of Chemical Sensing

Transducer Technologies

Chemical sensors have turned out to be a very powerful tool in analytical sciences, especially when small, rugged systems capable of on-line and remote measurements[2] are to be considered. A wide variety of transducers is proposed for this purpose, although the most prominent ones rely either on potentiometric, optical or acoustic effects. Similarly to chemical sensing, optical systems are mainly based on fiber optic setups, which are either used directly or by depositing a dye showing a response to the surrounding biological environment. Acoustic sensors, on the other hand, usually transform a mechanical movement of standing waves into an electronic signal, for the detection of biogenous matter usually quartz crystal microbalances (QCM[3]) and surface acoustic wave resonators (SAW[4]) are applied. An even more recent technology of transducers are surface plasmon resonators, where the electron gas in a thin gold layer is brought to resonance by polarized light with a defined angle of incidence. Naturally, as the excitation energy is introduced into the system by light and the reflectance is measured via a diode array detector, the signal is highly influenced by the dielectric properties of the surrounding medium. A comparative study of SPR and QCM for bioanalyte detection can be found in literature.[5] Different electrochemical and electronic devices are also used as transducers; they usually rely on measuring the capacitance or the conductance during cell growth. As every microorganism contains an outer membrane consisting of a lipid bilayer that acts as an insulator, biofilm growth significantly changes the electric properties on the electrodes within the sensing chamber. This effect usually can be detected when a certain threshold value of microbe surface concentration is exceeded. Naturally, during analysis one is interested in the initial cell concentration of a sample. Thus, if a sample is incubated in an electrochemical cell, the growing biomass will change the capacity and conductance and a sensor signal is observed. The time necessary for a distinct response to occur (the so called onset time of signal change) depends on the initial microorganism concentration in the sample. Of course, the more cells have been initially present the shorter this time will be.

Layer Design Strategies

Therefore, any of the transducer systems described here gives a detectable signal change when exposed to microorganisms, especially if these tend to form biofilms. In developing a sensor system for a defined analytical problem, however, it is necessary to generate a selectivity towards a specified analyte thus making it possible to discriminate between different types of cells.

Immunochemistry

Obviously, established analytical strategies for the discrimination between biological species, such as e.g., immunochemical methods, can be chosen for this purpose. One possibility to do so is to cover the sensitive area of a transducer with an antibody against the species to be detected. A variety of different methods has been proposed for this purpose, most of them having in common that a suitable antibody is immobilized on the surface of the transducer either directly or by linking it via a thin polymer coating (for more details see references 3 and 4 and the papers cited therein). Some authors, however, propose different strategies, e.g., by immobilising the sample cells and exposing them to antibodies[6] or by using sensitive coatings reacting with metabolic products of the analyte species,[7] for this latter purpose also entire viable or dead cells[8] can be deposited on the transducer.

Artificial Polymers—Imprinting

Although providing excellent sensitivity, biological recognition layers usually have the inherent disadvantage of comparably low long-term stability. In the case of living organisms, metabolic processes remove degraded enzymes and replace them by fresh ones forming an open system in this way. In a nonliving system, however, denaturizing strongly limits the amount of possible measuring cycles as well as the shelf-life of the respective sensor. Although it has been found that enzymes e.g., can be stabilized by caging them in the matrix of a sol-gel material, where they retain their biological activity, further improvement both in long-term stability as well as in reversibility would be highly desirable. A powerful strategy to overcome these limitations and to generate cavities ideally adapted to the analyte-to-be is molecular (or in this case better: supramolecular) imprinting into a highly cross linked polymer matrix. The method combines a quite straightforward synthesis (especially compared with the production of supramolecular hollows for host-guest-chemistry) with an outstanding variability and flexibility in application. The main idea is to polymerize the material in the presence of the analyte-to-be, which can either be covalently linked to a monomer (covalent imprinting) or be mixed with the starting material but not interfering with the polymerization reaction (noncovalent imprinting). Especially in the latter case the polymer morphology is determined by weak, noncovalent interactions between the template and the monomer compounds ending up in the optimal sterical arrangement. The template is thus incorporated into the three-dimensional polymer network and can be removed from the matrix once the reactions have finished, leaving behind diffusion pathways. As a result of the high content of cross linking agents, the structure does not collapse upon the removal of the printing molecule, but the shape is retained therefore leading to ideally adapted pores ranging from nanometers to micrometers. The the templates perfectly fit into the holes in a selective manner both in geometrical and enthalpic respects. Aside of the comparably simple and therefore very elegant way to generate the interaction sites, another advantage of the method is given by the outstanding variety of polymeric systems that can be used. These cover both organic polymers as well as inorganic ones being synthesized via a variety of polyreactions, such as polyadditions, polycondensations and radical polymerizations.

Surface Imprinting with Bioanalytes

For analytes of molecular size usually bulk imprinting procedures are used, as the small particles diffuse through the network rather fast and therefore can also reach interaction sites deep within the bulk in a reasonable time. Of course, this results in comparably high mass effects for the materials. This strategy, however, can not be applied for biological samples due to their size; in this case surface imprinting procedures are to be used: Nonetheless, as microorganisms are much bulkier than molecules, this easily makes up for the restriction. The resulting functional surfaces show very strong interactions with the templating species and can therefore be regarded as artificial antibodies.

Yeast

Early work done in this field was accomplished by imprinting polyurethane with yeast cells,[9,10] which were chosen as a model template due to their robustness and availability. Figure 1 depicts the principal procedure used in this case: a stamp containing the microorganisms is pressed into a prereacted polymer mixture. The first step involves producing a suitable stamp. For this purpose a glass slide is covered with yeast and then pressed against a Teflon plate to achieve a perfectly flat surface. Meanwhile, a suitable monomer mixture is prepolymerized and deposited onto the transducer by spin-coating. In this case highly cross linked polyurethane consisting of diisocyanatodiphenylmethane, bisphenol A and phloroglucinol (serving as cross-linker) is used, the polymer contains a double molar excess of the alcoholic compounds to prevent covalent binding between the microorganisms and the forming polymer. Of course, other macromolecular systems such as sol-gel glasses can also be used.[11] Finally, the stamp is pressed onto the transducer followed by polymer curing usually taking place overnight. After the reactions have finished, the stamp is removed and adhering cells are washed from the surface by hot water leaving behind their cast in the material (see Fig. 2; here some of the hollows are occupied by cells). The resulting cavities show hexagonal, honeycomb-like packing, thus indicating that the cells adopt the most densely packed surface structure during stamp production. Some experimental details have to be taken into account: the quality of the imprinted surface depends not

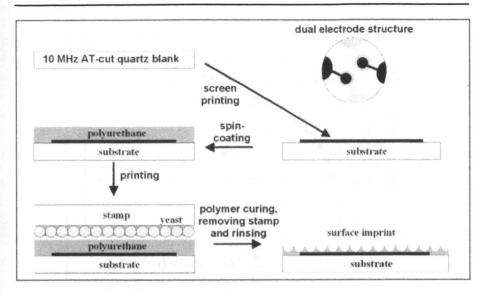

Figure 1. Imprinting procedure for cells.

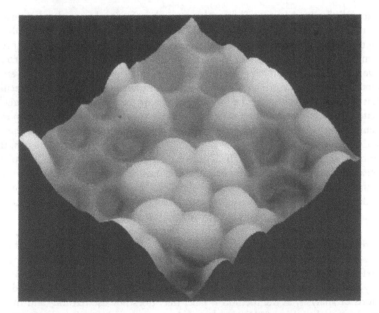

Figure 2. Poylurethane surface imprinted with yeast cells, reinclusion of cells.

only on the stage of prepolymerization before stamping but also on the morphological and functional properties of the microorganism cell walls. While mobile oligomeric chains grow during film synthesis, a wide variety of noncovalent interactions influences their arrangement around the cells: phenolic monomers form hydrogen bonds with the cell surface, additionally there are π-π-interactions, Van-der-Waals as well as hydrophobic interactions. Obviously, the growing polymer partly engulfs the stamp cells, as the resulting structures are rather deep and show sharp ridges. All these interactions leading to the ideal arrangement of the film around the microorganisms occur in an interfacial layer being only a few micrometers thick. Usually,

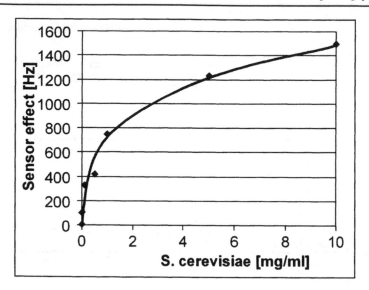

Figure 3. Sensor calibration curve for an imprinted polyurethane layer exposed to yeast cells.

the template cells have to be removed from the matrix by a fast washing pulse that pushes them away from the surface, as their interactions with the structured polymer are comparably strong. Producing templated polymers on transducers is compatible to industrial standard procedures of layer generation and can readily be extended to the manufacturing of wide-stretched surfaces, as we succeeded in producing good quality imprints covering an area of several square centimeters. However, imprinting polymers with cells rather than with small molecules leads to a further difference: in this case the building blocks of the polymer are much smaller than the templates, therefore the resulting cavities fit exactly for the cell used. When molecules are used for templating, on the other hand, the monomers have about the same size as the analytes. In this case the exact morphology of the pores depends on a variety of parameters, the most important of which is temperature.[12] In Figure 3 the sensor characteristic of a two electrode QCM is given, where one electrode is coated with a yeast-imprinted layer and the other contains a nonimprinted layer and thus serves as reference. The data shown actually represents the frequency difference between the two electrodes. It can clearly be seen that the signal increases monotonously with growing exposition to yeasts thus proving the potential of the sensor system. When changing from pure phosphate buffer to a suspension containing yeasts, the device frequency on the selective channel decreases as a result of cell incorporation into the cavities, whereas the reference signal remains (almost) unaffected. As soon as the surrounding media is switched back to pure buffer, the frequency reaches the initial value thus proving the excellent reversibility of our sensor system. This overcomes many of the limitations associated with current methods of analysis, as the method is label-free, does not use natural (and thus fragile) antibodies, no special washing and drying steps are necessary and therefore regeneration can be avoided. Thus, imprinting polymers with microorganisms by making use of self-organization effects yields materials with excellent sensing abilities.

Even biological processes can be cast into the material: Figure 4 shows an inverted image of a yeast imprinted layer (the cavities appear as elevations in the picture, the effects can be seen much better this way). In the region marked, an ongoing budding process of a cell can clearly be seen. Another fact worth mentioning is the size distribution of the imprinted cavities; the variation in dimensions depicts the distribution of cell ages within the population. Therefore, the resulting sensors are able to incorporate a yeast cell at any stage of living, which greatly enhances method sensitivity.

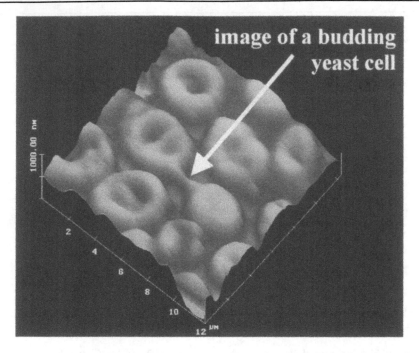

Figure 4. Imprint of budding yeast cells.

Selectivity

Selectivity, however, is a major question not yet addressed. For this purpose the sensors prepared are exposed to different strands of yeasts, but also to bacteria, while recording the frequency shifts on the QCM (see Fig. 5). The analytes in this case are *Saccharomyces cerevisiae* cells (provided both in compressed as well as in active dry form), *S. bayanus*, Gram positive *Leuconostoc oenus* and Gram negative *E. coli*. The three yeast suspensions contain the same amount of microorganisms; the bacteria samples surpass this by two orders of magnitude. First of all, the sensor shows the same response for the two differently pretreated *S. cerevisiae* samples, which is an indicative that the interaction between layer and analyte is independent of possible surface artifacts resulting from drying procedures. The frequency shift for *S. bayanus*, however, reaches only about half the value compared with the template species. Therefore, the properties of the material in fact strongly depend on the surface structure of the templating microorganism, which points to the presence of not only a microstructure but also a noticeable amount of patterning on a molecular scale. Thus, not only the microscopic shape of the cell is cast into the material, but obviously also details of the outer cell membrane in nanometer dimensions are correctly reproduced indeed suggesting effective molecular printing. Born this in mind, it is not surprising that the two different bacteria strains do not show gravimetric sensor effects even in a hundredfold higher concentration. Of course, microorganisms can also be detected by bare transducer surfaces without the necessity of an interaction layer, but in this case an appreciable sensor response only occurs if cell concentration is suitably high for biofilm formation. Within the film the individual cells are closely confined in a small space defined by the packing and thus show only minor mobility. In case the individual microorganism moves freely on the transducer device, nonSauerbrey effects can be observed. *L. oenus* and *E. coli*, as representatives of Gram-positive and Gram-negative bacteria, respectively, also show different adhesion phenomena on the imprinted and the nonimprinted polymeric sensor coatings, as can be seen in Figure 5. All columns represent the signal of the templated channel on the quartz corrected by the nontemplated reference sensor. Negative frequency responses represent Sauerbrey

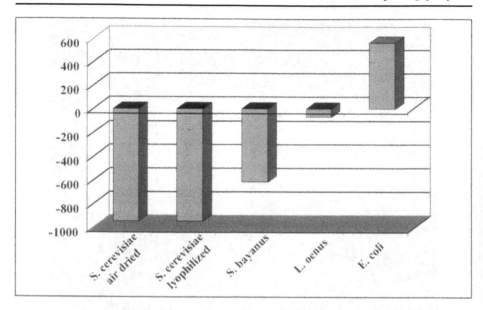

Figure 5. Cross sensitivities of a 10 MHz QCM sensor coated with a yeast-imprinted layer towards different species, data are already modified by the values of the reference QCM.

behavior (which is the usual phenomenon), thus positive effects signify that the bacteria more readily interact with the nonimprinted material. The Gram-positive *L. oenus* does not adhere at all on the reference channel but in fact shows a small but significant amount of interaction with the selective polymer, whereas the Gram-negative *E. coli* reacts completely differently. The details of this behavior of the latter species are a result of the known fact that it has strain- and material-dependent adhesion properties. Another point is worth mentioning: all inclusion phenomena observed are reversible, i.e., adherent cells can be washed away from the sensor surface by very easy means. This makes another fundamental difference between these artificial antibodies and their natural analogues, as the latter usually bind irreversibly with their respective antigen, which imposes a further limitation onto the use of natural compounds for sensing purposes (reversibility actually is a fundamental condition for a chemosensor). The artificial materials on the contrary interact weakly with the analyte by forming e.g., OH-bridges or undergoing other noncovalent interactions.

As mentioned earlier, not only organic polymers but also sol-gel materials can be surface-templated to yield sensor layers for cells. The main difference between the two materials is given by the different mechanical stabilities: in this case the inorganic materials are much more stable against mechanical and chemical impact than their organic counterpart. Therefore, whenever ruggedness is required, sol-gel procedures are favored over other polymerization procedures. For the use with biological samples, materials based on titanium have proven to be ideally suited, as they show more polar surfaces than the respective silica polymers thus better interacting with matrices under physiological conditions (e.g., contact lenses are usually made from titanium-based sol-gel materials).

When shear wave SAW resonators (STW) are used as transducer elements, method sensitivity is greatly increased. In Figure 6 the STW sensor responses of a polystyrene microsphere with a diameter of approximately 5 μm and of a yeast cell on the sensor are given. The deposition of the microspheres is controlled via light microscopy; therefore the short frequency decrease can be traced back to the sedimentation of a single polymer bead. Comparing the amount of frequency shift for the polymer and the yeast cells and calculating the respective masses, the frequency shift in Figure 6B can clearly be traced back to the interaction of a single yeast cell with the imprinted polymer surface.

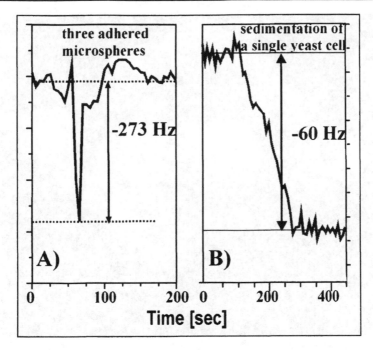

Figure 6. STW sensor effect of a silica microsphere with approximately 5 μm in diameter (A) and a yeast cell (B).

Although surface imprinting procedures in principle are a very straightforward and elegant method to generate cavities, a variety of parameters has to be taken into account to realize them. Factors expected to influence the interaction strength are e.g., prepolymerization status, humidity of the template cells, reaction time, reaction temperature, and others. As the templating procedure includes the pressing of a stamp into the forming polymer, the cells undergo mechanical stress. Yeast cells are very rugged and therefore can be directly used for imprinting procedures. These conditions, however, are too severe e.g., for erythrocytes: in this case the cells are easily osmotically destroyed impairing proper film formation. In this case the use of red cell ghosts might be an alternative.

Bacteria Sensors

Early reports of using bacteria as templates during a polymer synthesis were given by the group of Vulfson in 1996/97.[13,14] The authors self-assembled bacteria at the interface between the hydrophilic and the hydrophobic compound of a surfactant-stabilized emulsion. At this phase boundary a polyamide film is formed around the bacteria that are actually covalently included into the forming polymer network. This is followed by photopolymerizing a hydrophobic material within the organic phase leading to microbeads. After hydrolytic cleavage of the bonds between the bacteria and the polymer, functional hollows remain on the particle surfaces that are also capable of reincluding the template species. The main differences between this procedure and the one previously described for yeasts are the formation of microbeads instead of films and the covalent binding of the microorganisms to the polymer.

Templates for bioimprinting to generate sensor layers via the stamping method thus are not restricted to yeast cells, but also a variety of (much) smaller particles can be used for templating, as can be seen e.g., in Figure 7, where an AFM images of *E. coli* cells on an imprinted polyurethane surface can be seen. To prevent covalent linking between the bacteria and the forming polymer, an excess of phenol functionalities is used during synthesis, additionally it has been found to be useful to lyophilize the bacteria prior to molding. In this case again the surface

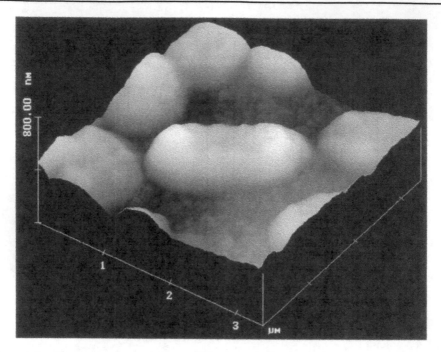

Figure 7. *E. coli* imprint, surface is partly occupied by re-included bacteria.

imprinting procedure already described for the yeasts is utilized, however the production of the stamp requires thorough tuning of the chemical parameters involved. A clear difference compared with yeast imprints can be found, anyway, by regarding the reversibility of the sensor signals: although both types of microorganism can be eliminated from their respective sensor materials, removing the yeast requires a strong washing pulse. This is not necessary for the bacteria, because they are much smaller in size than the *Saccharomyces* species thus offering a much lower interaction area with the forming polymer and the final layer, so it behaves more like a small molecule within the imprint material. Figure 8 shows the sensor responses of a QCM coated with such a layer when exposed to an *E. coli* suspension. Whereas the frequency of the reference channel remains almost unaffected, only a very slight decrease can be observed, the imprinted layer shows exclusively positive frequency shifts. This is remarkable, as it contradicts the premises given by the Sauerbrey equation, namely that increasing the mass on the electrode decreases the resonance frequency of the device. However, the phenomenon can be explained when regarding analyte mobility on the surface: According to Sauerbrey an ideally rigid mass is required for the validity of the correlation between mass and frequency. When bulky analytes such as bacteria are not tightly bound, the mechanical properties of the adherent layers change from rigid to viscoelastic, leading to the anomalous positive frequency shifts observed in this case. The slightly negative response of the reference channel can be traced back to the formation of bacteria aggregates: *E. coli* bacteria can be regarded as "sticky" and therefore tend to form bigger clusters that are no longer mobile on the surface and form a film if the concentration of the bacteria in the surrounding medium is high enough. The question arises why this effect can not be observed on imprinted layers. First, obviously the individual bacteria are still separated from each other as every single one occupies a cavity on the imprinted surface. Thus any aggregation is hindered and forming of a film is not possible. Second, the ridges between the imprinted holes are apparently low enough for the bacteria to roll over them. Therefore the bacteria retain their mobility on the surface leading to very high nonSauerbrey responses. Nonetheless, sensor curves can be recorded for these species and therefore bacterial concentrations can be determined.

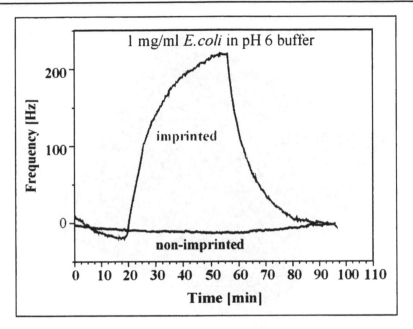

Figure 8. *E. coli* sensor effects on an *E. coli*-imprinted and a non-imprinted polyurethane layer.

Viruses

Stepping down the size scale for biological species, the next possible analytes for the detection with imprinted sensor layers are viruses. In this case a sensor would be even more favorable as viruses can not be detected by microscopes and therefore no easy and straightforward method for their determination exists. The tobacco mosaic virus (TMV) is not only one of the simplest viruses known but also imposes substantial threat for agriculture, as it does not only infect tobacco plants but also e.g., cucumber and pumpkin cultures. It consists of a helical strand of RNA covered with a protein shell; the resulting aggregate has a cylindrical shape with a length of about 200 nm and a diameter of about 20 nm. Although already very small in size, this species is still too large to be used for a bulk imprinting; therefore, once again the known surface grafting procedure has to be applied, where a monolayer of the virus on a stamp is pressed into the surface of a polymerizing material. In this case thermally prereacted styrene-methacrylate copolymers are used. The stamp consists of a glass plate covered with maltose that is dissolved in hot water after the polymerization has finished enabling removal. Self-organization processes control the polymerization reaction around the surfaces and lead to the hollows. Afterwards, the template viruses are washed from the surface by a 0.2% (w/w) solution of sodium dodecyl sulfate in water leaving behind the adapted cavities (see also Fig. 9). In the AFM image the resulting pits can clearly be seen, their size excellently agrees with the known dimensions of the TMV. Once again, mass-sensitive measurements prove the ability of selective reinclusion rendered possible by the imprinting procedure: Figure 10 shows the sensor effects of an imprinted and a nonimprinted layer on a QCM towards TMV in buffer. Clearly, the imprinted layer incorporates the viruses from the solution and yields a Sauerbrey-like mass effect.

Biomacromolecules

The last step down in size scale for surface imprinting procedures is given by (bio-) macromolecules. These usually can not be used for bulk imprinting procedures, as they are not removable from the inside of a polymeric matrix and thus no diffusion pathways can be generated. In surface imprinting procedures a variety of biopolymers, such as e.g., lysozyme or trypsin,

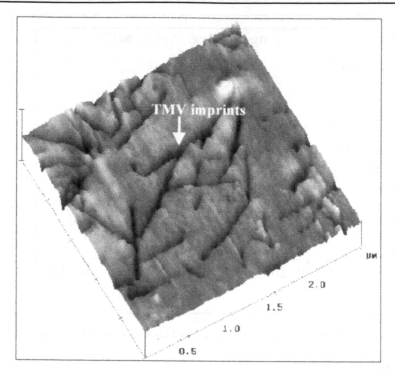

Figure 9. AFM image of a TMV-imprinted polymer layer.

has successfully been used as templating agent.[15] In this case the stamp for surface imprinting is produced by crystallizing the respective template protein on a glass slide. Radically polymerized materials turned out to be the most suitable polymeric system for this purpose; the prereacted mixtures are spin-coated onto the transducer of interest and cured under UV-irradiation after applying the stamp. The resulting polymers are moderately hydrophobic and should therefore cause hydrogen bonding between different carboxylic functionalities in the protein;

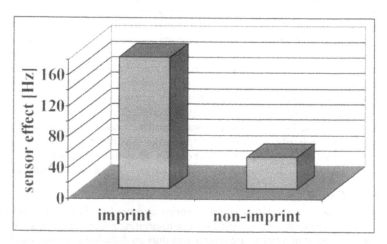

Figure 10. Sensor response pattern for imprinted and non-imprinted polymer layers towards TMV.

Figure 11. Sensor response of a QCM with trypsine-imprinted layer.

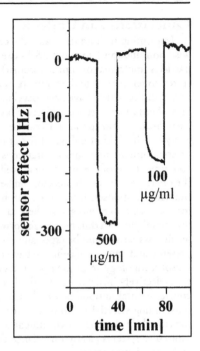

nonetheless they yield reliable sensor responses when applied on a QCM (Fig. 11). A sensor characteristic of this material is shown in Figure 12, where the strictly monotonic increase in sensor response with concentration can be seen. This opens the way to a straightforward and elegant method for the determination of proteins that can be performed on-line and does not require sophisticated biochemical procedures to yield the results. Protein imprinted layers show an additional feature: the imprinted layers strongly enhance crystal formation as they obviously offer some type of nucleation centers. Compared with bare surfaces the templated materials show crystallization at much lower protein concentrations (down to 5 mg/ml) and remarkably faster (first crystals occur within one day for the low concentrations). Therefore, the materials could also be used for fast protein purification via crystallization and thus exhibit some catalytic activity.

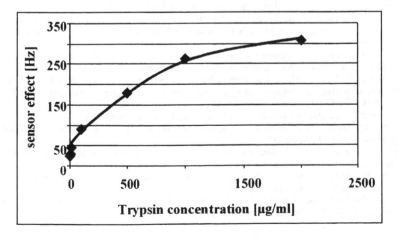

Figure 12. Sensor characteristic of a trypsin-imprinted material.

Conclusions and Outlook

Imprinting techniques enable the chemist to introduce chemical functionality into otherwise nonfunctional materials. Self-assembly of a forming macromolecule around biogenous particles (molecular or supramolecular) leads to cavities in the polymer surface that are ideally suited to reincorporate the template in an almost antibody-like manner. Most materials introduced in this article have been developed to form recognition layers for chemical sensing devices. Sensors are needed whenever fast, on-line detection of a specified analyte is required, therefore the main applications can be found in the fields of process control and environmental analysis. The field of industrial (i.e., process control) application includes e.g., determination of contaminant microbes in breweries or generally food-processing industry to avoid both contaminations of the fermenter as well as quality problems in the final product. Additionally, the microbial load of a bioreactor can be determined as the sensors show population-dependent frequency responses. It has to be emphasized that the method shown is especially interesting for the detection of viruses, as these can not be assessed by optical microscopy or light scattering techniques and thus no straightforward, easy-to-use analysis is yet available. Environmental sensing systems would be especially interesting for water monitoring applications, as e.g., the presence and amount of coliform bacteria is a fundamental parameter in water quality. Aside of sensor technology, imprinted polymers also have a high potential as filter membranes or beads that selectively incorporate exactly defined species and thus have antibody-like selectivity. Of course, natural antibodies are already successfully used in several fields stated, as they offer outstanding selectivity. However, they have a main drawback, namely their limited tolerance towards their chemical environment and the equally limited lifetime. Here, artificial macromolecular systems clearly outbalance their natural counterparts and open the way to robust economical applications.

Acknowledgement

This work was supported by FWF (P15512).

References

1. Kenndler E, Blaas D. Capillary electrophoresis of macromolecular biological assemblies: Bacteria and viruses. TrAC 2001; 20:543-551.
2. Dickert FL, Lieberzeit P. Solid state sensors for field measurements of gases and vapors. In: Meyers RA, ed. Encyclopaedia of Analytical Chemistry. Chichester: John Wiley and Sons, 2000:3831-3855.
3. Bunde RL, Jarvi EJ, Rosentreter JJ. piezoelectric quartz crystal biosensors. Talanta 1998; 46:1223-1236.
4. Cavic BA, Hayward GL, Thompson M. Acoustic waves and the study of biochemical macromolecules and cells at the sensor-liquid interface. Analyst 1999; 124:1405-1420.
5. Vikinge TP, Hansson KM, Sandström P et al. Comparison of surface plasmon resonance and quartz crystal microbalance in the study of whole blood and plasma coagulation. Biosens Bioelectron 2000; 15:605-613.
6. Howe E, Harding G. A comparison of protocols for the optimisation of detection of bacteria using a surface acoustic wave (SAW) biosensor. Biosens Bioelectron 2000; 15:641-649.
7. Qu X, Bao L, Su X et al. A new method based on gelation of tachypleus ambeocyte lysate for detection of Escherichia coliform using a series piezoelectric quartz crystal sensor. Anal Chimca Acta 1998; 374:47-52.
8. D'Souza SD. Microbial biosensors. Biosens Bioelectron 2001; 16:37-353.
9. Hayden O, Dickert F, Selective microorganism detection with cell surface imprinted polymers. Adv Mater 2001; 13:1480-1483.
10. Dickert FL, Hayden O, Halikias KP. Synthetic receptors as sensor coatings for molecules and living cells. Analyst 2001; 126:766-771.
11. Dickert F, Hayden O. Bioimprinting of polymers and sol-gel phases. Selective detection of yeasts with imprinted polymers. Anal Chem 2002; 74:1302-1306.
12. Dickert FL, Halikias K, Hayden O et al. Sensors based on fingerprints of neutral and ionic analytes in polymeric materials. Sensors and Actuators B 2001; 76:295-298.

13. Ahern A, Alexander C, Payne MJ et al. Bacteria-mediated lithography of polymer surfaces. J Am Chem Soc 1996; 118:8771-8772.
14. Alexander C, Vulfson EN. Spatially functionalized polymer surfaces produced via cell-mediated lithography. Adv Mater 1997; 9:751-755.
15. Hayden O, Bindeus R, Haderspöck C et al. Mass-sensitive detection of cells, viruses and enzymes with artificial receptors. Sensors and Actuators B2003; 91:316-319.

CHAPTER 6

A New Generation of Chemical Sensors Based on MIPs

Sergey Piletsky and Anthony Turner

Abstract

Molecular imprinting is a generic technology for the introduction of recognition properties into synthetic polymers. Over the last two decades, molecularly imprinted polymers (MIPs) have become a focus of interest for scientists engaged in the development of biological and chemical sensors. This is due to the many and considerable advantages they possess in comparison to natural receptors, enzymes and antibodies, such as superior stability, low cost and ease of preparation. This chapter will review recent achievements and potential applications of imprinted sensors.

Biosensors

According to the modern definition, biosensors are analytical devices comprising a biological or biologically derived sensing element either integrated within or intimately associated with a physicochemical transducer[1] (Fig. 1). The two broad classes of sensing elements are *catalytic* (enzymes, microorganisms, tissue slices and biomimetic catalysts) and affinity-based (antibodies, nucleic acids, receptor proteins and synthetic receptors).[2,3] These highly selective and sensitive sensing elements yield continuous or discontinuous electronic signals reflecting the concentration of an analyte or group of analytes, when combined with electrochemical, optical, piezoelectric, magnetic or thermometric transducers. Biosensor technology in general is a mature, fast-developing area, as evidenced by the relatively large number of the patents issued recently (200/year).

The majority of biosensor-related patents describe innovations in materials science rather than new types of transducers or detection principles. Particular attention has been paid to solving the most critical problems related to the application of biological molecules in sensing such as (a) low stability, (b) poor performance of biomolecules in organic solvents at low and high pHs and at high temperature, (c) absence of enzymes or receptors that are able to recognize certain target analytes, (d) problems with immobilization of biomolecules, and (e) poor compatibility with micromachining technology. The underdevelopment of the potentially huge biosensors market (Table 1) can be attributed to the above-mentioned problems. At present less than 10% of this market has been exploited with 90% of sales accounted for by glucose and BOD sensors.[4,5]

The search for possible solutions to the aforementioned problems has lead scientists to the development of stable synthetic analogues of natural receptors and antibodies. One of the most promising methods that, in theory, should be applicable for the design of affinity materials for most types of analyte is molecular imprinting.

Molecular Imprinting of Polymers, edited by Sergey Piletsky and Anthony Turner.
©2006 Landes Bioscience.

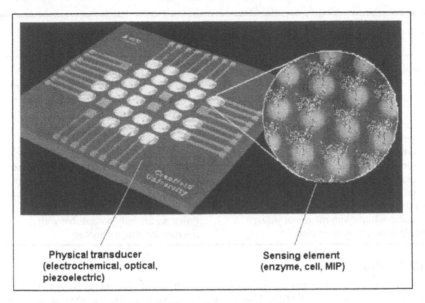

Physical transducer
(electrochemical, optical,
piezoelectric)

Sensing element
(enzyme, cell, MIP)

Figure 1. Schematic diagram showing the main components of a biosensor.

Molecular Imprinting—Introduction

The molecular imprinting approach involves formation of a complex between a given target (template) molecule and functional monomers in an appropriate solvent, which is then fixed by polymerization into a growing polymer chain. Subsequent removal of the template leaves binding sites within the polymer possessing both shape and the correct orientation of functional groups to allow selective recognition of the imprint species.[6,7] MIPs have a number of advantages in comparison with natural biomolecules (Table 2).

Imprinted polymers can in theory be prepared for any kind of substances. More than three hundred examples of successful imprinting have been reported including inorganic ions, drugs, nucleic acids, proteins and even microbial cells. The high specificity and stability of MIPs render them promising alternatives to the enzymes, antibodies, and natural receptors used in sensor technology.[8,9] However, there are limitations associated with the development of MIP sensors: (i) absence of a general procedure for MIP preparation; (ii) difficulty in integrating them with transducer; (iii) difficulty in transforming the binding event into an electric signal; (iv) generally poor performance of MIPs in aqueous solution.

Table 1. Potential market for biosensors

Application	Market, $ Billion
Microsystems market for in vitro diagnostics	19
Electronic noses and tongues (health care, testing of product quality, to establish authenticity of perfumes and wines)	4
Drug testing and drug delivery	2.9
DNA chips	1
Military (warfare agent detection)	0.64

Table 2. Comparison of natural biomolecules used in sensors and MIPs

Natural Biomolecules	MIPs
Low stability	MIPs are stable at low/high pHs, pressure and temperature (<180°C)
High price of the enzymes and receptors	Inexpensive and easy to prepare
Poor performance in non-aqueous media	MIPs can work in organic solvents
Different natural biomolecules have different operational requirements (pH, ionic strength, temperature, substrate)	Due to minimal operational requirements of MIPs, the design of MIP-based multisensor is relatively easy
Natural receptors and enzymes exist for limited number of important analytes	MIPs could be prepared for practically any compound
Poor compatibility with micromachining technology and miniaturization	Polymers are fully compatible with micromachining technology

MIP Design

One of the major problems in MIP design is the choice of an optimal polymerization protocol for the development of MIPs. This is mainly because of several variable parameters such as the range of monomers that can be used (more than 4000 polymerizable compounds are commercially available), possible solvents, temperature and pressure under which the polymerization is performed etc. The most advanced approaches available for the selection of appropriate functional monomers include combinatorial and computational methods. In the combinatorial approach the best composition is selected on the basis of simultaneous synthesis and testing of tens of hundreds of imprinted polymers prepared on a small scale.[10,11] In the computational approach, the monomer screening is performed virtually.[12] Computationally designed MIPs often possess affinity comparable with antibodies (Table 3).

Polymer-Detector Integration

The most direct way to integrate a MIP with a transducer is electropolymerization. Substrate-selective polyaniline electrodes with molecular-recognition properties in relation to the monomers were prepared by Vinokurov and coauthors.[13] Boyle and coauthors prepared a selective sensor by electropolymerizing pyrrole in the presence of adenosine tri-phosphate in water solution on a platinum electrode.[14] The resulting polypyrrole-ATP film exhibited reversible electrochemical behavior, depending on concentration of ATP in solution. A similar result was demonstrated for electropolymerized phenol, formed in the presence of phenylalanine, which was able to retain a "memory" for a templating amino acid.[15] Imprinting of a neutral compound, glucose, has been achieved successfully by electropolymerization of o-phenylenediamine.[16] The big advantage of electropolymerization in comparison with other

Table 3. Affinity and sensitivity range of computationally designed molecularly imprinted polymer in comparison with antibodies

Receptor	K_d, nM	Sensitivity Range (μg l^{-1})
Computational MIP	0.3 ± 0.08	0.1-100
Monoclonal antibody	0.03 ± 0.004	0.025-5
Polyclonal antibody	0.5 ± 0.07	0.05-10

immobilization techniques lies in the ability to deposit a recognition film at a precise spot on the detector surface. It is possible to coat an electrode with complex geometry with a homogeneous film. The polymer thickness and deposition density is regulated by polymerization conditions (e.g., applied voltage).

Another approach consists of self-assembly of a MIP layer on the surface of a physical transducer. In the first such example, Tabushi et al performed chemosorption of octadecylchlorosilane in the presence of n-hexadecane onto tin dioxide or silicon dioxide.[17] Following removal of the hosts, electrodes were used for electrochemical detection of phylloquinone, menaquinone, tocopherol, cholesterol and adamantane. A similar approach was followed for the development of an ellipsometric two-dimensional MIP sensor for phylloquinone.[18] This method was expanded further for the preparation of monolayers imprinted with water-soluble templates. The methodology comprised two steps: (a) adsorption of the template on the SiO_2 or InO_2 surface and (b) treatment of the electrode with adsorbed template by trimethyl chlorosilane from the gas phase. This method was successfully used for the development of sensors for nucleic acids, cholesterol[19] and catechol derivatives.[20] Mirsky and coauthors proved that the stability of the sensor could be improved by coimmobilization of the template in an imprinted layer.[21] A stable monolayer, consisting of template (thiobarbituric acid) and functional monomer (hexadecylmercaptane) was coimmobilized on a gold surface with template forming depressions in a hexadecylmercaptane layer. These depressions were able to accommodate barbituric acid, changing the electrode/monolayer capacitance in the process of binding. Despite some advantages, including fast sensor response and easy preparation, these 2-D systems in general suffer from lack of stability as compared with conventional 3-dimensional polymers.

Thin MIP films can be deposited on a solid support by surface grafting using chemical, UV or plasma initiation.[22,23] The advantage of this approach lies in the possibility of modifying very inert surfaces (polystyrene, polypropylene etc.) with specific polymers. MIP synthesis and immobilization is performed as a one-step procedure, directed by an applied potential or by exposing the monomer mixturecoated detector to UV light. Most frequently however, MIPs are deposited on the detector surface by in situ UV or thermoinitiated polymerization.[24,26] The following sections present an overview of the development such sensors.

Principal Types of MIP Sensors

Detection of binding has been realized using electrochemical, optical and piezoelectric transducers.[1,2,27,28] Two principal types of MIP sensors could be developed: (i) affinity sensors (immunosensor and receptor-type sensor devices) and (ii) catalytic sensors. Immunosensor-type devices are the most common form of MIP sensor. The detection in these devices is based on the measurement of the concentration of template adsorbed by the MIP immobilized on the detector surface. Receptor sensors explore a MIP's ability to change conformation upon binding with the template, which leads to a change in a measurable property such as conductivity, permeability or surface potential.[8] Alternatively, sensors can be constructed which exploit the ability of a functional monomer to change its property upon interaction with template, most frequently fluorescence.[29]

MIP Based Affinity Sensors

Affinity sensors measure the concentration of the template (preferably electroactive or fluorescent) adsorbed by a MIP immobilized on the detector surface.

Affinity Piezoelectric Sensors

Different electrochemical, piezoelectric and optical sensors have been developed using MIPs. The simplest combination of MIP with sensor explores the gravimetric detection principle. Piezoelectric sensors have advantages such as: (a) relative simplicity of the sensor design; (b) easy interpretation of the sensor response; (c) compatibility with a variety of solvents and a

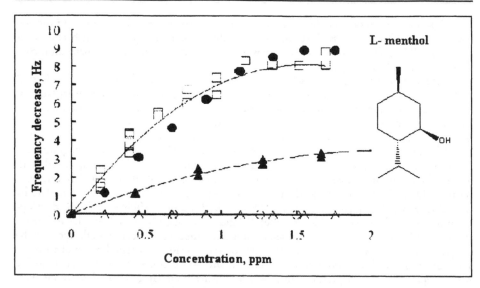

Figure 2. Response of MIP-coated quartz crystals to monoterpene analogues: L-menthol (squares), D-menthol (solid triangles), citronellol (solid circles), citronellal (triangles), and menthone (circles).[25]

variety of templates. A piezoelectric MIP sensor for the determination of L-menthol in the liquid phase was reported by Percival and coauthors.[25] A MIP was cast in situ on to the surface of a gold-coated quartz crystal microbalance (QCM) electrode as a thin permeable film. Selective rebinding of the target analyte was observed and quantified as a frequency shift in the QCM (Fig. 2). The sensor was able to distinguish between D- and L-enantiomers of menthol and other terpenes (in 0.2-1 ppm concentrations). A bulk acoustic wave MIP sensor for measuring paracetamol in real samples, with a high selectivity and sensitivity, was fabricated by Tan and coauthors.[30] A noncovalent MIP was synthesized using two functional monomers: 4-vinylpyridine and methacrylic acid. The sensor was stable and exhibited good reproducibility. The same group reported a biomimetic quartz crystal thickness-shear-mode (TSM) sensor, using a methacrylic acid based MIP as the sensitive material for the determination of nicotine in human serum and urine.[31] The sensor showed high selectivity and a sensitive response to nicotine in aqueous system. Ji and coauthors demonstrated that the sensitivity of QCM could be significantly increased by increasing surface area available for binding the analyte.[32] They designed a sensor selective for 2-methylisoborneol (MIB) by integrating a MIP with a QCM sensor precoated with nylon film. The response of the imprinted sensor was significantly higher than the response of the nonimprinted sensor at MIB concentrations above 10 ppb.

Molecularly imprinted polyurethanes were used as sensor materials for monitoring the degradation of automotive engine oils.[33] Imprinting with characteristic oils permits the analysis of these complex mixtures without accurately knowing their composition. Willner and coauthors developed a piezoelectric sensor for NAD(P)$^+$/NAD(P)H cofactors suitable for the analysis of biocatalysed oxidation of lactic acid and ethanol.[26] Chianella and coauthors developed a microcystin-LR sensor where detection process involved a combination of a preconcentration stage, using a MIP solid-phase extraction cartridge, and measurement by MIP based piezoelectric sensor device.[34] This approach allowed the detection limit for the toxin to be decreased to as low as 0.35 nM, thus meeting the requirements of the EU Drinking Water Directive. An interesting example of a piezoelectric sensor capable of selective detection of whole cells was demonstrated by Dickert and Hayden.[35] The polymer surface imprinted with yeast cells and integrated with a sensor was capable of detecting yeast cells and cell membrane fragments in growth media.

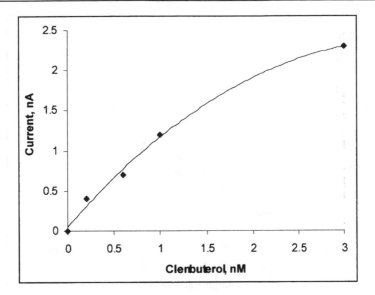

Figure 3. Calibration curve for clenbuterol, displaced by excess of electroinactive isoxsuprine.[39]

As a rule the sensitivity of a piezoelectric sensor is lower than optical and electrochemical devices. The sensitivity of QCM sensors may be enhanced in two ways. It may be possible to increase the concentration of binding sites in the MIP by optimizing the monomer composition and polymerization conditions. Alternatively, the mass sensitivity of the acoustic device may be improved. This latter aim could be achieved by increasing the resonant frequency of the sensor, as the sensor response to mass loading is proportional to the square of the operating frequency. Alternatively, surface acoustic wave devices may be employed that extend the range of operating frequencies from 10 MHz (traditional for bulk QCM devices) to over tens and even a hundred MHz thus facilitating detection in liquids.[36]

Affinity Electrochemical Sensors

Amperometric and optical sensors generally possess higher sensitivity than piezoelectric sensors. One of the first MIP based amperometric devices was developed by Piletsky and coauthors for detection of electroactive aniline and phenol.[37] Kriz and Mosbach developed an amperometric sensor for morphine based on competition between an electroinactive competitor (codeine) and morphine for a morphine-selective MIP immobilised onto an electrode surface.[38] The sensor showed reasonable sensitivity for morphine (0.1-10 mg/l) and good stability over time. It was recently shown that a similar approach can be used for the detection of clenbuterol in bovine liver samples using differential pulse voltammetry.[39] Here the electroinactive analogue-isoxsuprine competitively displaced clenbuterol that was specifically adsorbed by a MIP (Fig. 3). Murray and coauthors developed potentiometric sensors for the analysis of lead and uranil ions in complex media (Fig. 4).[40]

Affinity Optical Sensors

One of the first MIP-based optical sensors specific for dansyl-L-phenylalanine was developed by Kriz and coauthors.[24] Fluorescent template, accumulated in the polymer matrix, was detected by a fibreoptic sensing device. An interesting variant of an optical sensor based on a MIP was proposed by Steinke and coauthors.[41] The MIPs prepared had anisotropic properties and provided specific orientation of bound template molecules. Therefore the MIPs showed a pronounced dichroism under UV light which depended on specific binding. In another example, Dickert and coauthors demonstrated the detection of fluorescent polycyclic aromatic

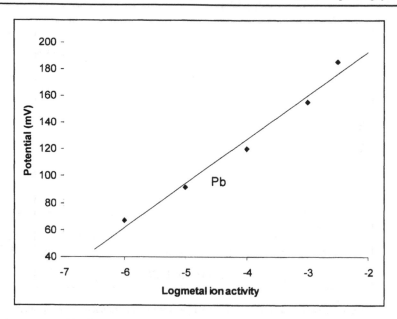

Figure 4. Response of lead (II) ion templated electrode. Ions such as Ca, Cd, Cu, Ni, Zn and La had negligible interference.[40]

hydrocarbons using optical sensors with imprinted polyurethanes (Fig. 5).[42] Jakusch and coauthors developed an infrared evanescent wave sensor for 2,4-dichlorophenoxyacetic acid with detection limit 4.1 µM.[43] It is interesting that infrared spectroscopy provided an additional element contributing towards selectivity of the sensor response.

A serious limitation to the broad applicability of immunosensor-type devices is the limited number of practically important electroactive or fluorescent templates. A solution to this problem is the development of sensors that can operate in a competitive mode by using binding competition between template and its fluorescent or electroactive labeled analogue. Competitive assays with enzyme-labeled templates were developed for epinephrine,[22] and 2, 4-dichlorophenoxyacetic acid.[44] A MIP sensor for chloramphenicol (CA) was reported by Levi and coauthors.[45] The sensor included a HPLC column with CA-specific MIPs. A constant flow of dye-labeled CA (chloramphenicol-Methyl Red) was run through the column at a concentration of 0.5 µg/ml. Analyte containing free CA displaced the adsorbed conjugate, giving a peak with an area that was proportional to CA concentration. CA in blood serum samples was analyzed successfully.

The quantification of ligand-polymer binding events can be achieved also through the displacement of nonspecific dyes from a MIP by template.[46] In this work the dye solution of rhodamine-B was passed through a MIP-HPLC column specific to L-Phe-amide. When the template was injected, part of the dye was competitively replaced by the analyte from the MIP. This displacement peak was three times higher for the template than for the opposite enantiomer. Kroger and coauthors reported a similar displacement principle in combination with electrochemical measurements for template detection.[47] The displacement of nonspecific indicator molecules from a set or array of MIPs throws open possibilities for the development of multisensors.

Receptor Sensors

The affinity sensors described above are able to detect templates that possess a specific property such as optical absorbance, fluorescence or electrochemical activity. Direct detection

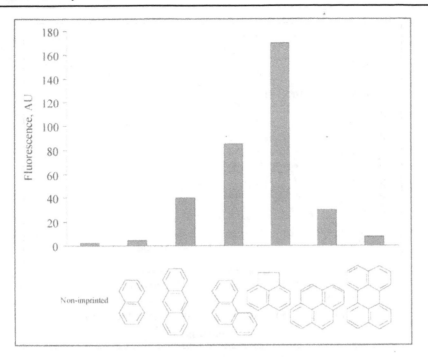

Figure 5. Selectivity pattern of pyrene detection by fluorescence, using polyurethanes imprinted with polyaromatic hydrocarbons.[42]

of "inert" templates can be realized in receptor sensors. Broadly receptor based MIP sensors can be divided into two groups. The first group explores a MIP's ability to change conformation upon binding with template, leading to change in measurable property such as conductivity, permeability or surface potential.[8] The second group explores the ability of a functional monomer to change its property upon interaction with the template, e.g., fluorescence.[29]

Receptor Electrochemical Sensors

Early work which demonstrated the direct detection of an "inert" template was reported by Piletsky and coauthors.[48] They explored the MIP's ability to change the conformation or surface potential upon binding with template. Template molecules such as amino acids, nucleic acids and cholesterol changed the polymer conformation and as a result also increased the transport of ions passing through the imprinted membranes.[8,49,50] This "gate effect" has been used for quantification of the concentration of templates. There have been a number of publications related to exploiting the "gate effect" in sensor development.[51-53] Sensors specific for sugars,[8] L-phenylalanine, cholesterol[50] and atrazine[54] show high selectivity and sensitivity in the micromolar-nanomolar range (Fig. 6).

Preparation of potentiometric MIP sensors, based on electropolymerized materials, was first described by Vinokurov.[13] Here the monomers themselves reacted as templates forming specific polymers. Sensors for pyrrole, aromatic amines and substituted phenols, based on polypyrrole, polyaniline and aniline-p-aminophenol copolymers, respectively, were prepared. A successful potentiometric sensor was later reported for the detection of glucose. This was based on the measurement of the concentration of protons released during interaction of metal-complexing imprinted polymer with glucose.[55] A clinically relevant measurement range of glucose concentration in plasma was reported (0 to 25 mM).

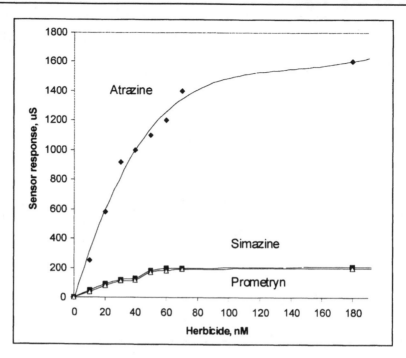

Figure 6. Sensor response to herbicides obtained with a polymer imprinted with atrazine.[54]

Receptor Optical Sensors

The "gate effect" can also be used for the development of optical sensors. This possibility was illustrated using a MIP specific for sialic acid.[56] A fluorescent complex was formed when a polymer suspension was brought into contact with OPA reagent, a mixture of o-phthaleic dialdehyde and mercaptoethanol. The kinetics of the complex formation depended on the presence of the template, sialic acid, which modulated the diffusion of soluble components to the reactive sites (Fig. 7). The polymer was able to discriminate sialic acid from other sugars such as glucose and mannose.

Receptor sensors can also be constructed by introducing signaling monomers into the polymer structure. Thus Cooper and coauthors integrated a functional monomer into a cross-linked matrix, which was able to change its fluorescence properties in the presence of compounds which are proton donors.[57] Polar templates were recognized by strong quenching of fluorescent emission induced by hydrogen bonding.

Dickert and coauthors showed a similar effect by using betaine dyes (phenol blue) with strong hypsochromic effects for protic solvent gas-phase analysis (Fig. 8).[58]

A fluorescent sensor for cAMP detection was constructed using an environmentally sensitive dye trans-4-[p-(N,N-dimethylamino)styryl]-N-vinylbenzylpyridinium chloride).[59] The resulting polymer displayed both functions of template recognition and sensing (Fig. 9).

Ye and Mosbach reported a new type of proximity scintillation assay for (S)-propranolol. During the imprinting reaction they covalently incorporated a scintillation monomer (4-hydroxymethyl-2,5-diphenyloxazole acrylate) into MIP microparticles.[60] This monomer was capable of transforming β-radiation from the bound tritium-labeled template, into a fluorescent signal.

Highly specific MIPs that are based on group specific fluorescent reporters have been reported for sugars,[61] carboxylic acids[62] and primary amines.[63] In these works the generally nonspecific signal generated by the chemical reaction of a fluorescent reporter became selective as a result of the imprinting effect.

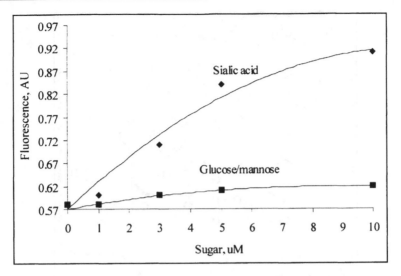

Figure 7. Influence of sugars on the formation of the fluorescent isoindole complex between OPA reagent and amino-functionality in a polymer imprinted with sialic acid.[56]

Catalytic Sensors Based on MIPs

Although immense progress has been made in the field of MIP catalysts[64,65] there has been virtually no published work on catalytic sensors based on MIPs. Recently, in what could be the first example of a catalytic MIP sensor, Piletsky and coauthors integrated MIPs with sensors to produce a synthetic enzyme electrode.[66] They synthesized artificial tyrosinase using molecular imprinting of a transition stage analogue, representing a complex of polymerisable imidazole, copper and catechol (Fig. 10). The resulting polymer exhibited catalytic turnover, Michaelis-Menten kinetics and competitive inhibition, which were all similar to those of the natural enzyme (Table 4). Further developments in catalytic receptors based on MIPs will

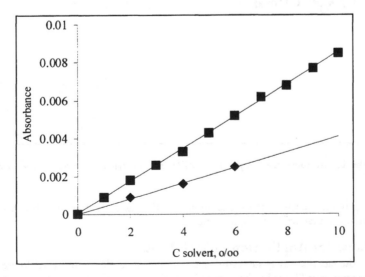

Figure 8. Absorbance versus solvent concentration in air for a polymer with polymer-immobilized phenol blue exposed to chloroform (♦) and ethanol (■).[58]

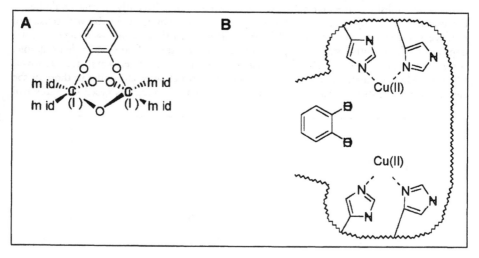

Figure 9. Schematic representation of the polymer binding site for cAMP with a signalling trans-4-[p-(N,N-dimethylamino)styryl]-N-vinylbenzylpyridinium monomer.[59]

Figure 10. Possible structure of the catalytic site of MIP mimicking tyrosinase and properties of synthesised polymers.[66]

depend largely on success in the preparation of MIP-based catalysts which can react with water-soluble and practically important analytes.

Niche Areas for Application of MIP Sensors

Despite the fact that many successful examples of the development of MIP-based electrochemical sensors exist (Table 5), the current level of commercial activity related to their development and marketing remains low. The remaining problems to be resolved continue to be

Table 4. Catalysis of catechol oxidation by natural and synthetic enzymes. Reaction conditions: 5 mM CuCl solution in 100 mM Tris-HCl, pH 8.0. For comparison mushroom tyrosinase (2000 U/mg) was used in 30 mg/ml concentration.[66]

Catalyst	Michaelis Constant Km, mM	Vmax × 10^{-7} Ms^{-1}
MIP (template – catechol)	4.3 ± 1.1	21.0 ± 2.6
Control (template – resorcinol)	3.9 ± 1.4	4.0 ± 0.8
Tyrosinase	0.9 ± 0.4	8.5 ± 2.1

Table 5. Sensing and detection with MIPs

Template	Detection	Reference
Amino acids and derivatives	Electrochemical, QCM, Optical	15,24,41,46,67-70
Aniline, phenol and derivatives	Electrochemical	20,37
Anions and cations	Electrochemical, Optical	40,71
Atrazine and other triazines	Optical	54,72
Automotive engine oils	QCM	33
Barbituric acid	Electrochemical	21
Caffeine	QCM, optical	73,85
Carboxylic acids	Optical	62
Chloramphenicol	Optical	45
Cholesterol	Electrochemical	74
Cinchola alkaloids	Optical	75
Clenbuterol	Electrochemical	39
2,4-Dichlorophe-noxyacetic acid	Electrochemical; Optical	44,47;76,77
Epinephrine	Optical	22
β-Estradiol	Optical	78
Flavinol	Optical	79
Gases	Electrochemical	80;81
2-MIB	QCM	32
Morphine	Electrochemical	38
Nicotine	QCM	31
Nitrobenzene	Amperometry	82
Nucleic acids and derivatives	Electrochemical; Optical	8,14;49,59,83
PAH	Optical	42
Paracetamol	QCM	84
Phenactin	QCM	30
Propranolol	Optical	60
Sarin and soman	Optical	9
Sugars and derivatives	Electrochemical; Optical	8,52,55,56,61
Theophylline and Xanthine	Optical	85
Terpene	QCM	25
Vitamin- K1	QCM	18

poor performance of MIPs in water and difficulty with integration of MIPs with transducers. With further advances in technology MIP sensors will find clear niches in the sensor market. The most promising areas of MIP sensor applications are (i) medical diagnostics; (ii) chemical and pharmaceutical manufacturing; (iii) application of MIPs mimicking natural receptors for drug screening and for in vivo monitoring; (c) environmental remote sensing; (d) rapid detection of chemical and biological warfare agents under battlefield and civil conditions (e) sensors for deep sea and space exploration. At the time of writing, it is clear that a number of commercial enterprises are focusing on the potential of MIPs. Start-up companies have already been formed which have identified MIP-based sensors as central to their business plan and the major diagnostic companies are watching such developments with interest. Turning exciting science into practical products is a long and hard path, but it is clear that MIPs have come of age and serious attempts are now being made to realize their huge potential benefits in the form of tangible products that will lead to wealth generation and improvement in the quality of life.

References

1. Turner APF. Biosensors- sense and sensitivity. Science 2000; 290:1315-1317.
2. Scheller FW, Wollenberger U, Warsinke A et al. Research and development in biosensors. Curr Opin Biotech 2001; 12:35-40.
3. Griffiths D, Hall G. Biosensors—what real progress is being made? Trends Biotoechnol 1993; 11:122-130.
4. Newman JD, Warner PJ, Tigwell L et al. Biosensors: Boldly going into the new millennium. Cranfield University 2000:84pp.
5. Newman J, Turner APF Sensors in medicine and health care (sensors applications) Wiley-VCH, ISBN: 3527295569 2002; 3.
6. Wulff G. Molecular imprinting in cross-linked materials with the aid of molecular templates - a way towards artificial antibodies. Angew Chem Int Ed Engl 1995; 34:1812-1832.
7. Mayes AG, Mosbach K. Molecularly imprinted polymers: Useful materials for analytical chemistry? TrAC Trends in Anal Chem 1997; 16:321-332.
8. Piletsky SA, Piletskaya EV, Panasyuk TL et al. Imprinted membranes for sensor technology-opposite behavior of covalently and noncovalently imprinted membranes. Macromolecules 1998; 31:2137-2140.
9. Jenkins AL, Uy OM, Murray GM. Polymer-based lanthanide luminescent sensors for detection of the hydrolysis product of the nerve agent soman in water. Anal Chem 1997; 71:373-378.
10. Lanza F, Sellergren B. Method for synthesis and screening of large groups of molecularly imprinted polymers. Anal Chem 1999; 71:2092-2096.
11. Takeuchi T, Fukuma D, Matsui J. Combinatorial molecular imprinting: An approach to synthetic polymer receptors. Anal Chem 1999; 71:285-290.
12. Piletsky SA, Day RM., Chen B et al. Rational design of MIPs using computational approach. WO-200155235 A1 2001.
13. Vinokurov IA. A new kind of redox sensor based on conducting polymer-films. Sensor Actuat B-Chem 1992; 10:31-35.
14. Boyle A, Genies EM, Lapkowski M. Application of electronic conducting polymers as sensors-polyaniline in the solid-state for detection of solvent vapors and polypyrrole for detection of biological ions in solutions. Synthetic Met 1989; 28:769-774.
15. Panasyuk TL, Mirsky VM, Piletsky SA et al. Electropolymerized molecularly imprinted polymers as receptor layers in capacitive chemical sensors. Anal Chem 1999; 71:4609-4613.
16. Malitesta C, Losito I, Zambonin PG. Molecularly imprinted electrosynthesized polymers: New materials for biomimetic sensors. Anal Chem 1999; 71:1366-1370.
17. Tabushi I, Kurihara K, Naka K et al. Supramolecular sensor based on SnO_2 electrode modified withoctadecylsilyl monolayer having molecular binding sites. Tetrahedron Lett 1987; 28:4299-4302.
18. Andersson LI, Mandenius CF, Mosbach K. Studies on guest selective molecular recognition on an octadecyl silylated silicon surface using ellipsometry. Tetrahedron Lett 1988; 29:5437-5440.
19. Piletsky SA, Starodub NF. Formation of selective surface of silica-based sensor for low-molecular-mass organic substances. Zh Anal Khim 1992; 47:623-629.
20. Morita M, Niwa O, Horiuchi T. Integrated array microelectrodes as electrochemical sensors. Electrochim Acta 1997; 42:3177-3183.
21. Mirsky VM, Hirsch T, Piletsky SA et al. Spreader-bar approach to molecular architecture: Formation of artificial chemoreceptors. Angew Chemie Intern Ed 1999; 38/8:1108-1110.
22. Piletsky SA, Piletska EV, Chen B et al. Chemical grafting of molecularly imprinted homopolymers to the surface of microplates. Application of artificial adrenergic receptor in enzyme-linked assay for β-agonists determination. Anal Chem 2000; 72:4381-4385.
23. Piletsky SA, Matuschewski H, Schedler U et al. Surface functionalization of porous polypropylene membranes with molecularly imprinted polymers by photo-graft copolymerization in water. Macromolecules 2000; 33:3092-3098.

24. Kriz D, Ramstrom O, Svensson A et al. Introducing biomimetic sensors based on molecularly imprinted polymers as recognition elements. Anal Chem 1995; 67:2142-2144.

25. Percival CJ, Stanley S, Galle M et al. Molecular-imprinted, polymer-coated quartz crystal microbalances for the detection of terpenes. Anal Chem 2001; 73:4225-4228.

26. Pogorelova SP, Zayats M, Bourenko T et al. Analysis of $NAD(P)^+/NAD(P)H$ cofactors by imprinted polymer membranes associated with ion-sensitive field-effect transistor devices and Au-quartz crystals. Anal Chem 2003; 75:509-517.

27. Wang J, Rivas G, Cai X et al. DNA electrochemical biosensors for environmental monitoring. A review Anal Chim Acta 1997; 347:1-8.

28. D'Souza SF. Microbial biosensors. Biosens Bioelectron 2001; 16:337-353.

29. Rathbone DL, Su D, Wang Y et al. Molecular recognition by fluorescent imprinted polymers. Tetrahedron Lett 2000; 41:123-126.

30. Tan Y, Peng H, Liang C et al. A new system for phenacetin using biomimic bulk acoustic wave sensor with a molecularly imprinted polymer coating. Sensor Actuat B-Chem 2001; 73:179-184.

31. Tan Y, Yin J, Liang C et al. A study of a new TSM bio-mimetic sensor using a molecularly imprinted polymer coating and its application for the determination of nicotine in human serum and urine. Bioelectrochemistry 2001; 53:141-148.

32. Ji HS, McNiven S, Yano K et al. A highly sensitive trilayer piezoelectric odour sensor. Anal Chim Acta 1999; 387:39-42.

33. Dickert FL, Forth P, Lieberzeit PA et al. Quality control of automotive engine oils with mass-sensitive chemical sensors-AQMs and molecularly imprinted polymers. Fresenius J Anal Chem 2000; 366:802-806.

34. Chianella I, Piletsky SA, Tothill IE et al. Combination of solid phase extraction cartridges and MIP-based sensor for detection of microcystin-LR. Biosensors Bioelectronics 2003; 18:119-127.

35. Dickert FL, Hayden O. Bioimprinting of polymers and sol-gel phases. Selective detection of yeasts with imprinted polymers. Anal Chem 2002; 74:1302-1306.

36. Jakoby B, Ismail GM, Byfield MP et al. A novel molecularly imprinted thin film applied to a Love wave gas sensor. Sensor Actuat A-Phys 1999; 76:93-97.

37. Piletsky SA, Kuris' YaI, Rachkov AE et al. Forming of imprinted polymers sensitive for aniline and phenol. Russ J Electrochem 1994; 30:1090-1093.

38. Kriz D, Mosbach K. Competitive amperometric morphine sensor based on an agarose immobilised molecularly imprinted polymer. Anal Chim Acta 1995; 300:71-75.

39. Pizzariello A, Stred'ansky M, Stred'anska S et al. A solid binding matrix/molecularly imprinted polymer-based sensor system for the determination of clenbuterol in bovine liver using differential-pulse voltammetry. Sensor Actuat B-Chem 2001; 76:286-294.

40. Murray GM, Jenkins AL, Bzhelyansky A et al. Molecularly imprinted polymers for the selective sequestering and sensing of ions. J Hopkins Apl Tech Dev 1997; 18:464-472.

41. Steinke JHG, Dunkin IR, Sherrington DC. Molecularly imprinted anisotropic polymer monoliths. Macromolecules 1996; 29:407-415.

42. Dickert FL, Tortschanoff M. Molecularly imprinted sensor layers for the detection of polycyclic aromatic hydrocarbons in water. Anal Chem 1999; 71:4559-4563.

43. Jakusch M, Janotta M, Mizaikoff B et al. Molecularly imprinted polymers and infrared evanescent wave spectroscopy. A chemical sensors approach. Anal Chem 1999; 71:4786-4791.

44. Surugiu I, Danielsson B, Ye L et al. Chemiluminescence imaging elisa using an imprinted polymer as the recognition element instead of an antibody. Anal Chem 2001; 73:87-491.

45. Levi R, McNiven S, Piletsky SA et al. Optical detection of chloramphenicol using molecularly imprinted polymers. Anal Chem 1997; 69:2017-2021.

46. Piletsky SA, Terpetschnig E, Andersson HS et al. Towards the development of multisensors based on molecularly imprinted polymers. Application of nonspecific fluorescent dyes for monitoring enantio-selective ligand-polymer binding. Fresenius J Anal Chem 1999; 364:512-516.

47. Kroger S, Turner APF, Mosbach K et al. Imprinted polymer based sensor system for herbicides using differential-pulse voltammetry on screen printed electrodes. Anal Chem 1999; 71:3698-3702.

48. Piletsky SA, Butovich IA, Kukhar VP. Design of molecular sensors on the basis of substrate-selective polymer membranes. Zh Anal Khim 1992; 47:1681-1684.

49. Piletsky SA, Dubey IYa, Fedoryak DM et al. Substrate-selective polymeric membranes. Selective transfer of nucleic acids components. Biopolym Cell 1990; 6:55-58.

50. Piletsky SA, Parhometz YuP, Panasyuk TL et al. Sensors for low-weight organic molecules based on molecular imprinting technique. Sensor Actuat B-Chem 1994; 18/19:629-631.

51. Hedborg A, Winquist F, Lundstrom I et al. Some studies of molecularly-imprinted polymer membranes in combination with field-effect devices. Sensor Actuat A-Phys 1993; 796:37-38.

52. Cheng Z, Wang E, Yang X. Capacitive detection of glucose using molecularly imprinted polymers. Biosens Bioelectron 2001; 16:179-185.
53. Yoshimi Y, Ohdaira R, Iiyama C et al. "Gate effect" of thin layer of molecularly-imprinted poly (methacrylic acid-coethyleneglycol dimethacrylate). Sensor Actuat B-Chem 2001; 73:49-53.
54. Sergeyeva TA, Piletsky SA, Brovko AA et al. Selective recognition of atrazine by molecularly imprinted polymer membranes. Development of conductometric sensor for herbicides detection. Anal Chim Acta 1999; 392:105-111.
55. Chen G, Guan Z, Chen CT et al. A glucose-sensing polymer. Nat Biotechnol 1997; 15:354-357.
56. Piletsky SA, Piletskaya EV, Yano K et al. Biomimetic receptor system for sialic acid based on molecular imprinting. Anal Lett 1996; 29:157-170.
57. Cooper ME, Hoag BP, Gin DL. Design and synthesis of novel fluorescent chemosensors for biologically active molecules. Abstr Pap Am Chem Soc 1997; 213:115.
58. Dickert FL, Geiger U, Lieberzeitv P et al. Solvatochromic betaine dyes as optochemical sensor materials: Detection of polar and nonpolar vapors. Sensor Actuat B-Chem 2000; 70:263-269.
59. Turkewitsch P, Wandelt B, Darling GD et al. Fluorescent functional recognition sites through molecular imprinting. A polymer-based fluorescent chemosensor for aqueous cAMP. Anal Chem 1998; 70:2025-2030.
60. Ye L, Mosbach K. Polymers recognizing biomolecules based on a combination of molecular imprinting and proximity scintillation: A new sensor concept. J Am Chem Soc 2001; 123:2901-2902.
61. Wang W, Gao S, Wang B. Building fluorescent sensors by template polymerization: the preparation of a fluorescent sensor for D-fructose. Org Lett 1999; 1:1209-1212.
62. Zhang H, Verboom W, Reinhoud DN. 9-(Guanidinomethyl)-10-vinylanthracene: A suitable fluorescent monomer for mips. Tetrahedr Lett 2001; 42:4413-4416.
63. Subrahmanyam S, Piletsky SA, Piletska EV et al. (2000). "Bite-and-switch" approach in creatine recognition by molecularly imprinted polymers. Adv Mater 2000; 12:722-724.
64. Ohkubo K, Sawakuma K, Sagawa T. Influence of cross-linking monomer and hydrophobic styrene comonomer on stereoselective esterase activities of polymer catalyst imprinted with a transition-state analogue for hydrolysis of amino acid esters. Polymer 2001; 42:2263-2266.
65. Wulff G. Enzyme-like catalysis by molecularly imprinted polymers. Chem Rev 2002; 102:1-27.
66. Piletsky SA, Nicholls IA, Rozhko MI et al. Molecularly imprinted polymer tyrosinase mimics. Organic letters, submitted 2003.
67. Liao Y, Wang W, Wang BH. Building fluorescent sensors by template polymerization: The preparation of a fluorescent sensor for L-tryptophan. Bioorg Chem 1999; 27:463-476.
68. Deore B, Chen Z, Nagaoka T. Potential-induced enantioselective uptake of amino acid into molecularly imprinted overoxidized polypyrrole. Anal Chem 2000; 72:3989-3994.
69. Cao L, Zhou XC, Li SF. Enantioselective sensor based on microgravimetric quartz crystal microbalance with molecularly imprinted polymer film. Analyst 2001; 126:184-188.
70. Peng H, Zhang Y, Zhang J et al. Development of a thickness shear mode acoustic sensor based on an electrosynthesized molecularly imprinted polymer using an underivatized amino acid as the template. Analyst 2001; 126:189-194.
71. Hutchins RS, Bachas G. Nitrate-selective electrode developed by electrochemically mediated imprinting doping of polypyrrole. Anal Chem 1995; 67:1654-1660.
72. Piletsky SA, Piletskaya EV, El'skaya AV et al. Optical detection system for triazine based on molecular-imprinted polymers. Anal Lett 1997; 30:445-455.
73. Kobayashi T, Murawaki Y, Reddy PS et al. Molecular imprinting of caffeine and its recognition assay by quartz-crystal microbalance. Anal Chim Acta 2001; 435:141-149.
74. Piletsky SA, Piletskaya EV, Sergeeva TA et al. Molecularly imprinted self-assembled films with specificity to cholesterol. Sensor Actuat B 1999; 60:216-220.
75. Matsui J, Kubo H, Takeuchi T. Molecularly imprinted fluorescent-shift receptors prepared with 2-(trifluoromethyl) acrylic acid. Anal Chem 2000; 72:3286-3290.
76. Haupt K, Mayes AG, Mosbach K. Herbicide assay using an imprinted polymer based system analogous to competitive fluoroimmunoassays. Anal Chem 1998; 70:3936-3939.
77. Lahav M, Kharitonov AB, Katz O et al. Tailored chemosensors for chloroaromatic acids using molecular imprinted TiO_2 thin films on ion-sensitive field-effect transistors. Anal Chem 2001; 73:720-723.
78. Rachkov A, McNiven S, El'skaya A et al. Fluorescence detection of beta-estradiol using a molecularly imprinted polymer. Anal Chim Acta 2000; 405:23-29.
79. Suarez-Rodriguez JL, Diaz-Garcia ME. Flavonol fluorescent flow-through sensing based on a molecular imprinted polymer. Anal Chim Acta 2000; 405:67-76.
80. Kodakari N, Sakamoto T, Shinkawa K. Molecular sieving gas sensor prepared by chemical vapour deposition of silica on tin oxide using an organic template. Bul Chem Soc Jpn 1998; 71:513-519.

81. Hernandez EC, Bachas LG. Biologically inspired recognition chemistry – for biosensors. In: Nicholelis DP, ed. Biosensors for direct monitoring of environmental pollutants in field. Netherlands: Kluwer Acad. Publishers, 1998:97-106.
82. Panasyuk T, DalOrto VC, Marrazza G et al. Molecular imprinted polymers prepared by electropolymerization of Ni-(Protoporphyrin IX). Anal Lett 1998; 31:1809-1824.
83. Spurlock LD, Jaramillo A, Praserthdam A et al. Selectivity and sensitivity of ultrathin purine-templated overoxidized polypyrrole film electrodes. Anal Chim Acta 1996; 336:37-46.
84. Tan YG, Zhou ZL, Wang P et al. A study of a bio-mimetic recognition material for the BAW sensor by molecular imprinting and its application for the determination of paracetamol in the human serum and urine. Talanta 2001; 55:337-347.
85. Lai EPC, Fafara A, Vandernoot VA et al. Surface plasmon resonance sensors using molecularly imprinted polymers for sorbent assay of theophylline, caffeine, and xanthine. Can J Chem 1998; 76:265-273.
86. Chianella I, Lotierzo M, Piletsky SA et al. Rational design of a polymer specific for microcystin-LR using a computational approach. Anal Chem 2002; 74:1288-1293.

CHAPTER 7

Molecularly Imprinted Membranes

Mathias Ulbricht

Abstract

This chapter provides an overview of the emerging and promising field of molecularly imprinted membranes (MIM). The focus is on solid membranes and the separation of molecules, predominately in liquid mixtures. In the first part, fundamentals of synthetic membranes and membrane separation technology are summarized, emphasizing that innovative principles for the preparation of membranes with improved or novel functionality via optimized membrane morphologies and functions include self-assembly or supramolecular aggregation as well as the use of templates. In the second part, MIM are outlined, starting with the main currently used preparation methods: simultaneous membrane formation and imprinting, and preparation of composite membranes. Then, the separation function of MIM is discussed for two different types as a function of their barrier structure. Microporous MIM can continuosly separate molecules based on facilitated diffusion of the template, or they can change their permeability in the presence of the template ("gate effect"). Macroporous MIM can be developed towards molecule-specific membrane adsorbers. Finally, the application potential for advanced MIM separation technologies is briefly evaluated.

Introduction

A membrane is an interphase between two adjacent phases acting as a selective barrier, at the same time organizing a system into compartments and regulating the transport between the two compartments. The main advantages of membrane technology as compared with other unit operations in (bio)chemical engineering are related to the unique separation principle, i.e., the transport selectivity of the membrane. Furthermore, separations with membranes do not require additives, and they can be performed isothermally and at very competitive energy consumption. Finally, both upscaling and downscaling of membrane processes as well as their integration into other separation or reaction processes is easy. The success of membrane technology has already been impressively demonstrated for the first industrial examples, water purification by reverse osmosis and blood detoxification by dialysis or ultrafiltration. In addition, other large scale applications have been realized in the last two decades, especially in the food and pharmaceutical industry and in the water treatment. Currently, applications of membrane technology are also emerging in the chemical industry. Serving these needs will require innovative research and development towards improved membrane materials and processes.

The development of synthetic membranes has always been inspired by nature, in particular by the fact that the selective transport through biological membranes is enabled by highly specialized macro- and supramolecular assemblies based on and involved in molecular recognition. In industrially established applications, state-of-the-art synthetic membranes have a much better overall performance than their biological counterparts. The very high salt rejections and fluxes through RO membranes obtained using operation pressures of up to 150 bar may serve as one example. Nevertheless, novel synthetic membranes with higher transport selectivity are

Molecular Imprinting of Polymers, edited by Sergey Piletsky and Anthony Turner.
©2006 Landes Bioscience.

Table 1. *Classification of membranes and membrane processes for molecular separations via passive transport**

Membrane Barrier Structure	Trans-Membrane Gradient		
	Concentration	Pressure	Electrical Field
non-porous	pervaporation (PV)	gas separation (GS) reverse osmosis (RO)	electrodialysis (ED)
microporous pore diameter $d_p \leq 2$ nm	dialysis (D)	gas separation nanofiltration (NF)	electrodialysis
mesoporous pore diameter $d_p = 2 \dots 50$ nm	dialysis	ultrafiltration (UF)	electrodialysis

*note that microfiltration membranes with selective pores in the range of 50 to 500 nm are not included because this barrier structure alone will not enable molecular separation

still of outstanding relevance in the field. Hence, for the development of a next generation of highly selective membranes, a "marriage" of the achievements of synthetic membranes with the "bio-inspired" concept of molecular imprinting is of particular interest.

This chapter will provide an overview of the emerging and promising field of molecularly imprinted membranes (MIM). Among the many different membranes and membrane processes, the selection will focus onto those where imprinting has already been implemented or where imprinting should or could be envisioned. Consequently, only solid membranes will be discussed, and the separation of molecules, predominately in liquid mixtures, by interactions with those membranes will form the core of the paper. Other ("nonseparation") applications of MIM, e.g., in sensors, will only be mentioned if a transport selectivity is also involved in the function of the material.

Membranes and Membrane Technology

Transport Processes through Membranes – Separation Mechanisms

Passive transport through membranes occurs as consequence of a driving force, i.e., a difference in chemical potential imparted by a gradient across the membrane in, e.g., concentration or pressure, or by an electrical field.[1] The barrier structure of membranes for molecule-selective separations can be classified according to their porous character (see Table 1).

For nonporous membranes, the interactions between permeand and membrane dominate transport rate and selectivity; the transport mechanism can be described by the solution / diffusion model.[2] For an estimation, the separation selectivity between two compounds is mainly influenced by the respective solubilities in the membrane. However, with real mixtures a strong coupling of transport rates for different components can occur, mainly via an increase of (nonselective) diffusibility in the membrane due to swelling of the membrane by the more soluble component.

For porous membranes, transport rate and selectivity are mainly influenced by sieving or size exclusion. Nevertheless, interactions of solutes with the membrane (pore) surface may significantly alter the membrane performance. Examples include gas separation using micro- and mesoporous membranes due to surface and Knudsen diffusion, and the rejection of charged substances in aqueous mixtures by microporous nanofiltration membranes due to their Donnan potential. Furthermore, with meso- and macroporous membranes, (selective) adsorption can be used for an alternative separation mechanism, membrane adsorbers are the most important example.[3]

Active development is concerned with the combination of membranes with further separation mechanisms, the most important are electrochemical potentials and affinity interactions.

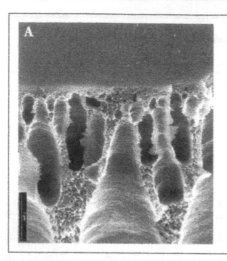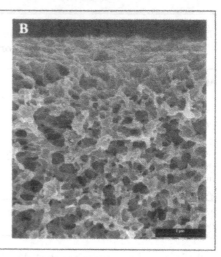

Figure 1. Synthetic separation membrane morphologies (pore structure and layer topology details in SEM, scale bar: 2 μm): A) integrally asymmetric membrane for UF (also relevant for NF, RO, PV and GS) – here made from polyacrylonitrile (GKSS, Geesthacht, Germany); B) symmetric macroporous membrane for MF – here made from polypropylene (Membrana GmbH, Wuppertal, Germany).

Membranes with novel architectures, e.g., "nano-tubule" or "supramolecular channel" membranes (cf. below), will in near future bridge the gap between a coventional membrane separation based on size and shape (MF, UF) and a more specific selection based on molecular properties (including size and shape). Membrane separations based on active transport have not yet been realized in technically feasible forms and processes, but should in the future provide opportunities for specific and efficient separations.

Preparation of Membranes and Technical Membrane Structures

Considering the diversity of membranes suited for technical applications, it will be useful to introduce the following main classifications:

- Membrane materials: organic polymers, inorganic materials (oxides, ceramics, metals), organic-inorganic composite materials.
- Membrane cross-section: symmetric, (integrally) asymmetric, bi- or multilayer, thin-layer or mixed matrix composite.
- Preparation method: phase inversion (PI; thermally induced - "dry PI", solvent induced - "wet PI"), sol-gel process, interface reaction, stretching, extrusion, track-etching, micro-fabrication.
- Membrane shape: flat-sheet, hollow fibre, hollow capsule.

As a rule, membranes for pressuredriven molecule-selective separations (UF, NF, RO, GS) have an asymmetric structure—integral or composite—with a thin (~ 100 nm to a few μm) mesoporous, microporous or nonporous selective layer on top of a macroporous support (100 to 300 μm thick) providing sufficient mechanical stability. By this means, the resistance of the barrier layer is minimized, thus ensuring a high membrane permeability (cf. Fig. 1A).

Macroporous membranes with a symmetric cross-section (100 to 300 μm thick) are the typical materials for MF, but become also increasingly relevant as base materials for composite membranes, e.g., for membrane adsorbers (cf. Fig. 1B). For niche applications, track-etched polymer membranes (8 to 35 μm thick) with quite well-defined cylindrical pores of even size are also available.

Currently, most of the technically used membranes are made from organic polymers via phase inversion methods. Using the casting / immersion precipitation approach, extensive

Table 2. Major applications for membrane processes and annual world market sales in year 2000 (million US $)

	Water Treatment	Food Industry	Medical Devices	Chemical & Pharma	Total
Microfiltration	310	95	20	35	460
Ultrafiltration	60	45	130	15	250
Reverse Osmosis	120	15	-	10	145
Electrodialysis	60	15	-	20	95
Dialysis	-	-	900	-	900
Gas Separation	-	-	-	45	45
Pervaporation	-	-	-	5	5
Total	550	170	1050	130	1900

knowledge exists on how to "finetune" the membrane's pore structure including it's cross-section morphology by the selection of polymer solvents and nonsolvents, additives, residence times and other parameters.[1] In addition, a significant number of composite membranes mainly prepared by interface polymerization reactions - on asymmetric or symmetric support membranes - have been established.[1]

Inorganic membranes, mostly prepared via sol-gel processes, steadily gain importance, especially due to their high stability under harsh process conditions, especially high temperature and organic solvents. However, limitations still exist with respect to molecule-selective separations as well as the high cost of inorganic membranes.

For special applications, unconventional formats of "membrane-filter" materials have been developed: An example are the Empore® "membrane-SPE discs" for solid-phase extraction (SPE) where adsorber particles are embedded in a very open polymer filter matrix.[4]

While flat-sheet is still the most important membrane shape, hollow-fibre membranes are the format of choice in order to increase the membrane area per volume of a separation unit. Their manufacturing is based on the same preparation mechanism as for flat-sheet membranes, but more complex challenges with respect to fibre spinning facility and process must be mastered in order to practically implement this technology.[1]

In summary, the established membrane materials and preparation technologies provide in many cases optimized solutions towards obtaining membranes with a desired separation capability—based on size selection, solution/diffusion, charge, or another mechanism—and with a high flux, both along with an adapted stability. Nevertheless, an improved or even tailored membrane separation selectivity will definitely enable more specialized membrane applications.

Current Applications of Membranes and Membrane Technology

In the last two decades membrane technology has been established in the market, in particular for tasks where no technically and/or economically feasible alternative exists. The current worldwide sales of synthetic membranes is estimated at over US $2 billion. Considering that membranes account for only 40% of the total investment for a membrane separation system, the total annual turnover for the membrane based industry can be considered as close to US $5 billion. The annual growth rate for all membrane products has been estimated at around 12-15%. The total sales of the membrane industry in different key application areas is shown in Table 2 (taken from ref. 5, as one representative compilation).

The successful implementation has been due to the unique separation principle based on using a membrane. Several completely different modes of separation can, in principle, all be done efficiently using membranes:

- removal of a small amount, e.g., a contamination, from a large feed stream yielding a large amount of purified product, by either:
- retention of the small fraction by the membrane, e.g., desalination of water by RO,
- selective permeation of the small fraction through the membrane, e.g., solvent dehydratation or azeotrope separation by PV,
- enrichment of a small amount of a product by selective permeation of the solvent, if desired including other components, through the membrane, e.g., concentration or/and desalting of valuable proteins by UF,
- separation of two or more components, present in low to moderate amounts in a solution, by their selective permeation or retention through or by the membrane, e.g., fractionation of biomolecules by UF, NF, D or ED.

It must be noted that both membrane permeability and selectivity can be completely controlled by concentration polarization or membrane fouling, and these phenomena can significantly reduce the performance which would be expected based on intrinsic membrane properties. A high product purity and yield (by selectivity) and a high throughput (by permeability), i.e., the optimum membrane separation's performance, can only be achieved by process conditions adapted to the separation problem and the membrane material. Therefore, before it can come to real applications, optimizations of the membrane module configuration and design as well as of the process conditions will be most important.[1]

Membrane separation technologies commercially established in large scale are (cf. Table 2):
- D for blood detoxification and plasma separation ("Medical devices"),
- RO for the production of ultrapure water, including potable water ("Water treatment"),
- MF for particle removal, including sterile filtration (various industries),
- UF for many concentration or fractionation processes (various industries including "Water treatment").

Technically mature membrane separations with a large growth potential in the next few years especially include UF and NF for concentration, fractionation and purification in the food and pharma industries.[6] Here, the selectivity of separation is still often limited, especially due to an uneven pore size distribution of the membranes. Emerging applications based on partially "mature" membranes and processes which still need to demonstrate commercial viability are: GS, PV, and ED. Here, main limitations are due to limited membrane selectivity and/or stability. Progress in these latter areas will open the doors into large scale membrane applications in the chemical industry (cf. Table 2).[7]

Furthermore, the presumably largest potential for membrane technology is in process intensification, e.g., via implementation of reaction / separation hybrid processes. Membrane reactors[8,9] are the most attractive examples, with the membrane being:
- selective – for product or byproduct removal, e.g., by coupling a reactor with PV or ED,
- catalytic – for enzyme catalysis, enabled by special composite membranes, or for (high-temperature) chemical catalysis, mainly based on inorganic membranes,
- catalytic and selective – e.g., composite membrane electrodes ("MEA") for fuel cells.

Finally, using specialized support and/or separation membranes in cell and tissue culture will pave the road towards biohybrid and artificial organs for medical and other applications.[9] Here, "biomimetic" synthetic membranes will be integrated into living systems, both supporting and facilitating biological processes for directly serving human needs.

Towards Improved and Novel Membranes for Future Applications

The large potential for membrane technologies in chemical and related processes is based on current and future needs in process technology, in particular for preserving ressources and intensifying processes, including saving energy. Further urgent requirements exist for reducing health risks, e.g., by removing toxins, by treating very large volume feed streams, e.g., water or air. Along with the implementation of biotechnology for production and therapy, the isolation and purification of high-value products and/or the removal of critical contaminations from complex mixtures is already on the agenda.[6]

Many technically challenging and commercially attractive separation problems can not be solved with membranes according to the state-of-the-art. Therefore, novel membranes with high (molecule-) selectivities for toxins, (chiral) drugs or biomolecules, or with a selectivity that can be switched by an external stimulus or that can adapt to the environment or process conditions are required. Such novel membranes developed for separations will immediately find applications also in other fields such as analytics, screening, membrane reactors or bio-artificial membrane systems.

Consequently, materials research and development should meet these demands for specialized ("tailor-made") membranes with significantly improved selectivity and/or flux along with a sufficient stability of membrane performance, and at a competitive cost. The following strategies will lead to a higher separation performance:

- nonporous membranes - composed of a selective transport and a stable matrix phase at an optimal volume ratio along with a minimal tortuosity of the transport pathways, thus combining high selectivity and permeability with high stability,
- porous membranes - with narrow pore size distribution, high porosity and minimal tortuosity.

In addition, minimizing the thickness of the membrane barrier layer will be essential. All these requirements can efficiently be addressed by various approaches within the field of nanotechnology.

Active research is focussed onto highly specific membrane separation based on molecular recognition in the nano-space; two recent examples may serve as an illustration. „Nanotubule" membranes with well-defined transmembrane pores having a diameter of a few nm had been developed by Martin et al.[10] The preparation had been based on controlled deposition of gold layers on the porewalls of track-etched membranes having pore sizes of about 10 nm. In combination with self-assembled functional monolayers on the thus obtained nano-tubules, selective membrane separation could be achieved using size and affinity selection of discrete molecules. "Supramolecular channel" membranes with pores mimicking biological ion-channels had been described by Möller et al.[11] Their approach had been based on the gelation of solutions by string-like supramolecular assemblies of functional gelator molecules, the subsequent fixation of these gels by an in situ polymerization followed by the removal of the gelator fibres yielding pore channels predetermined by the size and shape of the template.

Hence, innovative principles for the synthesis and/or preparation of membranes with improved or novel functionality via optimized membrane morphologies and functions include self-assembly or supramolecular aggregation as well as use of templates (molecules, micelles, particles, nano-structured matrices). Molecularly imprinted membranes are one very promising approach on this road.[12]

Molecularly Imprinted Membranes (MIM)

A high membrane performance depends on a well-defined membrane morphology with respect to pore structure and layer topology (cf. above). A general problem of the "conventional" MIP technology is the simultaneous and random fixation of the imprinted sites along with the formation of the polymer matrix including it's pore structure. As a consequence, random distribution and uneven accessibility of receptor sites in the volume of a MIP material —typically particles—are characteristic for the state-of-the-art.[13] The most promising alternatives in MIP technology are thin MIP films, either formed at interfaces (e.g., ref. 14) or synthesized on solid supports (e.g., ref. 15).

MIM Preparation Strategies and Structures

Three main strategies can be envisioned for the preparation of MIM, with a three-dimensional and flat-sheet shape:

1. simultaneous formation of MIP structure and membrane morphology,
2. sequential approach – preparation of membranes from previously synthesized "conventional" MIPs, i.e., particles,

3. sequential approach – preparation of MIPs on or in support membranes with suited morphology.

Preparation of Self-Supported MIM – Simultaneous Formation of MIP Structure and Membrane Shape

Self-supported flat-sheet membranes should be at least 10 μm thick in order to have sufficient stability (cf. above). Hence, for simultaneous MIM preparation, control of film thickness, e.g., by solution casting or using moulds, is essential. Also, when established MIP synthesis protocols are to be applied, the "synchronization" of imprinting and film solidification are of critical importance for MIM shape, structure and function.

Sol-Gel Processes towards Inorganic or Inorganic / Organic Hybrid Materials

After the first demonstration of molecular imprinting by the synthesis of silica networks via a sol-gel process, imprinting attempts with purely inorganic materials have been very much focussed onto creating well-defined micropores by using templates, thus also preparing inorganic membranes.[16,17] However, inorganic MIM with molecular recognition function have not yet been reported.

In Situ Crosslinking Polymerization

Mathew-Krotz and Shea had prepared free-standing, but brittle membranes by thermally initiated cross-linking copolymerization of one of the "standard" monomer mixtures (MAA/EDMA) for molecular imprinting.[18] SEM studies revealed a regular porous structure built up by 50 to 100 nm diameter nodules. Sergeyeva et al have introduced an improvement by using an oligourethane-acrylate macromonomer in imprinting polymerization mixtures in order to increase the flexibility and mechanical stability of the membranes; self-supported MIM with a thickness between 60 and 120 μm could be prepared.[19] Kimaro et al have developed a cross-linking copolymerization of styrene monomers followed by leaching of a polyester present in the reaction mixture.[20] Based on SEM and permeation data, it was speculated that "trans-membrane channels" had been obtained, induced by the removable macromolecular pore former.

Polymer Solution Phase Inversion ("Alternative Imprinting")

Phase inversion (PI), the main approach towards technical polymeric membranes (cf. above), can also be applied for molecular imprinting; i.e., the solidification of a polymer is used instead of an in situ polymerization. Yoshikawa et al have used polystyrene resins with peptide recognition groups, in a blend with a matrix polymer, for MIM formation via a "dry PI" process.[21-24] The permeability was much higher for the MIM as compared with the blank membranes. Kobayashi et al have used functional acrylate copolymers for a "wet PI" process yielding asymmetric porous MIM.[25] Recently, the polymer selection for "wet PI imprinting" has been extended to most of the commonly used membrane materials, e.g., cellulose acetate,[23] polyamide,[26,27] polyacrylonitrile[27] and polysulfone.[24,27] The formation of porous MIM from a compatible blend of a matrix polymer—for adjusting a permanent pore structure—and a functional polymer—for providing binding groups—could provide even more alternatives.[28]

Considering the limitations faced with the conventional in situ crosslinking polymerisation approach towards MIP materials, it is remarkable, that most MIM prepared via "alternative imprinting" had at least acceptable binding performance in aqueous media. However, such MIM lost their "template memory" when exposed to a too organic environment where swelling and chain rearrangement seemed to "erase" the imprinted information.[22]

In conclusion, for all simultaneous preparations, the limited accessibility of imprinted sites due to a random distribution inside and on the surface of the bulk polymer phase remains a major unsolved problem. Thus, the advantage of membrane preparation technologies to provide well-defined pore structures is not yet fully exploited for obtaining self-supported micro- and macroporous MIM.

Preparation of Composite MIM – Sequential Approach from Presynthesized MIPs

MIP particles had been used to provide coatings for MIP sensors, but only few attempts towards processing presynthesized MIPs to free-standing separation membranes had been reported yet. An example is an arrangement of MIP nanoparticles as a filter cake on one or between two MF membranes; these flat-sheet filters had been evaluated with respect to their flow and binding properties.[29,30] Embedding MIP particles into a suited porous polymer matrix, in analogy to the "membrane-SPE discs" (cf. above), could be an alternative.

Preparation of Composite MIM – Sequential Approach by MIP Synthesis on/in Membranes

The preparation of composite membranes allows one to adjust membrane pore structure and MIP recognition sequentially and by two different materials. The following examples illustrate that only the very first steps towards composite MIM have been made to date.

Porefilling MIP Composite Membranes

In early work, established MIP synthesis mixtures, e.g., MAA/EDMA, have been polymerized in mm-thick glass filters to fill their pores.[31,32] Later, reaction mixtures have been casted into the pores of a symmetric MF membrane and a cross-linking copolymerization of a functional polyacrylate has been performed.[33] In both cases, thick "symmetric MIM" have been obtained.

Thin Film MIP Composite Membranes

Thin film MIP composite membranes have been first prepared by Hong et al using photo-copolymerization of a MAA/EDMA mixture on top of an asymmetric 20 nm pore size alumina membrane.[34] Hattori et al have used a cellulosic dialysis membrane as matrix and applied a two-step grafting procedure yielding a MIP by in situ copolymerization in the thin active layer of the base membrane.[35]

Thin-Layer MIP Porous Composite Membranes

Thin-layer MIP porous composite membranes have been developed to achieve high performance MIM adsorbers.[36-39] The structure of the base membrane can be used as a means to adapt both pore size—permeability—as well as internal surface area—binding capacity—to the desired application. Using a coated photoinitiator, a photo-initiated crosslinking graft copolymerization yielded very thin MIP films which were covalently anchored and covered the entire surface of the base membrane.[37] Sergeyeva et al have discovered that a previously prepared hydrophilic layer on the support membrane can have two functions: (i) matrix for the crosslinking polymerization and limiting monomer conversion to "filling" the layer thus forming an interpenetrating network, (ii) minimizing nonspecific binding.[38] A superior MIM performance, especially a high template specificity, could be achieved.

In conclusion, the sequential approach will allow the use of the base membrane pore structure (barrier pore size) and layer topology (symmetric vs. asymmetric) as well as the location of the MIP—on top of ("asymmetric") or inside ("symmetric") the support membrane—to prepare different MIM types, with the MIP either as selective barrier or transport phase or as an affinity adsorber layer (cf. below).

Selective Binding and Transport in MIM

As a consequence of the binding selectivity of the template versus other species, two main categories of MIM function with respect to membrane transport selectivity can be distinguished: retardation or facilitation for the selected species (see Fig. 2). For MIM function, it is critically important to control both MIP specificity and membrane pore structure. With exclusively microporous MIM, template binding to imprinted sites can either change the pore network thus altering membrane permeability in general ("gate effect") or the permeation rate is controlled by the interaction with the micropore "walls". In MIM with larger trans-membrane

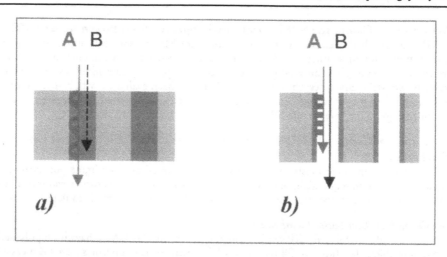

Figure 2. Separation mechanisms for MIM, as consequence of a binding selectivity obtained by imprinting for a substance A: a) transport of A is facilitated via binding / desorption to MIP sites, while the nonspecific transport of another substance B by diffusion is hindered by the micropore structure of the membrane ("fixed carrier" membrane); b) transport of A is retarded either by binding or binding / desorption to MIP sites on the surface of trans-membrane pores, while another substance B which has no specific interactions with the membrane surface will be transported by diffusion or convection (membrane adsorber).

pores, nonselective transport by diffusion or convection can only be compensated by binding to accessible imprinted sites, causing a retardation which can be used in membrane adsorbers.

Microporous MIM—MIP as Barrier or Transport Phase

Triggered Response to Template Binding – "Gate Effect"

Studies with porefilling MIP composite filters indicated an alteration of MIM permeability / conductivity due to binding of the template. The opposite behaviour of noncovalently and covalently imprinted membranes was explained by the effect of template binding onto MIP swelling; e.g., a strong shrinking due to binding of template to the covalently imprinted material could be detected even macroscopically.[32] For noncovalently imprinted materials, was much more complicated to correlate microscopic and macroscopic changes.[32] Studies with much thinner self-supported MIM via in situ polymerization and noncovalent interactions with the template provided clear evidence for this "gate effect". A most remarkable template specificity could be observed: The conductivity reponse to the template atrazine was more than 6 times higher than for other triazine herbizides.[19] Another proof for the "gate effect" was obtained with thin-film MIP composite membranes: The diffusive transport rate of another solute (creatinine) increased 1.23 fold in the presence of the template (theophylline) while without any additive or with caffein the fluxes were the same.[35]

Facilitated or Retarded Template Transport (See Table 3)

Self-supported or composite MIM prepared by in situ polymerization with different templates all showed a similar diffusive transport behaviour because a faster transport of the template could be observed. However, only in one study has a facilitated transport via "fixed carrier" MIP sites been demonstrated by the increase of transport selectivity with decreasing solute concentration.[34] The remarkably high selectivities and permeabilities for the "trans-membrane channel" MIM, prepared with a polymer porogen,[20] will definitely need further verification. MIP membranes prepared via "alternative imprinting" ("dry PI") showed a more complex transport behaviour, especially as a function of the applied driving force for transport. The MIM behavior—for dialysis and electrodialysis—was summarized in a phenomenological

Table 3. Examples for microporous MIM preparation, structure and separation performance

MIM Matrix	MIM Functionality	Template	Membrane MIM Preparation	Thickness (μm)	Source Separation by	Conc. (mmol/l)	Solvent	Flux (nmol·cm^{-2}·h^{-1})	Perm-Selectivity from Competition Experiments	Ref.
Poly(EDMA-co-MAA)		9-EA	in situ p. (>100)	not given	diffusion	0.076	CHCl$_3$/MeOH, 94/6	0.2	$\alpha_{As/Gs} \sim 3.4$	18
PSt-co-DVB-co-UO$_2^{2+}$ Vinylbenzoat			in situ p. (+porogen)	100	diffusion	0.2	H$_2$O	2.7	$\alpha(UO_2^{2+}/Ni^{2+})$ 20, >100	
Poly(EDMA-co-MAA)		Tho Caf	in situ p. composite	~ 0.05 (barrier in composite)	diffusion	0.010 0.001 0.010	MeOH	17 18	$\alpha_{Tho/Caf} \sim 2.6$, $a_{Tho/Caf} \sim 5.0$, $a_{Caf/Tho} \sim 3.0$	34
PAN-co-St	PSt-DIDE	Boc-L-Trp	dry PI	~ 145	electro-dialysis diffusion	1.0 1.0	H$_2$O/EtOH 50/50	~ 3 < 1	$a_{I/D} \sim 6.0$, $a_{I/D} \sim 0.8$	22
cellulose acetate		D-Glu L-Glu	dry PI	105	electro-dialysis	1.0	H$_2$O/EtOH 50/50	10	$\alpha_{D/L} \sim 2.3$, $\alpha_{L/D} \sim 2.3$	23

9-EA: 9-ethyl adenine; As: Adenosine; Boc: Tert.-butyloxycarbonyl; Caf: Caffein; co: ... co (polymer); DIDE: Tetrapeptide: H-Asp(OcHx)-Ile-Asp(OcHx)-Glu(Obz)-CH$_2$; DVB: Divinylbenzene; EDMA: Ethylenglycol dimethacrylate; Gs: Guanosine; Glu: Glutamine; MAA: Methacrylic acid; PAN: Polyacrylonitrile; PSt: polystyrene; St: tyrene; Tho: Theophylline; Trp: tryptophan

relationship where the flux monotonically increased with the difference in chemical potential while the selectivity was around 1 at about 20 kJ/mol (corresponding to a concentration difference of 1 mmol/l), showed a pronounced maximum in the range of 200 kJ/mol and levelled off again to about 1 at very high (electrical) potential values.[22]

Mechanisms for Transport and Selectivity

A detailed pore morphology analysis had not yet been performed for microporous MIM. Permeability data for MIM and blank membranes indicated the absence of large transmembrane pores, and that imprinting creates a specific micropore fraction and contributes to the connectivity of pores.[12,21,32,34] Hence, two models could explain MIM transport selectivity. A static model will be based on affinity binding to the "walls" of permanent pores which could either facilitate or retard the transport of the template. The critical parameters are the affinity and the density of imprinted sites: With increasing site density, the contribution of facilitated transport via "fixed carrier" sites will also increase (cf. Fig. 2a).[40] A dynamic model considering the adaptation of the micropore structure to environmental conditions due to interactions with solutes - in particular the template - might be much more realistic for understanding liquid separation with MIM. Solid porous polymers, prepared via in situ crosslinking polymerization or phase inversion, have a structural flexibility as a function of their solvation. For MIPs, significant template-induced polymer shrinking or swelling have been observed, and the "gate effect" for MIM has been confirmed with charged and uncharged species. Therefore the possible impact on other permeation data should be (re)analyzed. Nevertheless, facilitated transport could also occur in the dynamic model, but the carrier sites may have a certain mobility.

In conclusion, microporous MIM's permselectivity is based on preferential and reversible binding and exchange between template and MIP sites in the membrane thus providing pathways for selective trans-membrane transport. However, the different behaviour of membranes from different materials and preparation methods, imprinted for various templates and studied under various conditions, demonstrates the need for further detailed investigations of membrane structure as well as detailed transport characterization of well-defined membranes from controlled preparations, with a particular focus on dynamic effects on micropore structure.

Macroporous MIM – MIP as Affinity Adsorber Layer

With macroporous membranes, molecular separations can only be achieved via interactions with the membrane material. Convective flow through the membrane can be used as a means to improve separation performance via elimination of diffusion resistances. The advantages of membranes in comparison with other adsorbers such as beads are a high selective binding capacity at a high throughput.[3] With MIM, molecule selectivity could be tailored by the binding affinity of imprinted sites (cf. Fig. 2b). However for MIM adsorbers, membrane morphology is of major importance: The micropore fraction will determine the binding capacity, and a connected macropore fraction will be essential for efficient transmembrane transport and elimination of diffusion resistance.

MIM Adsorbers Prepared via "Alternative Imprinting"

MIM adsorbers prepared via "alternative imprinting" ("wet PI") showed in some cases very impressive binding selectivities, e.g., a separation factor of 50 for theophylline vs. caffein.[25] However, these data have been measured for single solutes only, i.e., real selectivities under competivite conditions are missing. Furthermore the data were measured at very low flow rates where the intra-membrane transport occured mainly via diffusion. The reason was the asymmetric pore structure with a microporous skin layer, created by the immersion step, which largely reduced the membrane permeability.[25,36] A significantly improved MIM permeability could be obtained by adapted PI conditions for a polymer blend.[28] Nevertheless, further work is necessary to achieve an acceptable membrane adsorber performance for phase inversion MIM.

MIP Particle Composite Membranes

MIP particle composite membranes, with a macroporous void fraction and a rather symmetric layer topology, could be developed towards competitive adsorbers. Currently, however, both binding capacities and permeabilities are still low.[30]

Thin-Layer MIP Composite Membranes

Due to the macroporous structure of the support MF membrane, MIM for herbicides could be characterized at very high flow rates:[37-39] The dynamic binding capacities, normalized to the amount of functional polymer, were similar to the static binding capacities for the best phase inversion MIM.[25] For the advanced composite MIM a very high selectivity, e.g., a separation factor of 15 for terbumeton vs. atrazine, had been achieved.[38] Furthermore, quantitative template recovery by elution from the MIM was possible, and the MIM were reusable in several subsequent bind-wash-elute cycles.[37] Currently, the main objective is further improving the MIM binding capacities.[41] High MIM permeabilities would enable an efficient isolation or removal of a dilute valuable or toxic compound from a very large volume.

Current Separation Performance and Potential of MIM

The empirical data from the last decade can be considered as the "proof-of-feasibility" for separations with MIM, but much further work will be necessary to really explore their potential. Nevertheless, based on fundamental knowledge about membrane materials and technology, guide-lines for a rational development of improved MIM with tailored and stable selectivities for diverse separations can now be envisioned.

Microporous MIM must be compared with established membranes, mainly for UF, D or NF. With state-of-the-art membranes, a continuos separation of two isomers with a permselectivity of 5 (cf. Table 3) can not be achieved. If the fluxes through MIM could be increased by a factor of 10 without compromising the selectivity (of course, a further increase would be desirable!) and if this performance could be maintained for a long time under technical conditions, such novel materials could immediately gain practical relevance. Imprinting efficiency, membrane morphology and separation conditions can be further optimized in order to improve the selective flux. It is most promising that significant binding and transport selectivities can also be achieved by imprinting with rather common functional polymers.[23,27,28] In terms of membrane morphology, the potential of thin-layer composite MIM for increasing permeability has already been indicated.[34,35] Imprinting efficiency and membrane morphology can most efficiently be addressed by tailored composite membranes, i.e., using the sequential preparation approach. An example, following the guide-lines towards a higher membrane separation performance, is filling the straight and regular pores of thin track-etched membranes with MIPs.[41] Also, the evidence for a positive impact of a higher driving force onto flux and selectivity is most interesting.[21,22] In conclusion, advanced MIM which enable a truely molecule-selective separation based on affinity interactions could have a very large application potential.

Macroporous MIM are a sub-group of affinity membrane adsorbers which directly compete with other affinity materials, either established, e.g., particles, or alternative ones, e.g., monoliths. For the first high-flux composite MIM, binding selectivities are promising but the capacities must be improved.[37-39] When compared with commercial affinity membranes using, e.g., ion-exchange groups, MIM—due to the higher spatial order of functional groups in the imprinted sites on the accessible surface—will per se have somewhat lower capacities. However, when compared with immobilized proteins, receptor site density may even be higher for MIP layers. In order to achieve the performance goals, further improvements of the (sequential) preparation of composite MIM will be the most effective approach. Hence, tailored materials for MIM-SPE could already be envisioned.

Once MIM materials with attractive intrinsic properties have been obtained, module and process design will be the next critical issues. In particular, for separations by microporous MIM with low permeabilities, the preparation of hollow-fibre membranes could serve as a means to increase the membrane area per volume of a separation unit. For higher driving forces and long term operations, problems with concentration polarization and membrane fouling must be solved.

Possible Applications of MIM

The application potential for MIM will be based on the success of their further development, driven by tackling those problems which can not be solved by state-of-the-art separation membranes. Of course, separations using improved or novel membranes must then still be compared with other unit operations.

Separations Based on MIM

The vision of a tailored and truely molecule-selective separation for a wide range of target molecules is the strongest motivation for MIM development. MIM for chiral separations may, similar to MIP particles, be the first examples for practical applications. In comparison with chromatography, the upscaling of a membrane separation should be much easier. Such success could serve as a "door opener" for other MIM. An increased fractionation selectivity in comparision with conventional UF, NF or D membranes would be very attractive, especially for many biotechnology processes. Furthermore, ED and gas or vapour separation—for functional target molecules—are further processes where selective MIM could yield significant improvements. For all the above cases, MIM with a microporous barrier enabling facilitated trans-membrane transport using imprinted sites would enable continuous separations. "Gate MIM" could be developed towards environment-sensitive or switchable membranes. All technical areas with pure or purified special target molecules as products will in the future benefit from such novel MIM separations (cf. Table 2). Alternatively, MIM adsorbers will be used mainly for isolation and removal of small molecular fractions, especially from a large volume. Such MIM will be applied instead of conventional adsorbers or in combination with other membrane separation steps, especially in water treatment and in the food and pharma industry (cf. Table 2).

Integrated Processes Based on MIM

Once the potential of MIM for special separations has been realized, their application for process intensification can be forseen. In membrane reactors, the selective removal of products or byproducts could be perfomed, with stable MIM also for organic reaction mixtures where conventional separation membranes currently often fail. As a next step, the development of catalytic MIM is also already on the way.[42]

The integration of a MIM into a system where membrane transport selectivity is used indirectly has already been demonstrated, the conductometric sensors based on the "gate effect" of MIM are examples.[19,32] Finally, other nonseparation applications of synthetic membranes, e.g., controlled release, could benefit from novel MIM, when a combination of molecular recognition and compartmentalization or transport will yield a superior performance.

Conclusions

The unique feature of MIM is the interplay of selective binding and permeation of molecules, making them potentially superior to state-of-the-art synthetic separation membranes already applied in various industries. Receptor and transport properties of microporous MIM can be based on template-specific binding sites in trans-membrane pores, which serve as fixed carriers for "facilitated" transport. Furthermore, template binding in microporous MIM can lead to a "gate-effect" which either increases or decreases membrane permeability. Alternatively, MIM can also function as adsorbers, leading to a retardation of template transport followed by breakthrough once the binding capacity has been saturated. In the last decade, the "proof-of-feasibility" has been shown for all MIM types. However, significantly advanced preparation methods, preferably towards composite membranes, and a much more detailed structural characterization will be necessary in order to be able to rationally design permselective

MIM. In general, MIM could serve as model systems for cellular transmembrane transport and natural receptors. Applications in sensors could be immediately derived from those models. However, an ultimate aim in membrane technology, the combination of molecular recognition and sieving in high performance membranes for challenging separation applications will in the future also be realized with advanced MIM.

References

1. Mulder M. Basic principles of membrane technology. 2nd ed. Dordrecht: Kluwer Academic Publishers, 1996.
2. Wijmans JG, Baker RW. The solution-diffusion model: A review. J Membr Sci 1995; 107:1-21.
3. Roper DK, Lightfoot EN. Separation of biomolecules using adsorptive membranes. J Chromatogr 1995; A702:3-26.
4. http://www.3m.com/empore
5. Srikanth G. Membrane separation processes - technology and business opportunities. Pune, India: Technology Information, Forecasting & Assessment Council (TIFAC), 2003.
6. van Reis R, Zydney A. Membrane separations in biotechnology. Curr Opinion Biotechn 2001; 12:208-211.
7. Nunes S, Peinemann KV eds. Membrane technology in the chemical industry. Weinheim: Wiley-VCH Verlag, 2001.
8. Sanchez Marcano JG, Tsotsis TT. Catalytic membrane reactors and membrane reactors. Weinheim: Wiley-VCH Verlag, 2002.
9. Drioli E, Giorno L. Biocatalytic membrane reactors. London: Taylor & Francis Ltd., 1999.
10. Martin CR, Nishizawa M, Jirage K et al. Investigations of the transport properties of gold nanotubule membranes. J Phys Chem 2001; B105:1925-1934.
11. Beginn U, Zipp G, Mourran A et al. Membranes containing oriented supramolecular transport channels. Adv Mater 2000; 12:513-516.
12. Piletsky SA, Panasyuk TL, Piletskaya EV et al. Receptor and transport properties of molecularly imprinted polymer membranes – a review. J Membr Sci 1999; 157:263-278.
13. Sellergren B, Hall AJ. Fundamental aspects on the synthesis and characterization of imprinted network polymers. In: Sellergren B, ed. Molecularly imprinted polymers – man-made mimics of antibodies and their application in analytical chemistry. Elsevier: 2001:21-57.
14. Mirsky VM, Hirsch T, Piletsky SA et al. A Spreader-bar approach to molecular architecture: Formation of stable artificial chemoreceptors. Angew Chem Int Ed 1999; 38:1108-1110.
15. Shi H, Tsai WB, Garrison MD et al. Template-imprinted nanostructured surfaces for protein recognition. Nature 1999; 398:593.
16. Raman NK, Anderson MT, Brinker CJ. Template-based approaches to the preparation of amorphous, nanoporous silicas. Chem Mater 1996; 8:1682-1701.
17. Mann S, Burkett SL, Davis SA et al. Sol-gel synthesis of organized matter. Chem Mater 1997; 9:2300-2310.
18. Mathew-Krotz J, Shea KJ. Imprinted polymer membranes for the selective transport of targeted neutral molecules. J Am Chem Soc 1996; 118:8154-8155.
19. Sergeyeva TA, Piletsky SA, Brovko AA et al. Conductometric sensor for atrazine detection based on molecularly imprinted polymer membrane. Analyst 1999; 124:331-334.
20. Kimaro A, Kelly LA, Murray GM. Molecularly imprinted ionically permeable membrane for uranyl ion. Chem Commun 2001; 1282-1283.
21. Yoshikawa M, Izumi J, Kitao T et al. Molecularly imprinted polymeric membranes for optical resolution. J Membr Sci 1995; 108:171-175.
22. Yoshikawa M, Izumi J, Kitao T. Alternative molecular imprinting, a facile way to introduce chiral recognition sites. React Funct Polym 1999; 42:93-102.
23. Yoshikawa M, Ooi T, Izumi J. Alternative molecularly imprinted membranes from a derivative of a natural polymer, cellulose acetate. J Appl Polym Sci 1999; 72:493-499.
24. Yoshikawa M, Izumi J, Guiver MD et al. Recognition and selective transport of nucleic acid components through molecularly imprinted polymeric membranes. Macromol Mater Eng 2001; 286:52-59.
25. Wang HY, Kobayashi T, Fuji N. Molecular imprint membranes prepared by the phase inversion technique. Langmuir 1996; 12:4850-4856.
26. Reddy PS, Kobayashi T, Fujii N. Molecular imprinting in hydrogen bonding networks of polyamide nylon for recognitions of amino acids. Chem Lett 1999; 293-294.
27. Reddy PS, Kobayashi T, Fujii N. Recognition characteristics of dibenzofuran by molecularly imprinted polymers made from common polymers. Eur Polym J 2002; 38:779-785.

28. Ramamoorthy M, Ulbricht M. Molecular imprinting of cellulose actetate sulfonated polysulfone blend membranes for rhodamine B by phase inversion technique. J Membr Sci 2003; 217:207-219.

29. Lehmann M, Brunner H, Tovar G. Enantioselective separations: A new approach using molecularly imprinted nanoparticle composite membranes. Desalination 2002; 149:315-321.

30. Lehmann M, Brunner H, Tovar G. Molekular geprägte nanopartikel als selektive phase in kompositmembranen: Hydrodynamik und stofftrennungen in nanoskaligen schüttungen. Chem Ing Techn 2003; 75:149-153.

31. Piletsky SA, Dubey IY, Fedoryak DM et al. Substrate-selective polymeric membranes. Selective transfer of nucleic acid components. Biopolim Kletka 1990; 6:55-58.

32. Piletsky SA, Panasyuk TL, Piletskaya EV et al. Imprinted membranes for sensor technology: Opposite behavior of covalently and noncovalently imprinted membranes. Macromolecules 1998; 31:2137-2140.

33. Dzgoev A, Haupt K. Enantioselective molecularly imprinted polymer membranes. Chirality 1999; 11:465-469.

34. Hong JM, Anderson PE, Qian J et al. Selectively-permeable ultrathin film composite membranes based on molecularly-imprinted polymers. Chem Mater 1998; 10:1029-1033.

35. Hattori K, Yoshimi Y, Sakai K. Gate effect of cellulosic dialysis membrane grafted with molecularly imprinted polymer. J Chem Eng Jpn 2001; 34:1466-1469.

36. Wang HY, Kobayashi T, Fuji N. Surface molecular imprinting on photosensitive dithio-carbamoyl polyacrylonitrile membrane using photo graft polymerization. J Chem Technol Biotechnol 1997; 70:355-362.

37. Piletsky SA, Matuschewski H, Schedler U et al. Surface functionalization of porous polypropylene membranes with molecularly imprinted polymers by photografting polymerization in water. Macromolecules 2000; 33:3092-3098.

38. Sergeyeva TA, Matuschewski H, Piletsky SA et al. Molecularly imprinted polymer membranes for substance-selective solid-phase extraction from water by surface photo-grafting polymerisation. J Chromatogr 2001; A907:89-99.

39. Kochkodan V, Weigel W, Ulbricht M. Thin layer molecularly imprinted microfiltration membranes by photofunctionalization using a coated α-cleavage photoinitiator. Analyst 2001; 126:803-809.

40. Noble RD. Generalized microscopic mechanism of facilitated transport in fixed site carrier membranes. J Membr Sci 1992; 75:121-129.

41. Ulbricht M, Belter M, Langenhangen U et al. Novel molecularly imprinted polymer (MIP) composite membranes via controlled surface and pore functionalizations. Desalination 2002; 149:293-295.

42. Brüggemann O. Catalytically active polymers obtained by molecular imprinting and their application in chemical reaction engineering. Biomol Eng 2001; 18:1-7.

CHAPTER 8

Recognition of Enantiomers Using Molecularly Imprinted Polymers

Börje Sellergren

Introduction

With the increasing structural complexity of new drugs, the importance of enantiomerically pure compounds is growing.[1] Resolution of racemates is often the first step in this process. Conventionally, preparative optical resolution is performed by fractional crystallization, microbiological methods, kinetic enzymatic resolution or by chromatography. Methods allowing continuous production of pure enantiomers such as simulated moving bed (SMB) chromatography[2] or counter current distribution[3] or chromatography[4] as well as techniques to rapidly analyse enantiomeric purity are increasing in importance. In the case of phases exhibiting particularly high enantio-selectivities, batch-,[5] membrane-,[6] or bubble-based[7] separation techniques may be more attractive.

Polysaccharide-based phases (modified amylose or cellulose) are, due to their high site density and broad applicability, the most common chromatographic phases used for preparative scale separations.[8] A problem with these as well as other common CSPs is the limited predictability of elution orders and separability. Thus, screening of stationary phase libraries is often a necessary step in the method development. This is not the case for molecularly imprinted CSPs (MICSPs) where the elution order is known beforehand. These are also attractive due to their high enantioselectivity and stability. To date, MICSPs have been used in liquid chromatography,[9] capillary electrochromatography,[10] supercritical fluid chromatography,[11] thin layer chromatography[12] and solid phase extraction.[13] However, in analytical and preparative HPLC, they have sofar been unable to compete with traditional chiral stationary phases. This is due to a number of intrinsic limitations related to the imprinted phases (Table 1). The most important are probably the limited site capacity and poor efficiency of the bulk imprinted materials, which limits the amount of loadable racemate and leads to broad and strongly tailing peaks (for a typical elution profile see Fig. 1). Secondly, there is a need for preparative amount of pure enantiomer in order to produce one batch of polymer. Hence, this often requires the template to be recovered and recycled, complicating the production. Nevertheless, apart from the benefits mentioned above, the classical benefits of imprinting still apply i.e., polymer robustness and reproducibility, ease and cost of preparation.

This review will report some recent developments in the area of molecular imprinting aimed at recognizing enantiomers and discuss approaches to overcome the above limitations and thus to improve their performance to a competitive level. Recent advances in the analytical application of these recognition elements will also be discussed. For a more comprehensive coverage the reader is refered to other reviews.[9,14]

Molecular Imprinting of Polymers, edited by Sergey Piletsky and Anthony Turner.
©2006 Landes Bioscience.

Table 1. MIPs in chiral chromatography

Benefits	Limitations
• High selectivity	• Low sample load capacity*
• Ease of preparation	– 1-2 mg/g dry weight
• Predictable elution order	• Poor efficiency (N, A_s, R_s)
• Reproducibility	• Preparative amount of chiral
– Batch to batch	template required
– Column to column	• High selecivity**
• Robustness of packing	
– T< 120°C	
– Organic solvents	
– Extreme pH values	
• Cost	

* Preparative application; ** Analytical applications

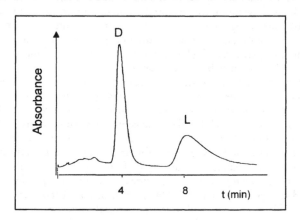

Figure 1. Typical elution profile for a racemate (D,L-phenylalanine anilide (D,L-PA)) resolved on an imprinted CSP (template: L-PA). Sample: 10 nmole D,L-PA; Eluent: MeCN / 0.05M potassium phosphate, pH 4 : 7/3 (v/v), Temperature: 60°C.

Enantiomers as Model Templates

Single enantiomers were originally used as model templates to facilitate the evaluation of the memory effects observed in the corresponding imprinted polymer.[15] Since mirror image molecules have identical physical properties, enantioselectivity exhibited by an imprinted polymer made of achiral monomer units can only be due to structural changes caused by the chiral template. Most often these structural changes are ascribed to imprinted sites or cavities complementary to the template in terms of size, shape and functional groups (see other chapters in this book). According to a more general interpretation, the enantio-selectivity may be the result of chiral surfaces induced by clusters of templates or a template induced chirality in the polymer main chain, due to induced tacticity or helical structures (Fig. 2).

Most evidence today however, supports the existance of discrete binding sites highly complementary to the template enantiomer. This is based on the use of model templates producing polymers with high affinity and selectivity for the template. Extensive structural and

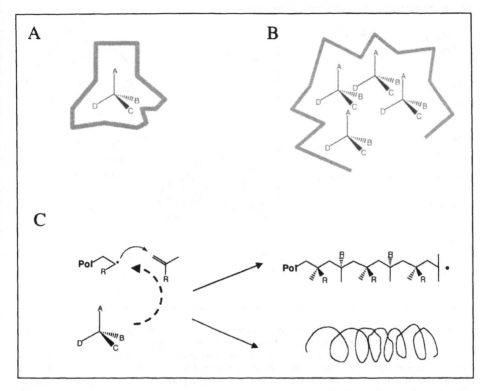

Figure 2. Possible origins of enantioselectivity in polymers imprinted with pure enantiomers. A) monomolecular binding sites; B) the cluster model; C) main chain chirality.

thermodynamic characterisation of the corresponding materials have improved the understanding of their chromatographic behaviour and the molecular recognition mechanism.

One extensively studied system uses L-phenylalanine anilide (L-PA) as template and methacrylic acid (MAA) as functional monomer (Fig. 3).[16,17] In the elucidation of retention mechanisms, the use of enantiomers as templates has the benefit of cancelling out non-specific interactions, which affects both enantiomers equally. Therefore the separation factor (α (=k'_L/k'_D)) uniquely reflects the contribution to binding from the enantioselectively imprinted sites. As an additional comparison the retention factors (k') on the imprinted phase is compared with the retention factors on a nonimprinted reference phase. The efficiency of the separations is routinely characterized by estimating a number of theoretical plates (N), a resolution factor (R_s) and a peak asymmetry factor (A_s).[18] These quantities are affected by the quality of the packing and mass transfer limitations as well as of the amount and distribution of the binding sites.

As commonly observed for the MAA based imprinting protocol, the resulting materials exhibit pronounced selectivities for the structures used as template (Table 2). The racemate corresponding to the template is well resolved on the corresponding MICSP whereas the analogue racemates are less retained and only poorly resolved. This ability to recognize subtle structural differencies has been attributed to the combination of functional group and shape complementarity between the binding site and the substrate.

In order to elucidate the influence of template shape and conformational entropy on the molecular recognition properties of MIPs, Spivak and Campbell[19] proposed the use of chiral monoamines as templates. These provide only one strong binding interaction for MAA and the association energy should be similar for all monomer template complexes studied. This allows

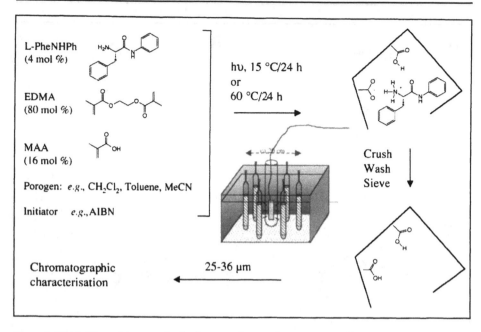

Figure 3. The L-PA model system. In the first step, the template (L-PA), the functional monomer (MAA) and the crosslinking monomer (EDMA) are dissolved in a poorly hydrogen bonding solvent (porogen) of low to medium polarity. The free radical polymerization is then initiated with an azo initiator, commonly azo-N,N'-bis-isobutyronitrile (AIBN) either by photochemical homolysis below room temperature or thermochemically at 30°C or higher. In the final step, the resultant polymer is crushed by mortar and pestle or in a ball mill, extracted using a Soxhlet apparatus, and sieved to a particle size suitable for chromatographic (25-38 μm) or batch (150-250 μm) applications.[17]

Table 2. MIP resolves the template racemate ... but not that of a close structural analogue

![Table 2 structures showing template and analogue molecules, with "or" between the two right-hand top structures]

Table 3. Separation factors (α) for the different chiral amines on each imprinted polymer

MIP template	Substrate					
	1	2	3	4	5	6
1	1.33	1.20	1.00	1.00	1.00	1.00
2	1.23	1.58	1.14	1.16	1.00	1.07
3	1.00	1.00	2.26	1.78	1.00	1.00
4	1.00	1.00	1.65	3.25	1.00	1.00
5	1.05	1.03	1.00	1.05	1.44	1.01
6	1.00	1.01	1.00	1.00	1.00	1.00
NIP	1.00	1.00	1.00	1.00	1.00	1.00

the influence sterics and conformational entropy of differently sized groups surrounding the chiral center on the recognition by the MIP to be studied (Table 3). It would also reveal how the enantioselectivity responds to the distance between the chiral center from the binding group interaction.

The template library shown in Table 3 was used to prepare imprinted polymers using the conventional poly(MAA-co-EDMA) procedure with dichloromethane as porogen. In view of the similar pK_a-values of the templates and their similar ^{1}H-NMR complexation induced shifts vis a vis MAA, the degree of complexation should be similar for all templates. The MIPs were assessed as chromatographic stationary phases using acetonitrile/acetic acid (90/10) as mobile phase by comparing the retention factors and separation factors of all enantiomer pairs on all columns. The first comparisons concerned the influence of the steric contributions of the groups bound to the chiral center of the template. MIP 1 and 2 showed separation factors of 1.33 and 1.58 respectively for their own substrates. Thus the chiral discrimination improves when increasing the aryl group size from phenyl to naphtyl. Both polymers showed crossreactivity with a separation factor of ca 1.2 for the opposite substrates. Whereas this was the only crossreactivity observed for MIP 1, MIP 2 showed crossreactivity for all templates except 5. This led to the important conclusion that the naphtyl group may serve as a "privileged" building block to widen the selectivity MICSPs. Among all templates, those giving the highest selectivity were 3 and 4 containing two chiral centers. The separation is here enhanced due to the larger shape differencies between the corresponding templates. These disubstituted amines also exhibited significant crossreactivity for the disubstituted counterparts whereas the monosubstituted amines where not separated on these MIPs. This confirms previous studies of the L-PA model system.

The influence of the conformational entropy of the imprinted molecule on molecular recognition, the conformationally locked template 5 was included in the comparison. The slightly higher enantioselectivity observed on MIP 5 compared to the MIP for the unlocked template 1 may suggest an effect of its lower conformational entropy. The unlocked substrate 1 was poorly recognized by MIP 5 and vice versa, 5 was poorly recognized by MIP 1. This indicates that these compounds exhibit different optimum conformations.

Finally the effect of the distance between the binding interaction and the chiral center is seen in the comparison between templates 1 and 6. As expected, MIP 6 showed a poorer enantioselectivity (α=1.13) than MIP 1 (α=1.33). This is probably the result of conformational flexibility which is expected to increase by inserting an additional free rotor between the binding interaction and the chiral center.

Use of Enantiomers as Templates to Mimic Natural Binding Sites

In view of the receptor like binding properties of some MIPs, it was proposed some years ago that MIPs could be used as a kind of molecular sieve to sort molecules on the basis of their biological activitiy.[20-22] It was assumed that the binding molecules would also exhibit enhanced affinity for the corresponding biological receptor. If such correlation would exist, the access to robust readily prepared synthetic receptors could become a powerful tool for the screening of combinatorial libraries. This would be of particular interest for receptors with unknown structure or that are too labile or costly to produce. Apart from isolating novel lead compounds such studies could also be more fundamental, directed towards obtaining insights into the nature of the synthetic or biological binding sites.

Several drugs interact enantiospecifically with their target receptor. In this context, the use of pure enantiomers as templates for producing MIPs has the benefit of facilitating the screening process in that nonspecific matrix interactions are canceled out when assessing the enantioselectivity of the material. In a study by Hart et al enantiomers of Benzodiazepines were used as templates to prepare synthetic receptors corresponding to a family of biological receptors, GABA, which structures are mainly unknown.[23] A series of benzodiazepine analogs were imprinted and the resulting MIPs evaluated as stationary phases in chromatography (Table 4). Similar to previous model systems, as the structural differencies between the template and the substrate increase the enantioselectivity and retention decrease. Also notable and in agreement with other studies is the increase in enantioselectivity with increasing size or increasing number of interaction sites of the perturbed side chains. This is seen in the low separation factor for the methyl derivative and the high separation factor for the benzyl and hydroxybenzyl derivatives. It was concluded that the benzodiazepine MIPs may prove useful for screening large libraries of compounds with similar or related affinities.

Table 4. Separation factors (α) for the different benzodiazepines on each imprinted polymer

MIP template	Substrate (R-group)				
	CH$_2$PhOH	CH$_2$Ph	CH$_2$Indol	CH(CH$_3$)$_2$	CH$_3$
CH$_2$PhOH	3.8	2.5	1.3	1.6	1.4
CH$_2$Ph	2.3	3.0	1.7	1.6	1.7
CH$_2$Indol	1.5	1.8	2.3	1.3	1.4
CH(CH$_3$)$_2$	1.2	1.3	1.3	2.2	1.6
CH$_3$	1.0	1.1	1.1	1.1	1.3

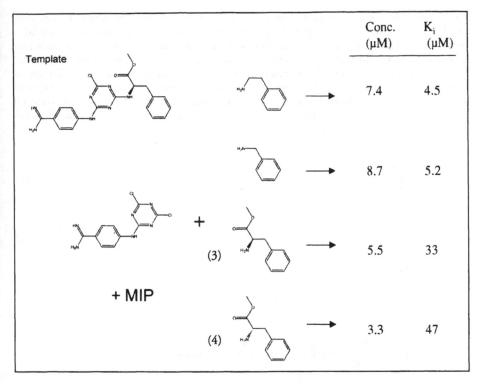

Figure 4. Use of polymers, imprinted with inhibitor for the enzyme kallikrein, to direct the synthesis towards biologically active substances. The approximative product concentration obtained after extraction from the imprinted polymer (Conc) and the inhibition constant (K_i) for kallikrein have been indicated.

A correlation between MIP binding affinity and biological affinity was reported by Yu et al.[24] This group imprinted a known inhibitor of the protease enzyme kallikrein (Fig. 4). The resulting MIP was therafter assessed for its ability to direct the synthesis towards template like compounds in a simple substitution reaction. It was anticipated that the obtained yields of each product would reflect their affinity for the biological receptor. Interstingly a clear correlation between biological activity and yield for the two enantiomers 3 and 4 was obtained. Furthermore, this affinities agreed with the product yields obtained in presence of the native enzyme.

Binding Isotherms and Model Fitting

Most MIPs suffer from a heterogenous distribution of binding sites. In noncovalent imprinting, primarily two effects contribute to the binding site heterogeneity. Due to the amorphous nature of the polymer, the binding sites are not identical, somewhat similar to a polyclonal preparation of antibodies. Secondly, this effect is reinforced by nonstoichiometric monomer template complexation.[16] In most cases the major part of the functional monomer exists in a free or dimerized form, not associated with the template. As a consequence, only a part of the template added to the monomer mixture gives rise to selective binding sites. The poor yield of binding sites results in a strong dependence of selectivity and binding on sample load at least within the low sample load regime.

Further insight into the binding energies, modes of binding and site distributions in heterogenous adsorption experiments is gained from the corresponding binding isotherms. In the case of MIPs, obtained directly as chromatographic packing materials, frontal analysis has proven particularly valuable in this regard. This method allows accurate determination of adsorption and kinetic data from simple breakthrough experiments and the technique has proven its validity in a number of previous studies. The binding isotherms are plots of equilibrium concentrations of bound ligand (adsorbate) versus concentration of free ligand. The isotherms can be fitted using various models where different assumptions are made. The most simple is the Langmuir type adsorption isotherm (Eq. 1) where the adsorbent is assumed to contain only one type of sites, where adsorbate-adsorbate-interactions are assumed not to occur and where the system is assumed ideal. This isotherm depends on two parameters: the saturation capacity (site density), q_s, and the adsorption energy, b.[25,26]

$$q = \frac{a_1 C}{1 + b_1 C} \tag{1}$$

$$q = \frac{a_1 C}{1 + b_1 C} + \frac{a_2 C}{1 + b_2 C} \tag{2}$$

$$q = a C^{1/n} \qquad \text{(a and n=numerical parameters)} \tag{3}$$

$$q = \int \phi(\ln K) \frac{KC}{1 + KC} d(\ln K) \qquad \text{(K=association constant)} \tag{4}$$

The bilangmuir model (Eq. 2) or trilangmuir model, the sum of two or three Langmuir isotherms, correspond to models that assume the adsorbent surface to be heterogenous composed of two or three different site classes and finally the Freundlich isotherm model (Eq. 3) or the affinity spectrum model (Eq. 4) with no saturation capacity but instead a complete distribution of sites of different binding energies. Due to the above mentioned site heterogeneity, the isotherms obtained from MIPs prepared by the noncovalent imprinting route are usually modelled using equations 2-4 or a combination of the models.

As discussed earlier in this chapter, the use pure enantiomers as model templates facilitates the deconvolution of specific and non-specific contributions to the adsorption. This was used in a series of reports by the groups of Guiochon and Sellergren to obtain mechanistic aspects of the adsorption of substrates to MIPs.[26-29] The isotherms for the two enantiomers of phenylalanine anilide (PA) interacting with an L-PA imprinted stationary phase were determined by frontal analysis using an aqueous mobile phase composed of acetonitrile/potassium phosphate buffer (0.03M, pH 5.85): 70/30 (v/v) (Fig. 5).[26] These were best fitted with the Langmuir binary site or the Freundlich isotherm model. Using the former, the binding constants and site densities for L-PA at 40°C are respectively 84 M^{-1} and ca 90 µmol/g for the low affinity sites and 16000 M^{-1} and 1 µmol/g for the high affinity sites. For D-PA the respective values are 48 M^{-1} and 136 µmol/g for the low affinity sites and 5520 M^{-1} and 0.4 µmol/g for the high affinity sites. In view of the small saturation capacities observed for D-PA on these sites at the other temperatures studied (50, 60, 70°C) or after thermal annealing of the materials,[27] the second site class appears to be specific for L-PA. This was further substantiated by recent affinity spectrum analysis of the native and annealed material making use of the expectation-maximization method to fit the affinity distribution at higher resolution.[29] Particularly striking results were obtained for elevated column temperatures. Figure 6 shows a comparison of the affinity distributions for D- and L- PA adsorbed on an L- PA imprinted nontreated (A) and

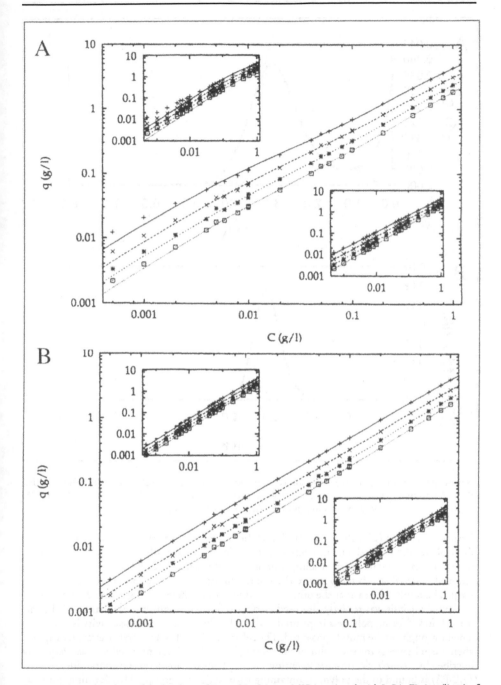

Figure 5. Frontal analysis of the binding of D- and L- PA to a MIP imprinted with L-PA. Fitting (lines) of the experimental isotherm data (symbols) for L-PA (A) and D-PA (B) to the Bi-Langmuir model (main figure), the Langmuir model (left inset) and the Freundlich model (right inset). For the runs at 40°C: solid lines and plus symbols, at 60°C: short dashed lines and stars, at 70°C: dotted lines and squares. Mobile phase: MeCN/potassium phosphate 0.05 M, pH 5.85: 70/30 (v/v). From Sajonz et al.[26]

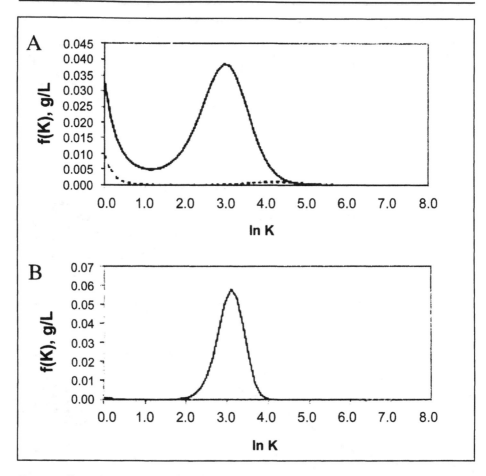

Figure 6. Affinity distributions of L-PA (solid curve) and D-PA (dashed curve) on native (A) and annealed (B) L-PA imprinted polymers at 70°C. Mobile phase: MeCN/potassium phosphate (KP) 0.05 M, pH 5.85: 70/30 (v/v). Reprinted with permission from the American Chemical Society.

thermally annealed (B) polymer at 70°C. For the nontreated material distributions appearing bimodal are seen for both enantiomers with considerably higher adsorbed amounts for L-PA. As seen in (B) the effect of annealing is dramatic. Wheareas no D-PA seems to bind to the annealed material at this temperature the site distribution for L-PA appears monomodal and sharp. The results obtained at the other column temperatures revealed broader distributions.

Frontal analysis was recently also used to obtain further insight into the nature of the imprinted sites.[28] Using polymers imprinted with L-PA, the retention and selectivity is known to depend strongly on the mobile phase pH. The selectivity is high at low pHs whereas it drops off when the pH exceeds the pKa value of the solute (Table 5). This retention effect was adequately described by a simple electrostatic retention model. Thus the amino group containing solute B (D,L-PA) is bound to the polymer containing carboxylic acid groups (HA) forming ion-pairs BH^+A^-. Assuming that ionexchange is the predominating retention mechanism the retention factor can be expressed as:

$$k'_B = K \alpha *_B \alpha *_A \qquad\qquad (5)$$

Table 5. Analytical retention of D-PA and L-PA on an L-PA imprinted polymer

Isomer	t_R (pH=3.0) min.	t_R (pH=5.8) min.	t_R (pH=7.0) min.
D-PA	3.81	7.66	3.30
L-PA	9.06	21.82	4.12
α_{app}	2.82	3.10	1.32
$\alpha*_A$	-	- - -	- - - - -
$\alpha*_B$	+1	≈ +1/2	0
Attraction	weak	strong	weak

Mobile phase: Acetonitrile/potassium phosphate buffer (0.03M) : 70/30 (v/v)

where $\alpha*_A$ and $\alpha*_B$ are the degree of ionization of the acid (A) and the base (B) respectively and K is a constant for a given column and ionic strength. The validity of this model is supported by data obtained by potentiometric titrations as schematically indicated in Table 5.

Although the model adequately describes the retention behaviour, the influence of pH on the enantioselectivity is more difficult to explain. Two scenarios may account for the decrease in selectivity with increasing pH (Fig. 7).

A. The first explanation is that the ratio of the numbers of nonselective and selective sites increases significantly with increasing pH, most likely due to an increased abundancy of the former type (Fig. 7A). This would lead to a dramatic decrease of the relative density of the enantioselective sites reducing their influence. Potentimetric titration data of the phases support this explanation. These indicated a small but significant difference in the average pK_a values of the imprinted (pK_a=8.9) and nonimprinted (pK_a=9.3) polymers. Thus the acid groups of the imprinted polymers are slightly more acidic than those of the nonimprinted polymer indicating that the imprinted sites are ionized at lower pH than the nonimprinted sites.

B. Structural changes at the selective sites may also contribute to the observed decrease in selectivity (Fig. 7B). Assuming binding sites containing two or more carboxylic acid groups positioned to interact by ion-pair and hydrogen bonding with the template, loss of hydrogen bond donors upon further ionization should cause a decrease in both binding affinity and selectivity of those sites.

Lacking molecular resolution structural data of the polymers, we reasoned that isotherm data at three different mobile phase pH would allow us to tell which one of the explanations are the most likely.[28] As seen in Table 6 an increase in pH from 3 to 5.8 leads to a more than 10 fold increase of the nonselective saturation capacity (q_{s1}) whereas only a ca 3 fold increase in that of the selective sites (q_{s2}). This provides clear support for explanation (A) but does not exclude influence of the second factor. The importance of this factor is illustrated by the values of the binding energy (i.e., coefficients b_i) in Table 6, showing an approximately five-fold decrease when the pH increases from 3 to 5.8. The above study is unique in the way it has shown that isotherm data can be used to gain valuable structural insight at the molecular level, not accessible by other techniques.

For preparative or semipreparative scale enantiomer separations the enantioselectivity and column saturation capacity are the critical factors determining the throughput of pure enantiomer that can be achieved. The above described MICSPs are stable, they can be reproducibly synthesized and exhibit high selectivities, attractive features for such applications. However most MICSPs have only moderate saturation capacities and isocratic elution leads to excessive peak tailing which precludes many preparative applications. Nevertheless with the L-PA MICSP described above, mobile phases can be chosen leading to acceptable resolution, saturation capacities and relatively short elution times also in the isocratic mode. Alternative means to enhance the efficiency and capacity of MICSPs will be discussed below.

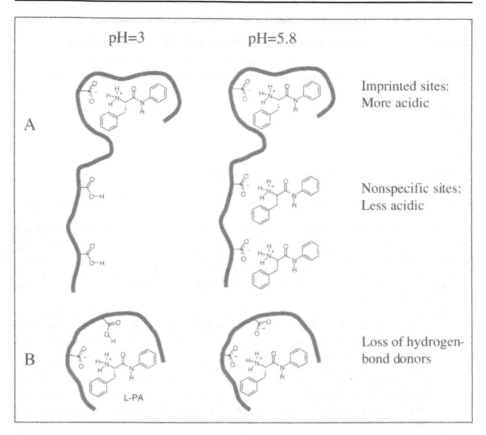

Figure 7. Models accounting for the decrease in enantioselectivity with increasing mobile phase pH.

Approaches to Binding Site Design

In spite of the fact that MAA can be used to generate CSPs showing high enantioselectivity for a large number of target enantiomers, for several targets it fails and other monomer combinations need to be found. Furthermore, as indicated in Table 1 the imprinted CSPs are associated with some more general drawbacks that may need to be addressed for these phases to offer benefits over alternative phases. It is clear that improvements aiming at increasing the yield of high energy binding sites or modifying the site distribution in other ways will have a large impact on the performance of the materials. The strategies adopted to achieve this have been focusing either on prepolymerization measures, aiming at correctly choosing monomers and stabilizing the monomer template assemblies prior to polymerization or postpolymerization measures (see previous section) aiming at modifying the distribution of binding sites by either chemical or physical means. The prepolymerization related strategies will be discussed in this section.

Combinatorial and Computational Techniques to Optimizing MICSPs

Due to the many parameters influencing the materials' properties at different length scales, as well as the absence of a clear understanding of how these parameters interplay, there are presently no well developed rules to follow for the design of materials exhibiting the desired recognition properties. Thus, combinatorial synthesis approaches or computational techniques,

Table 6. Results from bi-Langmuir model fittings of the frontal analysis adsorption isotherms of D- and L- PA on an L-PA imprinted stationary phase

pH=3.0T (°C)	L-PA						D-PA	
	a1	b1 (l/g)	qs1	a2	b2 (l/g)	qs2	a1	b1 (l/g)
40	2.10	1.17	1.8	5.13	47.3	0.11	2.00	1.17
50	2.00	1.08	1.8	4.22	29.2	0.14	2.00	1.08
60	1.95	0.88	2.2	3.96	28.2	0.14	1.95	0.88
70	1.88	0.78	2.4	3.49	24.7	0.14	1.88	0.78
pH=5.8T (°C)	**L-PA**						**D-PA**	
	a1	b1 (l/g)	qs1	a2	b2 (l/g)	qs2	a1	b1 (l/g)
40	6.5	0.36	18	4.7	10	0.45	6.5	0.36
50	4.55	0.27	17	2.4	8	0.3	4.55	0.27
60	2.73	0.05	50	1.9	6	0.3	2.73	0.05
70	2.02	0.01	na	0.93	4.4	0.2	2.02	0.01

allowing the main factors to be rapidly screened, have offered valuable tools in the development of new MIPs.

We and others recently introduced an in situ synthesis and evaluation technique for MIPs, resulting in libraries of mini-MIPs at the bottom of HPLC-autosampling vials.[30-32] With a final batch size of ca 40 mg of monomer the consumption of monomers and template is significantly reduced and the synthesis and evaluation can take place directly by HPLC. The recognition properties of the polymers could be assessed in situ by HPLC quantification of the non-bound fraction of the template at equilibrium (Fig. 8). These techniques were time consuming due to the slow removal of template and the need for serial analysis of the supernatant solutions. Recently this has been circumvented by the use of filter plates for rapid template removal and a multifunction plate reader for a parallel analysis of the supernatant fractions allowing the screening process to be rapidly performed.

The molecular modelling approach introduced by Piletsky et al is an alternative or complementary approach to find optimal monomer combinations.[33] A virtual library of functional monomers is created and screened for all possible interactions the individual monomers may engage in with the template. Monomers with the highest binding scores are subsequently selected to produce full scale MIPs with hopefully superior recognition properties. The approach was used for the optimization of MIPs for (-)-ephedrine (1). (Scheme 1) As expected for Brönsted-basic templates, best results were found using acidic functional monomers with the best binding scores found for itaconic acid and MAA. With more refined and affordable computational tools it is expected that this technique will play an important role in the design of imprinted polymers with improved properties.

MICSPs by Rational Design

One important limitation with the conventional imprinting protocol concerns the common use of low- or non-polar organic solvents in the imprinting step, e.g., dichloromethane and toluene. The choice of template is then restricted to those molecules soluble in such media. A further problem is that the use of commercially available functional monomers generally requires that a large excess of said monomers are employed to ensure that the template molecule is completely complexed. This, in turn, means that non-associated functional monomer is incorporated into the polymer matrix, leading to high levels of non-specific binding. One approach to improve this situation involves the preparation of functional monomers that

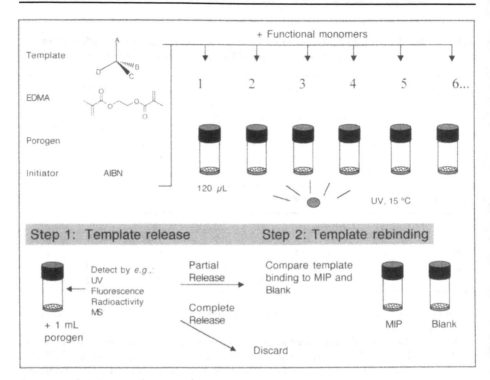

Figure 8. Combinatorial imprinting technique suitable for automation.

provide strong and stoichiometric interactions with a given template.[34-36] One of the more prominent examples comes from the group of Wulff who synthesised N,N'-substituted p-vinylbenzamidines (2) and showed that these monomers could be used to generate high fidelity sites for the molecular recognition of chiral carboxylic acids.[37]

Most of the reports on this topic are focused on co- or ter- polymers where the major part of the polymer matrix is composed of the crosslinking monomer, commonly EDMA. Although several crosslinking monomers have been tested in the past, EDMA has proven to be most widely applicable in molecular imprinting. However, it was noted by Spivak et al that only few studies have been devoted to improve the matrix properties of MIPs and thus that new rationally designed crosslinking monomers may offer additional benefits.[38] For this purpose EDMA was chosen as the lead compound. Bisacrylamides and bismethacrylamides have been successfully used for imprinting a wide variety of templates, but due to their poor solubility in organic solvents their use has been restricted to more polar solvent compositions.[39] Unfortunately, such conditions do not favor the formation of stable monomer template complexes. In order to enhance the solubility of the amide based crosslinkers, Spivak's group introduced hybrid monoamide based crosslinkers containing an additional ester functionality (NOBE) or keto functionality (NAG) (Fig. 9). The new crosslinkers could be synthesized in one (NOBE) or three (NAG) steps and were soluble in poorly polar organic solvents such as chloroform and methylenechloride. Apart from enhancing the solubility of amide based crosslinkers, the monomer size was an additional proposed design criterium. It was reasoned that smaller crosslinking monomers such as NAG would lead to a more snug wrapping of the polymer chains around the template during polymerization.

Dansyl-L-phenylalanine (3) was chosen as model template and polymers were prepared by photoinitiation using MAA as functional monomer and EDMA, NOBE or NAG as crosslinkers

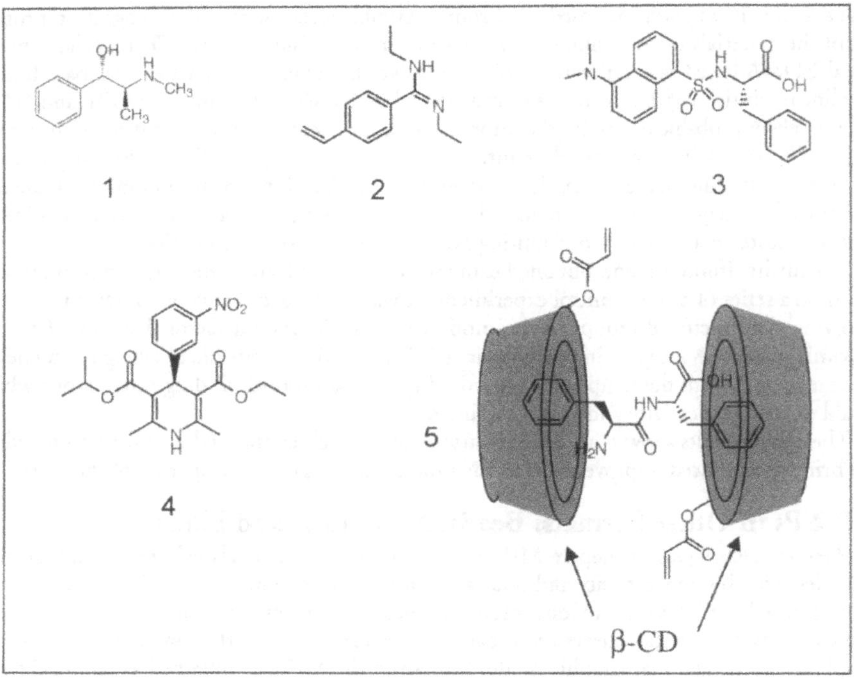

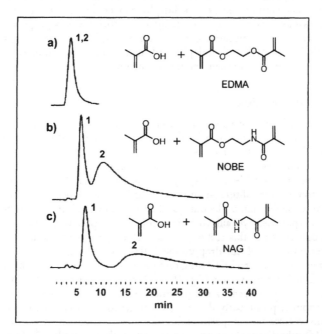

Scheme 1. Chemical structure of templates and monomers described in chapter.

Figure 9. Elution profiles of racemic dansyl-phenylalanine (3) on columns packed with MIPs prepared using the indicated monomer combinations. Mobile phase: Acetonitrile/acetic acid: 99/1 (v/v). Reproduced with permission from the American Chemical Society.

with acetonitrile as porogen. Based on chromatographic assessment of the recognition properties of the materials the new monomers showed very promising results. Whereas the conventional EDMA based material was unable to resolve the template racemate, near base line or base line resolutions of the racemates were achieved with the new monomers NOBE and NAG, respectively. A probable reason for the improved enantioselectivity is participation of the amide group of NOBE in hydrogen bonding interactions with the template. This is also supported by the previous finding that acrylamide is superior to MAA as functional monomer for the imprinting of carboxylic acids. The increased conformational rigidity of amide based crosslinkers may constitute an additional contributing factor to the improved properties.

The further improvements obtained using the crosslinker NAG is more difficult to explain. Based on a series of careful control experiments it was concluded that cooperative interactions involving the functional groups of the monomer is an important factor. Possibly, the close proximity of donor-acceptor interactions in a 1,3 disposition is capable of engaging in chelating interactions with the template. This would lead to additional binding interactions which would cause the selectivity and affinity to increase.

The above results show that small variations of the well established imprinting procedure can bring pronounced improvements of the molecular recognition properties of the materials.

MICSPs in Other Formats: Beads, Monoliths and Films

Previous techniques to prepare MIPs commonly led to materials exhibiting high affinity and selectivity, but low capacity and poor accessibility for the target molecule or molecules to the imprinted site. This leads to long response times when the materials are assessed as recognition elements in chemical sensors and broad, asymetric peaks when they are assessed as stationary phases in the chromatographic mode. Moreover, the MIPs are obtained as monoliths and useful particles can only be obtained after crushing and sieving cycles leading to a large loss of material. As a consequence, these materials are assessed mainly as molecular recognition elements for analytical quantifications, e.g., solid-phase extraction, in formats which are not dependent on high sample load capacity, chromatographic efficiency or large quantities of material.

In order to advance into preparative scale applications, high efficiency separations or fast sensing or catalysis, new MIP morphologies and manufacturing techniques showing promising improvements have recently been developed, the most recent being highlighted below.

Beads and Nanoparticles

MIPs in the bead format have previously been prepared through suspension polymerisation techniques,[40-43] core-shell emulsion polymerisation[44] or dispersion/precipitation polymerization techniques.[45-47] Much effort have been devoted to the development of a multi-step swelling polymerization technique using water as suspension medium.[48] This has resulted in polymers showing similar selectivities but slightly improved mass transfer characteristics compared with the corresponding monolithic polymers. Of particular relevance for bioanalytical applications was the functionalization of the outer surface of a polymer imprinted with (S)-naproxen with a hydrophilic polymer layer allowing direct injection of plasma samples on the columns.[43] More recent applications of this technique has yielded promising stationary phases for the separation of enantiomers of dihydropyridine (DHP) based drugs. In order to develop imprinted polymers for the achiral DHP drug nifedipine we recently screened a monomer library containing 14 functional monomers (Fig. 10).[32] Among the corresponding MIPs the highest imprinting factor was displayed by the polymer prepared using 4-vinylpyridine (4-VPy) as functional monomer, presumably due to a combination of weak hydrogen bonding and π-stacking. This was also the composition found to offer the highest enantioselectivities in the imprinting of (S)-nilvadipine (4) using the two step swelling procedure.[49] After optimization, baseline separation was achieved with column efficiencies comparable to commercially available CSPs.

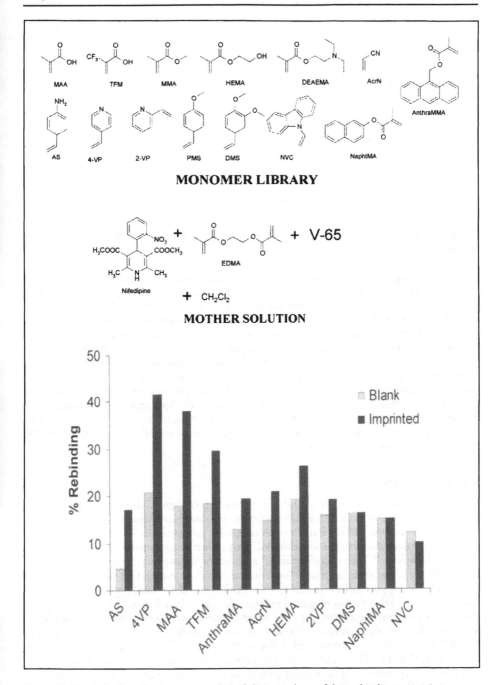

Figure 10. Search for functional monomers for nifedipine and test of their rebinding properties.

Nano- and micron-sized particles can be obtained by precipitation polymerization: essentially a stabilizer free dispersion polymerization under high dilution conditions.[45-47] This has the advantage over traditional suspension or emulsion polymerization in that it takes place in

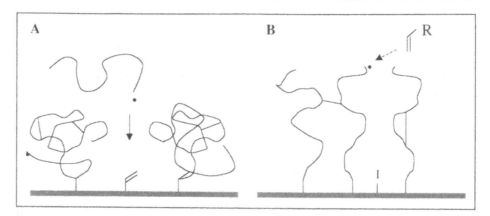

Figure 11. Schematic drawing showing the "grafting to" and "grafting from" approaches to graft polymers to supports.

the organic porogenic solvent system obviating the need for water to form the droplets. Thus in the context of molecular imprinting it is potentially a more general approach to form imprinted sites. Nevertheless, careful optimization is needed to achieve the desired particle size and dispersity. Several groups have however reported that spherical monodisperse particles can be obtained quickly, cleanly and in good yield.[46,47] These have found particular use as pseudostationary phases in capillary electrophoresis for enantiomer separations by the partial filling technique.[50,51] De Boer et al used 100-200 nm poly(MAA-co-TRIM) microspheres imprinted with (+)-ephedrine for the baseline resolution of racemic ephedrine with a 10 minute run time. Considerably shorter run times (< 2 min) was achieved by Schweitz et al in the resolution of racemic propranolol.[51] The capillary filling technique appears promising since it by passes the need for capillary packings and facilitates tuning of stationary phase selectivity. For instance packings imprinted with different targets can be mixed and thereby extend the range of racemates resolved in each run.

Layers and Films

Unfortunately, the conditions needed to generate sites of high affinity are often incompatible with the conditions needed to obtain the desired polymer morphologies. Therefore tedious trial and error is often needed to arrive at an acceptable compromise. These problems can be overcome by grafting techniques where the MIPs are grown on preformed support materials of known morphology.[52-58] The "grafting from" approach appears particularly promising in this regard (Fig. 11). This relies on immobilized radical initiators leading to chain growth mainly confined to the support surface. In this way the thickness of the grafted polymer can be better controlled and a higher density of grafted polymer chains can be achieved.[57] By producing thin grafted films we anticipated that the mass transfer problems associated with the majority of MIPs would be largely overcome.[58] These anticipated benefits we demonstrated by grafting poly(MAA-co-EDMA) imprinted with L-PA on the surface of silica supports modified with azoinitiators (Fig. 12). The materials could be prepared in a short time (1-2 hours) and exhibited dramatically superior mass transfer properties when compared to previously described monolith MIPs in liquid chromatography. Thus, 10nm pore size silica containing ultrathin grafted films ($\approx$ 1nm) exhibited the highest chromatographic efficiency with theoretical plate numbers (N) of ca 24000/m for the nonimprinted enantiomer (Fig. 13). This shows that the intrinsic efficiency of these phases is acceptable and comparable to conventional columns. Unfortunately, the peak width of the retained enantiomer is still broad, presumably mainly due to the heterogenous binding site distribution discussed above. Nevertheless, given that the

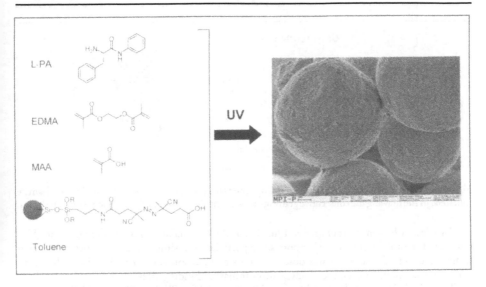

Figure 12. Procedure used to graft L-PA imprinted films onto the surface of silica supports and a SEM of a modified silica particle (Si100 with an average pore diameter of 10nm).

retention order can be easily programmed, the sharp band of one of the enantiomers should prove useful for analytical quantifications of enantiomeric excesses (in this context it should be mentioned that a rapid batch based technique to measure enantiomeric excesses using MIPs was recently proposed by Chen and Shimizu.[59]

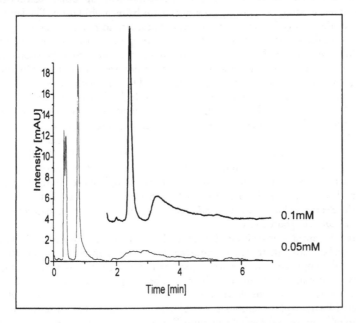

Figure 13. Elution profiles of D,L-PA injected on columns (33x4mm) packed with composite particles. These were composed of monodisperse silica particles (10nm average pore diameter) modified with a L-PA imprinted polymer film with an average thickness of 0.8nm. The mobile phase was in this case ACN/sodium acetate buffer, 0.01M, pH 4.8: 70/30 (v/v). The injeced amount of racemate has been indicated.

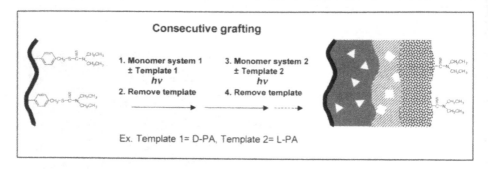

Figure 14. Principle of layer by layer grafting of imprinted layers on surfaces modified with dithiocarbamate iniferters. In the drawing the consecutive grafting of layers imprinted with optical antipodes of PA is shown.

Particles with even thinner grafted films (<1nm) were unable to resolve the racemate. This contrasted with the results for wide pore silica particles with similar graft densities but thicker films, were indeed resolution was observed. This comparison is informative about the minimum matrix volume needed to produce discriminating binding sites.

The composites were also suitable as packing material for CEC capillaries.[60,61] These exhibited enantioselectivies comparable with that showed in LC, high efficiencies, short analysis times (< 3min) and good reproducibility.

One problem with using immobilized symmetric azoinitiators is that decomposition leads to one soluble mobile initiating radical in addition to the desired immobilized intiating radical. This leads to premature gelation and precludes reuse of the rest unreacated monomers. In order to overcome this problem, initiators producing stable free radicals can be used. In this case only one of the radicals is capable of initiating polymerization, with the other radical being stable, but capable of terminating the growing polymer chains by recombination. The latter polymerization may exhibit living properties in the sense that a second polymer can be grafted to the first. Recently we showed that functional imprinted composite materials could be prepared by grafting of MIPs onto benzyl-N,N-diethyldithiocarbamate iniferter modified porous silica supports (Fig. 14).[62] The living properties of the latter system was demonstrated by the consecutive grafting of two polymer layers imprinted with two different enantiomers of the template or one imprinted and one nonimprinted layer in any order.[63] The success of the grafting was reflected in the separation of the two enantiomers obtained using the composite materials as chromatographic stationary phases. Table 7 lists the chromatographic properties of the materials after grafting of one or two layers of imprinted or non-imprinted layers. Materials containing an initial grafted layer of ca. 16nm prepared in presence of D-PA (P-D) exhibited pronounced D-selectivity. The living properties of the iniferter were then assessed by grafting of a second layer targeted towards the optical antipode of the template used in the first layer. Thus, grafting of an L-PA imprinted layer on the D-PA imprinted layer (P-DL1) resulted in reversal of the enantioselectivity. This shows that different molecular recognition features can be introduced in consecutively grafted layers.

MIP based chemical sensors is another area where enantioselective MIPs in layer or thin film format are becoming increasingly important (see other chapters of this book). The main problems with this application are the slow responses and poor sensitivities for the target analyte. Nevertheless, pronounced enantioselectivities have been reported for MIPs prepared as casted films on the surface of the sensor, commonly a quartz crystal microbalance (QCM). High enantioselectivities (ratio of the responses of ca 5) have been observed in the sensing of L-serine,[64] (S)-propranolol[65] and dansyl-L-phenylalanine.[66] Although the selectivity is high it should be noted that binding often is quite weak.

Mass transfer may be overcome by applying thin film grafting techniques and sensitivity by coupling the molecular recognition elements to a sufficiently sensitive signal transducer. Ul-

Table 7. Synthesis conditions and chromatographic characterisation of consecutively imprinted composite materials used as HPLC chiral stationary phases

Layer 1	Layer 2	Average Layer Thickness d (nm) Total	Layer 1	Layer 2	k'_L	k'_D	$\alpha\ (=k'_L/k'_D)$
L-PA	–	18	18	–	5.5	3.6	1.50
L-PA	D-PA	33	18	15	6.1	9.0	0.67
NIP	–	17	17	–	2.4	2.4	1.00
L-PA	NIP	31	12	19	6.5	3.2	2.03
NIP	L-PA	39	17	22	140	26	5.45

trathin films of metal oxides was used by Kunitake et al to produce such thin films exhibiting fast response and very high selectivity.[67] Based on thin films of the common matrix component, TiO_2, imprinting of a variety of Lewis basic chiral templates capable of coordination with Ti have been demonstrated. The films can be coated on metal or metal oxide substrates for use as sensing elements for QCM- or ISFET-based readings. Other reports confirm that sol gel films exhibit very promising features in terms of response times, selectivity and sensitivity, compared to organic polymer based coatings.[68]

Superporous Monoliths

Due to the absence of universal methods to produce MIPs in the shape of beads or to control their porous properties, in situ preparation techniques would be very attractive.[69] For instance, if the synthesis conditions could be chosen to create macropores in the monoliths, allowing convective mobile phase transport, they could be directly applied in the many chromatographic modes already demonstrated for MIPs. The in situ polymerized organic separation media introduced by Svec and Fréchet[70] acted as a catalyst for this work and the first in situ prepared MIPs appeared soon thereafter.[45,71,72] These relied on the use of mixtures of good and poor solvents to generate the flow-through pores. Due to the unsuitable porogen they exhibited much poorer enantioselectivities compared to the conventional crushed monoliths. However, for more strongly associating monomer-template systems, a higher selectivity was observed. This was the case in the imprinting of the bis-benzamidine pentamidine (PAM), that form strong complexes with MAA through hydrogen bonded ion pairs.[45]

As discussed in the previous paragraph, the use of aprotic less polar porogens may overcome the destabilizing effect on the monomer-template interactions typical of the polar porogen systems. This was demonstrated simultaneously by Nilsson[73] and Lin[74] with the aim at developing new chiral stationary phases for CEC. Schweitz et al used toluene[73] or isooctane/toluene mixtures[75] to achieve the convective pore system. Recently, a slightly modified approach has led to the first successful demonstration of imprinted flow through monoliths for liquid chromatographic enantiomer separations.[76] Thus, Huang et al observed that small amounts of toluene in dodecanol produced superporous packings exhibiting high enantioselectivities (Table 8). The complexity in finding suitable conditions for achieving flow through properties simultaneous to enantioselectivity appears clearly from the sensitive dependence of the separation factor and back pressure on the content of toluene in the porogenic mixture.

Hierarchical Imprinting Techniques

Another way to decouple the binding site from the pore formation process is to immobilize the template on the surface of porous, disposable solids that act as molds to create a desired porosity (Fig. 15).[77-79] In this way, the pore system is controlled by the solid mold regardless of the conditions applied to generate the imprinted sites. In addition, the imprinted sites are

Table 8. *Optimization of porogenic mixture in the synthesis of superporous monolithic stationary phases for chromatography*

Toluene Content in Porogen (% v)	Separation Factor (α)	Resolution Factor (R$_s$)	Surface Area (m²/g)	Pore Diameter (nm)
0	1.00	0.00	37	3213
5	1.66	0.70	45	1680
10	2.36	1.67	111	1081

The polymers were prepared using FMOC-L-tryptophan as template and a monomer mixture consisting of EDMA (90% v) and 4-vinylpyridine (10% v). The porogenicmixture was dodecanol containing the amounts of toluene indicated. The mobile phase was acetonitrile containing acetic acid (0.1%).

confined to the pore wall surface of the resulting material. So far the feasibility of this approach has been demonstrated in the imprinting of small molecules, i.e., nucleotide bases and small drugs. Recently, the benefits of confining the sites to the pore wall surface we demonstrated by using crude peptide solid phase synthesis products as epitope templates for the separation of larger peptides (Fig. 15).[79] The enantioselectivities observed using immobilized aminoacid derivatives were in general poorer than those observed using the template in soluble form. The latter approach was used by Yilmaz et al to produce spherical packing materials for the separation of the enantiomers of isoproterenol.[80] The procedure is attractive in view of the high yield of useful particles and the absence of water as common for the suspension or emulsion polymerization protocols.

Other Matrices for Imprinting of Enantiomers

Earlier in this chapter new imprinted material architectures have been described that exhibit superior mass transfer properties and saturation capacities. However, the heterogenous distribution of binding sites appears to be a more difficult problem to overcome. Hardly avoidable, the kinetically controlled formation of the polymer network leads to a statistical distribution of binding site microenvironments. One way to overcome this problem is to use polymer matrices formed by thermodynamically controlled polymerization reactions. This approach was suggested by Steinke et al who used ring opening methathesis polymerization (ROMP) to form networks under thermodynamic control in presence of a template.[81] The template (L-menthol) was linked via a sacrificial spacer to a monomer (Fig. 16). After polymerization the template and spacer were removed offering a binding site allowing the template to bind via noncovalent interactions. Although no evidence for reduced polyclonality was presented, the

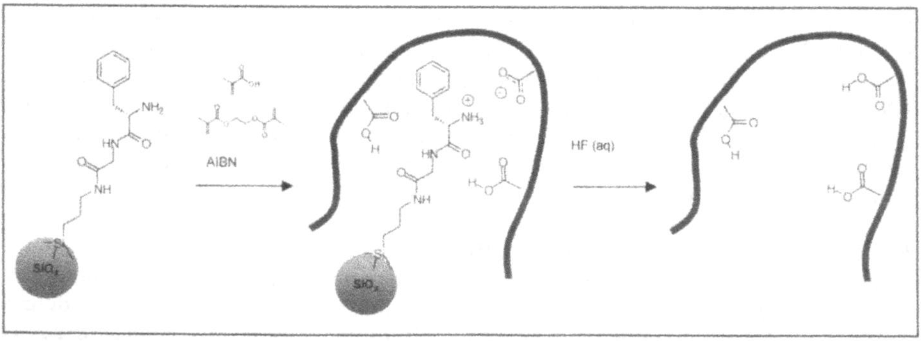

Figure 15. Principle of hierarchical imprinting using solid phase peptide synthesis products as templates.

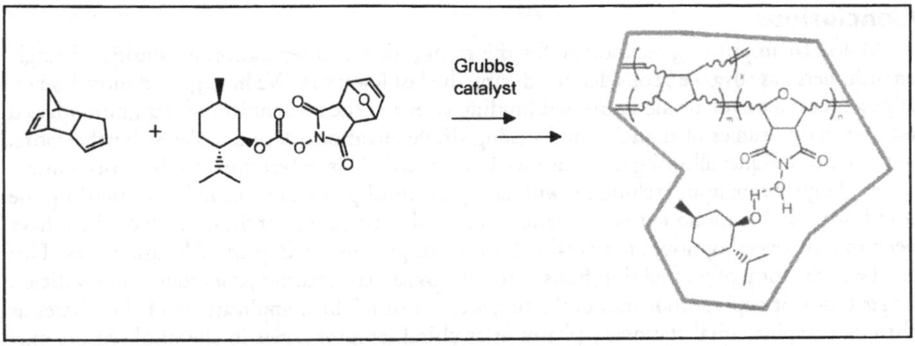

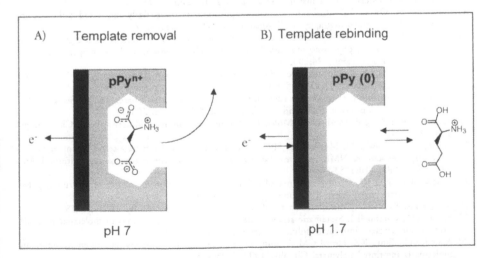

Figure 16. Synthesis of MIP ROMP using L-menthol as covalently linked template.

imprinted polymer recognized the correct enantiomer with high enantioselectivity (separation factor =2.1 obtained in batch experiments by equilibration of a ca 5mM solution of D,L-menthol in hexane/chloroform (1:1, v/v). Given that the template interacts with just one defined hydrogen bond, the results appear particularly promising.

Enantioselective imprinted polymers functioning in bulk water was achieved by Komiyama et al using polymerizable derivatives of cyclodextrins (5).[82] These were polymerized in presence of either the D- or the L- enantiomer of the dipeptide Phe-Phe in bulk water. Although cyclodextrin is a chiral selector per se, imprinting considerably enhanced the selectivity from a separation factor of 1.3 to a separation factor of 2.3 upon imprinting.

One approach which may have implications for design of enantioselective sensors is to imprint templates acting as dopants of conducting polymers. Thus, Nagaoka et al deposited a polypyrrole film on a quartz crystal in presence of L-glutamic acid acting as template (dopant) (Fig. 17).[83] Subsequent removal of the template from the polypyrrole film by overoxidation led to a film exhibiting very high enantioselectivities (uptake ratio, L/D=10) for the template enantiomer and negligable uptake of related amino acids (e.g., aspartic acid). Although the molecuar level origin of the successful imprinting remains largely unknown, the approach appears promising.

Figure 17. Model depicting the enantioselective uptake of glutamic acid (Glu) into an overoxidized polypyrrole. A) dedoping of Glu by overoxidation, and B) selective uptake of Glu upon charging/discharging the film.

Conclusions

Molecular imprinting technology for the recognition and separation or sensing of single enantiomers has advanced considerably during the last few years. We have gained more knowledge about the nature of the imprinted binding sites and the mechanism of recognition based on systematic studies of model systems using single enantiomers as templates. Furthermore, tools and techniques allowing new improved imprinted CSPs to be developed have been introduced. High throughput techniques with computational predictions promise to speed up the search for suitable monomer combinations and polymerization conditions. Once these have been found, several options are available for how to present the imprinted binding sites. This can be in the form of grafted thin films with improved mass transfer properties, nanoparticles, larger beads or superporous monoliths prepared in situ. Thus, applications of the phases as chromatographic chiral stationary phases or as chiral receptor layers in chemical sensors may soon become a reality.

References

1. McCague R, Casy G. Synthetic methods for enantiomers of drugs. In: Ellis GP, Luscombe DK, eds. Progress in Medicinal Chemistry. Vol. 34. Amsterdam: Elsevier, 1997.
2. Franco P, Minguilon C. Techniques in preparative chiral separations. In: Subramanian G, ed. Chiral Separation Techniques. 2nd Ed. Weinheim: Wiley-VCH, 2001.
3. Sellergren B, Ekberg B, Albertsson P et al. Preparative chiral separations in an aqueous two-phase system by a few counter-current extractions. J Chromatogr 1988; 450:277-280.
4. Armstrong DW, Menges R, Wainer I. Use of centrifugal partition chromatography and proteins in the preparative separation of amino acid enantiomers. J Liq Chromatogr 1990; 13:3571-3581.
5. Cao G, Garcia ME, Alcalt M et al. Chiral molecular recognition in intercalated zirconium phosphate. J Am Chem Soc 1992; 114:7574-7575.
6. Yoshikawa M. Optical resolution with molecularly imprinted polymeric membranes. Maku 2000; 25:280-282.
7. Armstrong DW, Schneiderheinze JM, Hwang YS et al. Bubble fractionation of enantiomers from solution using molecularly imprinted polymers as collectors. Anal Chem 1998; 70:3717-3719.
8. Miller L, Orihuela C, Fronek R et al. Chromatographic resolution of the enantiomers of a pharmaceutical intermediate from the milligram to the kilogram scale. J Chromatogr 1999; 849:309-317.
9. Sellergren B. Imprinted chiral stationary phases in high performance liquid chromatography. J Chromatogr A 2001; 906:227-252.
10. Schweitz L, Nilsson S. Capillary electrochromatography based on molecular imprinting. In: Sellergren B, ed. Molecularly Imprinted Polymers. Man-Made Mimics of Antibodies and Their Applications in Analytical Chemistry. Tech Instrum Anal Chem 2001; 23:377-393.
11. Ellwanger A, Owens PK, Karlsson L et al. Application of molecularly imprinted polymers in supercritical fluid chromatography. J Chromatogr A 2000; 897:317-327.
12. Suedee R, Saelim J, Thavornpibulbut T et al. Chiral determination of various adrenergic drugs by thin-layer chromatography using molecularly imprinted chiral stationary phases prepared with alpha-agonists. Analyst 1999; 124:1003-1009.
13. Adbo K, Nicholls IA. Enantioselective solid-phase extraction using Troger's base imprinted polymers. Anal Chim Acta 2001; 435:115-120.
14. Sellergren B. Enantiomer separations using designed imprinted chiral phases. In: Subramanian G, ed. Chiral Separation Techniques. 2nd Ed. Weinheim: Wiley-VCH, 2001.
15. Sellergren B, Ekberg B, Mosbach K. Molecular imprinting of amino acid derivatives. J Chromatogr 1985; 347:1-10.
16. Sellergren B, Lepistoe M, Mosbach K. Highly enantioselective and substrate-selective polymers obtained by interactions. NMR and chromatographic studies on the nature of recognition. J Am Chem Soc 1988; 110:5853-5860.
17. Sellergren B, Shea KJ. On the influence of polymer morphology on the ability of imprinted polymers to separate enantiomers. J Chromatogr 1993; 635:31.
18. Snyder LR, Kirkland JJ. Introduction to Modern Liquid Chromatography. Wiley, 1979.
19. Spivak DA, Campbell J. Systematic study of steric and spatial contributions to molecular recognition by non-covalent imprinted polymers. Analyst 2001; 126:793-797.
20. Allender CJ, Brain KR, Heard CM. Binding cross-reactivity of Boc-phenylalanine enantiomers on molecularly imprinted polymers. Chirality 1997; 9:233-237.

21. Bouman MAE, Allender CJ, Brain KR et al. A high-throughput screening technique employing molecularly imprinted polymers as biomimetic selectors. Methodol Surv Bioanal Drugs 1998; 25:37-43.
22. Ramstrom O, Ye L, Mosbach K. Screening of a combinatorial steroid library using molecularly imprinted polymers. Anal Commun 1998; 35:9-11.
23. Hart BR, Rush DJ, Shea KJ. Discrimination between enantiomers of structurally related molecules: Separation of benzodiazepines by molecularly imprinted polymers. J Am Chem Soc 2000; 122:460-465.
24. Yu Y, Ye L, Haupt K et al. Formation of a class of enzyme inhibitors (drugs), including a chiral compound, by using imprinted polymers or biomolecules as molecular-scale reaction vessels. Angew Chem 2002; 114:4640-4643.
25. Katti AM, Diack M, El Fallah MZ et al. Prediction of high concentration band profiles in liquid chromatography. Acc Chem Res 1992; 25:366-374.
26. Sajonz P, Kele M, Zhong G et al. Study of the thrmodynamics and mass transfer kinetics of two enantiomers on a polymeric imprinted stationary phase. J Chromatogr 1998; 810:1-17.
27. Chen Y, Kele M, Sajonz P et al. Influence of thermal annealing on the thermodynamic and mass-transfer kinetic properties of D- and L-phenylalanine anilide on imprinted polymeric stationary phases. Anal Chem 1999; 71:928-938.
28. Chen Y, Kele M, Quinones I et al. Influence of the pH on the behavior of an imprinted polymeric stationary phase—Supporting evidence for a binding site model. J Chromatogr 2001; 927:1-17.
29. Stanley BJ, Szabelski P, Chen YB et al. Affinity distributions of a molecularly imprinted polymer calculated numerically by the expectation-maximization method. Langmuir 2003; 19.
30. Lanza F, Sellergren B. Method for synthesis and screening of large groups of molecularly imprinted polymers. Anal Chem 1999; 71:2092-2096.
31. Takeuchi T, Fukuma D, Matsui J. Combinatorial molecular imprinting: An approach to synthetic polymer receptors. Anal Chem 1999; 71:285-290.
32. Lanza F, Hall AJ, Sellergren B et al. Development of a semiautomated procedure for the synthesis and of molecularly imprinted polymers applied to the search for functional monomers for phenytoin and nifedipine. Anal Chim Acta 2001; 435:91-106.
33. Piletsky SA, Karim K, Piletska EV et al. Recognition of ephedrine enantiomers by molecularly imprinted polymers designed using a computational approach. Analyst 2001; 126:1826-1830.
34. LŸbke C, LŸbke M, Whitcombe MJ et al. Imprinted polymers prepared with stoichiometric template-monomer complexes: Efficient binding of ampicillin from aqueous solutions. Macromolecules 2000; 33:5098-5105.
35. Quaglia M, Chenon K, Hall AJ et al. Target analogue imprinted polymers with affinity for folic acid and related compounds. J Am Chem Soc 2001; 123:2146-2154.
36. Hall AJ, Manesiotis P, Mossing JT et al. Molecularly imprinted polymers (MIPs) against uracils: Functional monomer design, monomer-template interactions in solution and MIP performance in chromatography. Mat Res Soc Symp Proc 2002; 723:M1.3.1-5.
37. Wulff G, Gross T, Schönfeld R. Enzyme models based on molecularly imprinted polymers with strong esterase activity. Angew Chem Int Ed Engl 1997; 36:1962-9164.
38. Sibrian-Vazquez M, Spivak DA. Enhanced enantioselectivity of molecularly imprinted polymers formulated with novel crosslinking monomers. Macromolecules 2003; 36:5105-5113.
39. Hart BR, Rush DJ, Shea KJ. Synthetic peptide receptors: Molecularly imprinted polymers for the recognition of peptides using peptide-metal interactions. J Am Chem Soc 2000; 122:460-465.
40. Mayes AG, Mosbach K. Molecularly imprinted polymer beads. Anal Chem 1996; 68:3769-3774.
41. Matsui J, Okada M, Tsuruoka M et al. Solid-phase extraction of a triazine herbicide using a molecularly imprinted polymer. Anal Commun 1997; 34:85-87.
42. Strikovsky AG, Kasper D, Gruen M et al. Catalytic molecularly imprinted polymers conventional bulk polymerization or suspension polymerization: Hydrolysis of diphenyl carbonate and diphenyl carbamate. J Am Chem Soc 2000; 122:6295-6296.
43. Haginaka J, Sanbe H. Uniform-sized molecularly imprinted polymers for 2-arylpropionic acid derivatives selectively modified with external layer and their applications to direct serum injection. Anal Chem 2000; 72:5206-5210.
44. Perez N, Whitcombe MJ, Vulfson EN. Molecularly imprinted nanoparticles prepared by core-shell emulsion polymerization. J Appl Polym Sci 2000; 77:1851-1859.
45. Sellergren B. Imprinted dispersion polymers: A new class of easily accessible affinity stationary phases. J Chromatogr A 1994; 673:133-141.
46. Lei Y, Cormack PAG, Mosbach K. Molecularly imprinted monodisperse microspheres for competitive radioassay. Anal Commun 1999; 36:35-38.

47. Ye L, Weiss R, Mosbach K. Synthesis and characterization of molecularly imprinted microspheres. Macromolecules 2000; 33:8239-8245.
48. Haginaka J, Takehira H, Hosoya K et al. Uniform-sized molecularly imprinted polymer for (S)-naproxen selectively modified with hydrophilic external layer. J Chromatogr 1999; 849:331-339.
49. Fu Q, Sanbe H, Kagawa C et al. Uniformly sized molecularly imprinted polymer for (S)-nilvadipine. Comparison of chiral recognition ability with HPLC chiral stationary phases based on a protein. Analytical Chemistry 2003; 75.
50. de Boer T, Mol R, de Zeeuw RA et al. Spherical molecularly imprinted polymer particles: A promising tool for molecular recognition in capillary elektrokinetic separations. Electrophoresis 2002; 23:1296-1300.
51. Schweitz L, Spegel P, Nilsson S. Molecularly imprinted microparticles for capillary electrochromatographic enantiomer separation of propranolol. Analyst 2000; 125:1899-1901.
52. Wulff G, Oberkobusch D, Minarik M. Enzyme-analog built polymers, 18. Chiral cavities in polymer layers coated on wide-pore silica. React Polym Ion Exch Sorbents 1985; 3:261-275.
53. Glad M, Reinholdsson P, Mosbach K. Molecularly imprinted composite polymers based on trimethylolpropanetrimethacrylate. React Polym 1995; 25:47-54.
54. Arnold FH, Plunkett S, Dhal PK et al. Surface modification with molecularly—Imprinted polymers for selective recognition. Polym Prepr 1995; 36:97-98.
55. Joshi VP, Karode SK, Kulkarni MG et al. Novel separation strategies based on molecularly imprinted adsorbents. Chem Engn Sci 1998; 53:2271-2284.
56. Piletsky SA, Matuschewski H, Schedler U et al. Surface functionalization of porous polypropylene membranes with molecularly imprinted polymers by photograft copolymerization in water. Macromolecules 2000; 33:3092-3098.
57. Prucker O, RŸhe J. Mechanism of radical chain polymerization initiated by azo compounds covalently bound tothe surface of spherical particles. Macromolecules 1998; 31:602-613.
58. Sulitzky C, RŸckert B, Hall AJ et al. Grafting of molecularly imprinted polymer films on silica supports containing surface-bound free radical initiators. Macromolecules 2002; 35:79-91.
59. Chen Y, Shimizu KD. Measurment of enantiomeric excess using molecularly imprinted polymers. Org Lett 2002; 4:2937-2940.
60. Quaglia M, De Lorenzi E, Sulitzky C et al. Surface initiated molecularly imprinted polymer films: A new approach in chiral capillary electrochromatography. Analyst 2001; 126:1495-1498.
61. Quaglia M, De Lorenzi E, Sulitzky C et al. Molecularly imprinted polymer films grafted from porous or nonporous silica: Novel affinity stationary phases in capillary electrochromatography. Electrophoresis. Electrophoresis 2003; 24:952-957.
62. RŸckert B, Hall AJ, Sellergren B. Molecularly imprinted composite materials via iniferter modified supports. J Mat Chem 2002; 12:2275-2280.
63. Sellergren B, RŸckert B, Hall AJ. Layer by layer grafting of molecularly imprinted polymers via iniferter modified supports. Adv Mat 2002; 14:1204.
64. Stanley S, Percival CJ, Morel T et al. Enantioselective detection of L-serine. Chemical 2003; B89:103-106.
65. Haupt K, Noworyta K, Kutner W. Imprinted polymer-based enantioselective acoustic sensor using a quartz crystal microbalance. Anal Commun 1999; 36:391-393.
66. Cao L, Li SFY, Zhou XC. Enantioselective sensor based on microgravimetric quartz crystal microbalance with molecularly imprinted polymer film. Analyst 2001; 126:184-188.
67. Lee S-W, Ichinose I, Kunitake T. Molecular imprinting of protected amino acids in ultrathin multilayers of TiO2 gel. Chem Lett 1998:1193-1194.
68. Marx S, Liron Z. Molecular imprinting in thin films of organic-inorganic hybrid sol-gel and acrylic polymers. Chem Mater 2001; 13:3624-3630.
69. Sellergren B. Imprinted monoliths. In: Svec F, ed. Monolithic Materials: Preparation, Properties and Applications. Amsterdam: Elsevier Science, 2003.
70. Svec F, Fr chet JMJ. Monolithic columns. Anal Chem 1992; 64:820.
71. Matsui J, Kato T, Takeuchi T et al. Molecular recognition in continuous polymer rods prepared by molecular imprinting. Anal Chem 1993; 65:2223-2224.
72. Sellergren B. Direct drug determination by selective sample enrichment on an imprinted polymer. Anal Chem 1994; 66:1578.
73. Schweitz L, Andersson LI, Nilsson S. Capillary electrochromatography with predetermined selectivity obtained through molecular imprinting. Anal Chem 1997; 69:1179-1183.
74. Lin J-M, Nakagama T, Uchiyama K et al. Enantioseparation of D,L-phenylalanine by molecularly electrochromatography. J Liq Chromatogr Relat Technol 1997; 20:1489-1506.
75. Schweitz L, Andersson LI, Nilsson S. Capillary electrochromatography with molecular imprint-based selectivity for enantiomer separation of local anesthetics. J Chromatogr 1997; 792:401-409.

76. Huang X, Zou H, Chen X et al. Molecularly imprinted monolithic stationary phases for liquid chromatographic separation of enantiomers and diastereomers. J Chromatogr 2003; 984:273-282.
77. Yilmaz E, Haupt K, Mosbach K. The use of immobilized templates—A new approach in molecular imprinting. Angew Chem Int Ed 2000; 39:2115-2118.
78. Titirici MM, Hall AJ, Sellergren B. Hierarchical imprinting using crude peptide solid phase synthesis products as templates. Chem Mat 2003; 15:822-824.
79. Titirici MM, Hall AH, Sellergren B. Hierarchically imprinted stationary phases: Mesoporous polymer beads containing surface-confined binding sites for adenine. Chem Mater 2002; 14:21-23.
80. Yilmaz E, Ramstr m O, Möller P et al. A facile method for preparing molecularly imprinted polymer spheres using spherical silica templates. J Mat Chem 2002; 12:1577-1581.
81. Patel A, Fouace S, Steinke JHG. Enantioselective molecularly imprinted polymers via ring-opening metathesis polymerisation. Chemical Communications 2003:88-89.
82. Asanuma H, Akiyama T, Kajiya K et al. Molecular imprinting of cyclodextrin in water for the recognition of nanometer-scaled guests. Anal Chim Acta 2001; 435:25-33.
83. Deore B, Chen Z, Nagaoka T. Potential-induced enantioselective uptake of amino acid into molecularly imprinted overoxidized polypyrrole. Anal Chem 2000; 72:3989-3994.

CHAPTER 9

MIP Catalysts:
From Theory to Practice

Michael J. Whitcombe

Abstract

The principles of the design of transition state analogues are discussed, illustrated with examples taken from the literature on catalytic antibodies. In the following discussion a number of imprinted polymer catalyst systems are described, including those catalyzing elimination reactions, hydrolyses and carbon-carbon bond formation, with particular emphasis on the template in each case and how it relates to the transition state for the reaction studied. Finally the use of imprints as sites for carrying out chemical transformations with some control over the regiochemistry and/or stereochemistry of the reaction is described.

Introduction

The purpose of this chapter is to describe how one might approach the design of an imprinted polymer catalyst and will be illustrated with examples from the literature. In addition, related systems for carrying out specific chemical transformations within the imprinted site, not necessarily in a catalytic manner, will be described.

From the earliest attempts at imprinting templates in synthetic polymers, a principal aim has been to mimic the exquisite selectivity and stereospecificity of the binding domains of enzymes, antibodies and biological receptors. One of the guiding motivations in understanding how to construct artificial binding systems has been the possibility of harnessing the power of biomimetic catalysis to create new and useful artificial enzymes. The complexity of this task can be considerably simplified if some of the elements of the active site can be optimally positioned by self-assembly, which is inherent in the imprinting method, hence molecular imprinting is seen as one of the more promising methods of creating artificial catalysts. Add to that the fact that MIPs are robust plastic materials, able to withstand harsh treatments that proteins never would,[1] and one can see that the potential applications of MIP catalysts are only limited by the imagination.

Transition State Theory

There are many aspects to the design of catalytic sites, functional group identity and placement being only one, but seeing as this is what imprinting does best, how to design a template to take advantage of this strength is of great importance. In order to understand what the template has to do, we need to consider transition state theory.

Any reaction that occurs spontaneously (has a negative free energy) may still proceed at an imperceptible rate if the activation energy for reaction ($\Delta G^{\ddagger}_{uncat}$) is too high to be acquired through the normal distribution of thermal energies. For bimolecular reactions the situation is even worse, as collisions between reactants not only need to be sufficient energetic, but if the orientation of the molecules is not appropriate, no reaction will take place. The highest point

Molecular Imprinting of Polymers, edited by Sergey Piletsky and Anthony Turner.
©2006 Landes Bioscience.

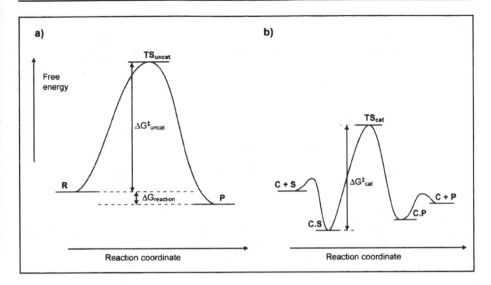

Figure 1. Reaction coordinate diagram for: a) uncatalyzed reaction. Reactant (R), is converted to product (P) via the high energy transition state (TS_{uncat}); b) The same reaction catalyzed by an enzyme-like species (C), capable of stabilizing the transition state (TS_{cat}) for the reaction leading from substrate (S) to product (P). The activation energy for the overall process $\Delta G^{\ddagger}_{cat}$ is less than $\Delta G^{\ddagger}_{uncat}$, resulting in an acceleration in the reaction rate.

in the reaction coordinate diagram (Fig. 1) is known as the transition state (TS) and exists on a knife-edge between products and reactants: bonds are being made or broken, partial charges may be developing and unusual coordination numbers (e.g., pentavalent carbon) may exist in the TS. It should be emphasized that the TS is not an intermediate, it has no chemical identity of its own and cannot be observed spectroscopically or by any other means, its structure can only be inferred by, for example, kinetic isotope effects or perhaps by computer modeling. If the energy of the reacting system can be modified by complexation with a catalyst, such that the pathway from reactants to the new TS requires a lower activation energy ($\Delta G^{\ddagger}_{cat}$), the reaction will proceed at a faster rate. It follows therefore that if an imprinted polymer can be prepared that stabilizes the TS for a reaction, then that imprinted material may be effective in increasing the rate of reaction.

As has been stated above, the TS may possess a rather unusual geometry and/or charge distribution, and it certainly is not available to be used as a template, therefore the concept of a transition state analogue (TSA) has been introduced, which is a stable species that mimics the geometry and other aspects of the assumed TS for the reaction under study. This approach has been widely used in the generation of catalytic antibodies,[2-6] where low molecular weight TSAs conjugated to a protein carrier are used as the inoculum for the generation of a population of (polyclonal) antibodies which are then screened for the required catalytic activity. The same concept of a transition state analogue can equally be applied to the generation of imprinted sites, in MIPs and imprinted sol-gel materials, to generate catalytic activity. It should be noted however that there is a subtle difference between generating catalytic antibodies and making a catalytic MIP using the same TSA as a template: antibodies are always selected from a (albeit vast) pool of possible peptide sequences, constrained by the structure of the immunoglobulin molecule and the availability of 20 amino acid monomers. Catalytic MIPs on the other hand, have to be designed; the molecular imprinter has to make rational choices about which monomer(s), crosslinker, porogen etc. will lead to an effective catalyst. We cannot afford to consider 10^9 possible combinations, but have to use our ingenuity and we have a lot more than 20 possible monomers to choose from!

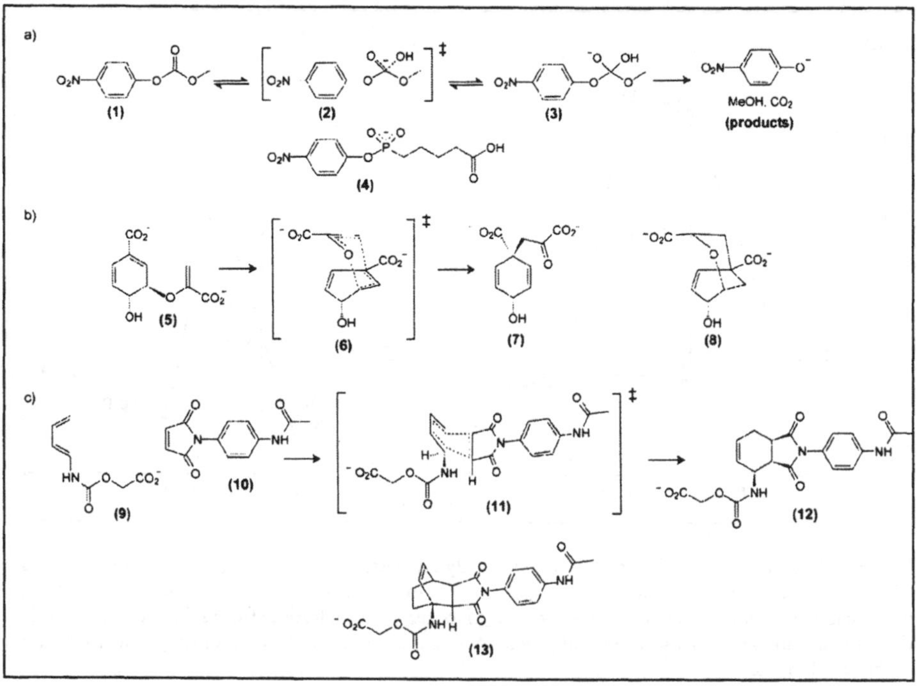

Figure 2. Some antibody catalyzed transformations, showing the relationship between the proposed transition states and the transitions state analogues (TSAs) used as haptens to raise the catalytic antibodies. a) Hydrolysis of a carbonate ester (1) via the transition state (2). The TSA (4) also resembles the tetrahedral intermediate (3). Adapted from reference 7. b) Claisen rearrangement of chorismate (5) to prephenate, (7), via (6) and the bicyclic TSA (8). Adapted from reference 8. c) Diels-Alder reaction of (9) and (10) proceeds via (11) to the product, (12). The TSA (13) mimics the unusual conformation of (11). Adapted from reference 9.

To understand how a TSA mimics the transition state of a reaction it will be necessary to consider some simple examples. Figure 2 depicts some transition states and the TSAs applied to the preparation of catalytic antibodies intended to catalyze the respective reactions.

In the first example (Fig. 2a) the hydrolysis of a carbonate ester (1) is considered. The tetrahedral transition state (2) assumes the nucleophilic attack of hydroxide ion, with a lessening bond order of the carbonyl group as a new bond between the carbonyl carbon and the attacking nucleophile is formed. The negative charge is also delocalized across the two oxygen atoms. This contrasts to the tetrahedral intermediate, (3) which is an observable species and has a fully developed charge on oxygen. The intermediate is unstable, either dissociating to products or reverting to starting material via the transition state. In order to mimic the structure and charge distribution in (2), the phosphonate salt (4) was used as the TSA in the raising of catalytic antibodies, with a reported rate acceleration of 810.[7]

The second example is of a unimolecular sigmatropic rearrangement, the Claisen rearrangement of chorismate (Fig. 2b). This reaction requires the reactant (5) to assume a conformation to allow orbital overlap and hence bond migration by a symmetry allowed process to occur. This gives rise to the "chair" form of the TS, (6) in which partial bond order exists throughout the transient ring structure, giving rise to the product, prephenate, (7). In this instance the TS can be mimicked by the stable fused ring compound (8), with a sigma bonded structure in place of the partially bonded TS structure. Antibody-catalyzed rate accelerations of up to 1×10^4 were seen when (8) was used as the hapten.[8]

The third example (Fig. 2c) is of a Diels-Alder reaction. In this case two reacting species (9) and (10) must be brought together in the correct orientation for reaction to occur. The transition state (11), which leads to (12), is mimicked by the fused ring adduct (13), which is itself a Diels-Alder adduct of (10) and the cyclohexadienyl analogue of (9). This strategy also gave rise to catalytically active antibodies.[9]

In all three cases above, the respective TSAs were seen to be potent inhibitors of the catalytic activity. This is expected behavior, and confirms that the antibodies raised were binding their respective haptens and that the binding domain is the site of catalysis. In addition the kinetics generally followed the Michaelis-Menten model, indicating that the catalysis was "enzyme-like" in nature. This is characterized by the following series of equations:

For a catalyzed reaction where, C is the catalyst, S is the substrate and P is the product:

$$C + S \rightleftharpoons C.S \rightleftharpoons C.P \rightleftharpoons C + P$$

$$\frac{d[P]}{dt} = -\frac{d[S]}{dt} = k_{cat}[C.S] = \frac{k_{cat}([C] + [C.S])}{1 + K_m/[S]} \qquad (1)$$

when [S] >> ([C] + [C.S]) and [S] << K_m

$$\frac{d[S]}{dt} = \frac{k_{cat}}{K_m}[S]([C] + [C.S]) \qquad (2)$$

The derived quantities k_{cat} and K_m are used to denote the efficiency of the catalytic process. K_m has the units of concentration, equivalent to a dissociation constant, and is a measure of how tightly the catalyst binds the substrate, k_{cat} is a measure of how rapidly the catalyzed reaction occurs. A further consequence of the enzyme-model is that saturation kinetics are seen—there are only a limited number of catalytic sites and when they are all active any further increase in the concentration of substrate will not increase the rate of reaction.

Catalytic MIPs

As we have seen above, the TSA hypothesis is a useful one in arriving at a structural model of the template required to prepare a MIP catalyst. However the imprinting methodology is primarily concerned with the placement of functional groups in the binding site and consideration must be taken as to how they will assist in the catalytic process. If proton transfer is required for the substrate to be converted to the product, then groups which facilitate this will be required in the imprint site. The well known example of the catalytic triad (serine, histidine and aspartic acid) of serine proteases[10] is an example of how evolution has coped with the problem of developing an effective hydrolytic enzyme. The efforts of molecular imprinters in their attempts to emulate the workings of enzymes are described in the following sections.

MIP-Catalyzed Elimination Reactions

A simple target for MIP-based catalysis is the β-elimination reaction of HF from (14) to give the conjugated double bond in (15). This problem was solved in two completely different ways by Beach and Shea[11] (Fig. 3a) and Müller et al[12] (Fig. 3b). Both groups had the same aim: general base catalysis of the elimination by siting a basic group adjacent to the hydrogen atom of (14). In the first case a basic monomer, 2-aminoethylmethacrylamide (17), serving as the functional monomer and catalytic group, was used with the malonic acid derivative (16).[11] This monomer may also have contributed an additional binding interaction with the ketone functionality of (14). The alternative approach[12] used a basic TSA, (18) and the acidic monomer methacrylic acid (MAA), (19), which is catalytically active as its conjugate base. This strategy, where specific groups are used to coordinate their complements in the imprint site

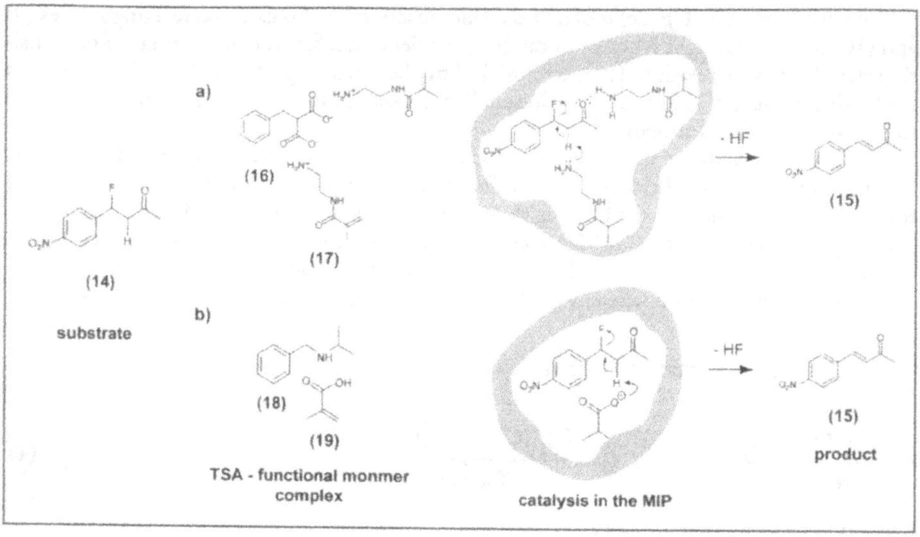

Figure 3. "Bait and switch" type strategies employed to synthesize MIPs catalyzing the dehydrofluorination of (14) by a general base mechanism. a) Benzylmalonic acid (16) imprinted with 2-aminoethylmethacrylamide (17). Adapted from reference 11. b) isopropyl-benzyl-amide (18), imprinted with methacrylic acid (19). Adapted from reference 12.

which subsequently take part in the catalytic process is known as the "bait and switch" approach. The template acts as "bait" to hook the appropriate functional monomers (or amino acid residues in the case of antibody production) in an effective conformation for proton transfer to occur.

A further example of an elimination reaction was published by Liu and Mosbach,[13] who showed that general base catalysis within a MIP can be used to catalyze the isomerization of benzisoxazole (20) to 2-hydroxybenzonitrile (21) in a 4-vinylpyridine based MIP, (Fig. 4). In this case the transition state (22) is mimicked by indole (23). Compared to the uncatalyzed reaction, a rate enhancement of 4×10^4 was reported, although the MIP-catalyzed reaction was only 7.2 times faster than with the blank polymer.

MIP-Based Hydrolytic Catalysts

The generation of MIP-based catalysts for the cleavage of esters, amides, carbonates and carbamates and related transesterification catalysts has received a lot of attention. This is partly because this class of reaction is relatively important synthetically, especially if regio- and

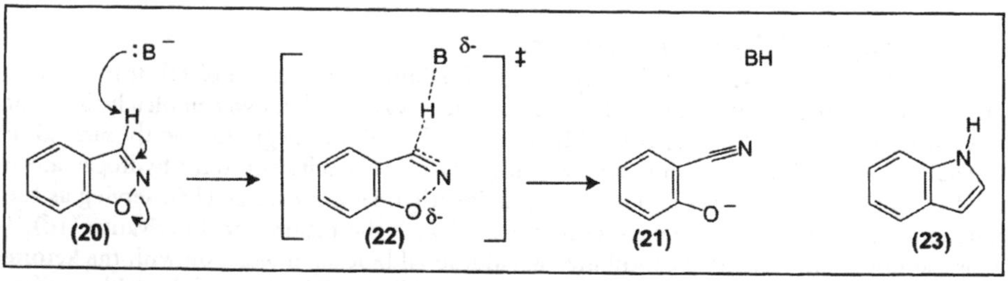

Figure 4. Benzisoxazole (20) isomerization to (21), catalyzed by an imprinted polymer catalyst. The transition state (22) is sufficiently substrate-like for (23) to be an effective TSA. Adapted from reference 13.

Table 1. Hydrolytic enzyme-mimicking MIPs taken from the literature

Polymer System	TSA Structure	Catalytic Activity	Refs.
4-(5)-vinylimadzole with Co2+, DVB.	(substrate mimic)	Hydrolysis of	14
4-(5)-vinylimadzole polymers with Co²⁺, crosslinked with ethylene-*bis*-acrylamide or with 1,4-dibromobutane.		Hydrolysis of	15
4-(5)-vinylimidazole, ethylene-*bis*-acrylamide copolymer with Co²		Hydrolysis of	16
Z-histidinyl-derivatised poly(ethyleneimine) with Co²⁺, crosslinked with 1,6-dibromohexane.		Hydrolysis of	17
Methyl-*N*-acryloyl-L-histidinate, acrylamide, ethylene-*bis*-acrylamide based copolymers with Co²⁺.		Hydrolysis of	18,19
4-(5)-vinylimidazole, DVB copolymer.		Hydrolysis of	20
Co2+ and *N*-methacryloyl-L-serine, *N*-methacryloyl-L-aspartic acid, *N*-methacryloyl-L-histidine copolymer, grafted on a poly (glycidyl methacrylate-co-ethyleneglycol dimethacrylate) crosslinked support.		Hydrolysis of	21
Surface imprinting on an O/W emulsion using a histidine-based emulsifier and Co²⁺ host system.		Hydrolysis of	22

Table continued on next page

Table 1. Continued

Polymer System	TSA Structure	Catalytic Activity	Refs.
Covalent attachment of phosphonate TSA to imidazole-bearing phenol monomer.	See Figure 5 and text, below.	See Figure 5 and text, below.	23,24
N,N'-diethyl (4-vinylphenyl) amidine-based polymers.	See Figure 6 and text, below.	See Figure 6 and text, below.	25
DVB, stryrene copolymer.	See Figure 7 and text, below.	See Figure 7 and text, below.	26
N,N'-diethyl (4-vinylphenyl) amidine-based polymers.		Hydrolysis of	27
4-vinylphenyl-benzamide, ethyleneglycol dimethacylate, methyl methacrylate copolymer with Co²⁺.		Hydrolysis of	28
Surface imprinting in an W/O emulsion using a histidine-based emulsifier and Co²⁺ host system.		Hydrolysis of	29
10% crosslinked (EGDMA) hydrogel copolymer of HEMA, MAA and N-methacyloylhistadine, with Co²⁺.		Hydrolysis of	30
"Footprint" catalysts, imprinted mixed silica alumina gel materials.	Various	Various hydrolysis and transesterification reactions	For a review, see ref. 31.

stereo-specific catalysts can be prepared, but also because a clearly defined strategy in terms of the TSA analogue structure (phosphate and phosphonate esters) has been well established. The ways in which polymers have been imprinted against these molecules are rather varied and some examples[14-30] are summarized in Table 1. A few of the more interesting hydrolytic MIPs are described in more detail in following text.

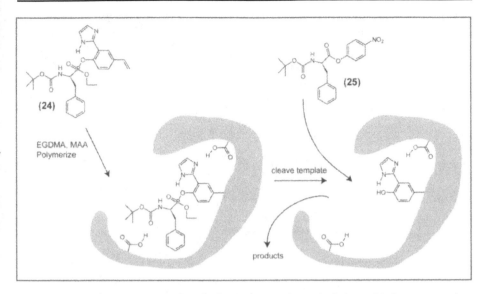

Figure 5. Scheme for the synthesis of a MIP for the enantioselective hydrolysis of (25), using a covalent template (24) approach. Methacrylic acid (MAA) is used to position the substrate through coordination with the Boc-group and also facilitates proton transfer through the imidazole function by coordination with the unprotonated nitrogen. Adapted from reference 23.

An Enantioselective Esterolytic MIP

An interesting attempt to assemble a catalytic triad in an esterolytic polymer was published by Sellergren and Shea in 1994,[23] with a follow-up paper in 2000.[24] This is illustrated in Figure 5. The authors used a mixed covalent and noncovalent strategy which involved the covalent TSA:functional monomer species (24) as the template. After polymerization and hydrolysis of the template, this left a phenolic group bearing an imidazole in the imprint site, positioned to interact with the carbonyl group of the substrate, (25). Additional interactions were provided by the inclusion of methacrylic acid (MAA), which was expected to coordinate to the basic nitrogen of the imidazole group and provide a "proton shuttle" to assist in the hydrolysis of (25). A second MAA residue, hydrogen bonding to the t-Boc carbonyl (as illustrated) may also be present, helping to correctly orient the substrate in the catalytic site. This polymer catalyst was reported to be the first example of an enantioselective imprinted hydrolytic enzyme mimic.

Polymers with Strong Esterase Activity

A significant step forward in noncovalent imprinting in recent years has been the introduction of monomers which form near stoichiometric complexes with templates in a entirely noncovalent sense.[32] Amongst these, the amidines, introduced by Wulff,[33] have the ability to bind carboxylic acids and phosphonate esters with very high affinities, such that the complexes are nearly completely in the associated form, even in water. This makes them very well suited to the stabilization of phosphonate TSA structures (Fig. 6) and their structure also facilitates in proton transfer, making them near ideal catalytic groups as well. In this example, taken from reference 25, the TSA (26) interacts with two molecules of the amidine monomer (27), to create a well-defined imprinted site following template removal. Substrate (28), is cleaved by the enzyme mimic to its constituent parts (29) and (30). The rate enhancement of up to 235 times is remarkable, especially when the one considers the phenyl ester is not activated by the presence of a nitro group, as so many of the other examples are. One drawback of this system is that the homoterephthalic acid product (29), is strongly bound to the polymer and competes

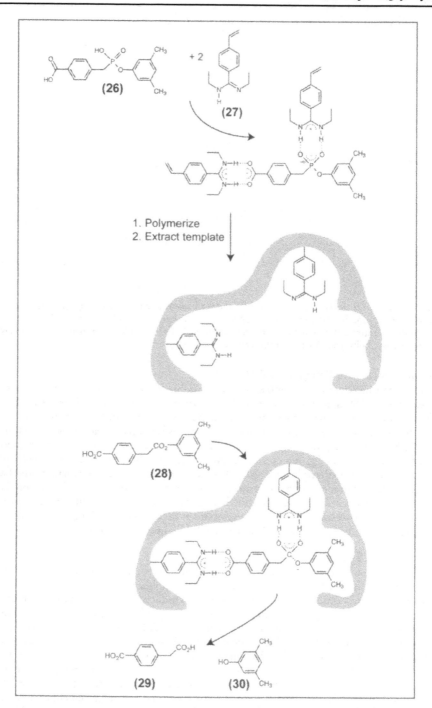

Figure 6. MIP catalyst prepared using stoichiometric binding interactions. The phosphonate TSA (26) is imprinted with the amidine-based monomer (27). After template removal the polymer stabilizes the transition state for the hydrolysis of the carboxylic ester (28) to (29) and (30). High catalytic activity was seen, despite the nonactivated nature of the ester. Adapted from reference 25.

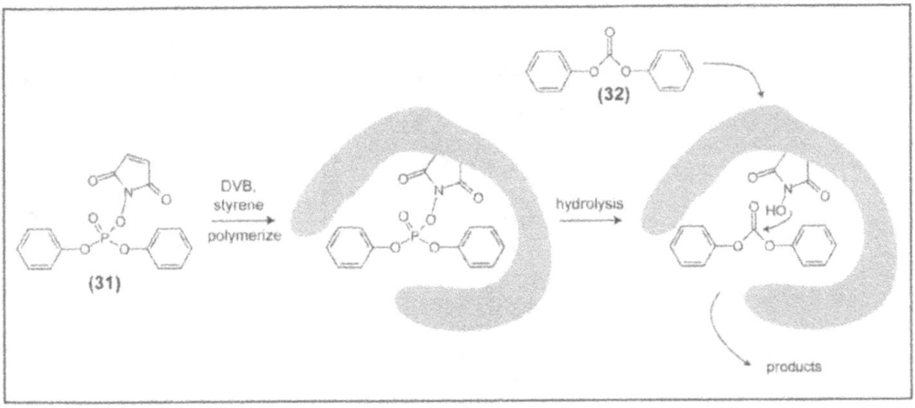

Figure 7. Covalent approach to the introduction of a catalytic group. In this example a phosphate ester of N-hydroxymaleimide (31) is used to introduce a catalytic hydroxyl group into the active site of a MIP capable of hydrolyzing diphenylcarbonate (32). Adapted from reference 26.

with substrate for the catalytic sites. This is an example of product inhibition, which can also be a problem when using enzymes in the laboratory. When carbonate[27,34,35] and carbamate (urethane)[34,35] substrates are used with an appropriately imprinted amidine-based polymer, the products do not bind to the active site, product inhibition is avoided and even greater rate enhancements can be seen.

A labile Covalent Bonding Approach to an Imprinted Polymer Catalyst

A simple approach, to the introduction of a catalytic group was used by Kim et al[26] who prepared the phosphate ester (31) as an analogue of the transition state for diphenyl carbonate (32) hydrolysis, (Fig. 7), bearing N-hydroxymaleimide. This monomer will copolymerize readily with styrene, so the covalent template-monomer was polymerized in a styrene/divinylbenzene (DVB) copolymer. A relatively facile cleavage gave the polymer with a hydroxyl group arranged to facilitate cleavage of (32) with rate enhancements of up to 120-fold.

In general the phosphonate and phosphate TSAs described above resemble the tetrahedral intermediates (see 3, Fig. 1a for an example). This is understandable, given that we have to use a stable compound as a TSA, but it will also be valid if the transition state is close in energy (and therefore structure, in accordance with the Hammond Postulate[36]) to this intermediate. Similarly (23), (Fig. 4), is substrate-like, indicating an early transition state.

MIP Catalysis of Carbon-Carbon Bond Formation

The formation of carbon-carbon bonds is often seen as one of the more difficult of the chemical transformations to achieve, nevertheless there are some examples of MIPs catalyzing these transformations.

An Artificial Aldolase Mimic

Condensation reactions between carbonyl compounds are one method of carbon-carbon bond formation. These reactions tend to be reversible, however dehydration of the intermediate product in the Aldol reaction tends to "lock" the product in its final form. This reaction has been the target of a MIP catalyst, in this case (Fig. 8), Matsui et al[37] produced a catalyst using (33) as the template, polymerized as its Co^{2+} complex with 4-vinylpyridine (34) in a DVB/styrene copolymer. The polymer, in the presence of the coordinating metal ion Co^{2+}, binds the reactant species acetophenone (35) and benzaldehyde (36) and catalyzes the condensation via the enolate of (35) and facilitates the dehydration to (37). The template (33) resembles the intermediate condensation product (before dehydration) and is another example of a product-like TSA.

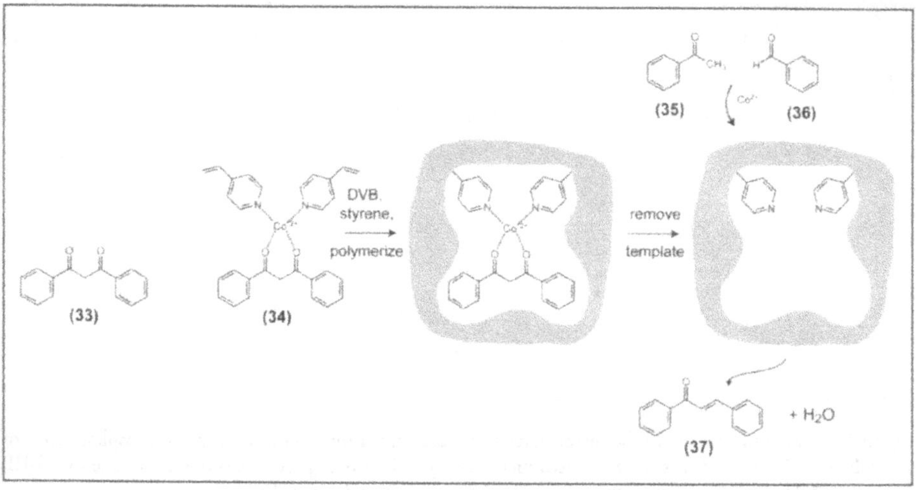

Figure 8. Carbon-carbon bond formation by MIP-catalyzed Aldol condensation. The diketone template (33) is imprinted as the 4-vinylpyridine – Co^{2+} complex (34) in a DVB/styrene polymer. The resultant polymer catalyzed the condensation of acetophenone (35) and benzaldehyde (36) and the dehydration of the intermediate product to form chalcone (37). Adapted from reference 37.

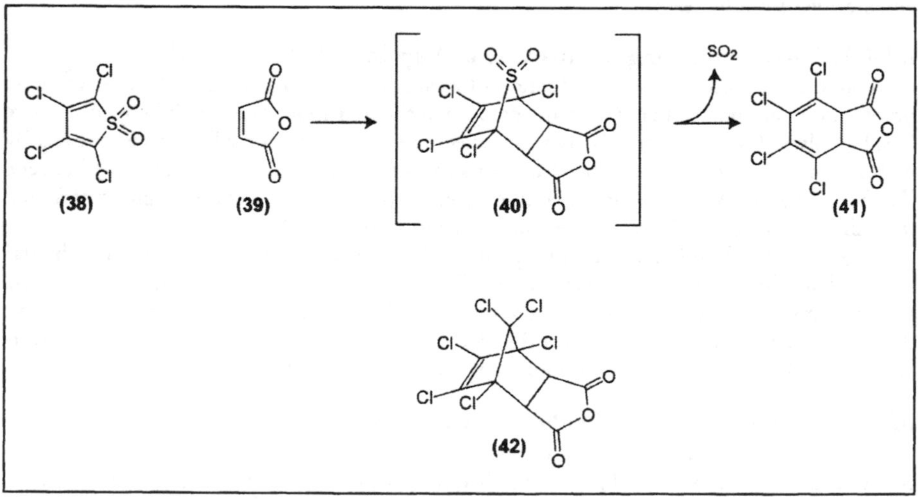

Figure 9. An artificial Diels-Alderase. The TSA (42) was imprinted with methacrylic acid as the functional monomer to give a polymer capable of catalyzing the reaction of (38) and (39). The initially formed product (40) spontaneously loses SO_2 by a second sigmatropic rearrangement to give the product (41). In this example the TSA closely resembles the product. Adapted from reference 39.

MIP That Catalyzes a Diels-Alder Reaction

We have already seen an example of a Diels-Alder reaction catalyzed by an antibody[9] (Fig. 1c). Another example of an antibody-catalyzed Diels-Alder reaction[38] was the inspiration for Liu and Mosbach[39] in their synthesis of a MIP catalyst for a similar reaction sequence (Fig. 9). The reaction between (38) and (39) to give (40) is followed by a spontaneous secondary sigmatropic rearrangement, with the loss of SO_2, to give the final product (41). In this case an

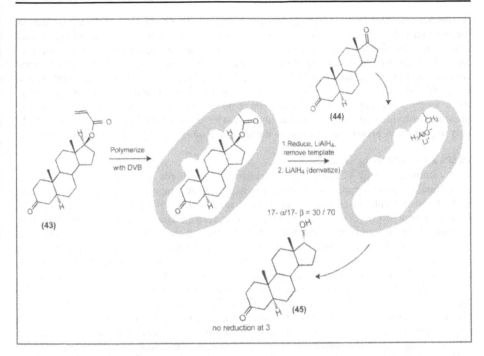

Figure 10. Imprinted reducing agents. The ester (43) is imprinted in a DVB matrix. The template is removed by reduction with lithium aluminum hydride. Treatment with further LiAlH₄ creates an immobilized reducing agent within the imprint site capable of regioselective and stereoselective reduction of the diketone (44). Adapted from reference 39.

analogue of the intermediate product (42) was used as the template in an MAA/EGDMA copolymer. Note the use of chlorine as a substitute for carbonyl oxygen in the TSA.

MIPs as Adjuncts to Synthesis

While catalytic turnover may be the ultimate goal in the use of MIPs in synthesis, the complementary binding sites of an imprinted material may be utilized in other ways to great effect. Some examples of this work are given in the following section and show the potential for imprinted polymers to influence the outcome of a reaction due the constraint of carrying out that reaction in a site imprinted with an appropriate template.

MIPs as Selective Polymer-Supported Reagents

Polymer-supported reagents are frequently used in organic synthesis where a clean separation may otherwise be difficult or impossible to achieve. The advantage of the heterogeneous reagent is that it can be simply filtered from the product, which is uncontaminated with excess reagent or by-products. If, however the reagent is attached to the polymer support within an imprint site it is possible to exercise a further degree of control over the reaction. This was the aim of Byström et al[39] who prepared an imprinted reducing agent capable of the selective reduction of steroidal ketones (Fig. 10). In their system, the ester (43) was imprinted in a DVB matrix, removal of the template was achieved by reduction of the ester bond with lithium aluminum hydride. Treatment with further LiAlH₄ resulted in the formation of active hydride site within the polymer at the former point of attachment of the template ester group. Reduction of the diketone (44) with this imprinted reagent occurred exclusively at the 17-position, whereas in free solution or with a nonimprinted polymer both the 3- and 17-positions would be affected. Furthermore some stereoselectivity was evident with the ratio of α- to β-isomers in the product (45) indicating that some hydride delivery on the hindered face of the steroid (consistent with the template structure) had occurred, differing again from the control reaction, where almost exclusively (96%) the β-isomer was formed. Using a polymer reagent similarly imprinted with a cholesterol derivative (3-β hydroxyl) an even greater stereoselectivity was seen, with 70% of the α-isomer being formed. The very high regioselectivities of these polymeric reagents was explained by the fact the approach of substrate ketones to the reducing agent is constrained by the shape of the imprint, with the axial methyl groups being particularly important in preventing reaction of the substrate when misaligned with the imprint site.

MIPs as Protecting Groups

A common strategy in many organic transformations is the use of protecting groups, to mask some functional groups while other chemical transformations are carried out elsewhere in the same molecule. Their great advantage is that once they have done their job, they can be selectively removed to reveal the original functional groups which are then available for further reaction. Protection and deprotection must be very efficient reactions if the extra steps involved are not going to deplete the final yield in a multi-step synthesis. In addition protecting groups cannot normally be reused, adding to the cost of the final product. What if an imprinted polymer could be used as a protecting group, would it overcome some of these problems?

We prepared a number of polymers imprinted with hydroxysteroids, such as (46) and (47), using the boronophthalide monomer (48), a form of covalent imprinting.[40] The isomeric templates in this example had a *t*-butyl ester group at the 24-position, to define a "pocket" in the imprint site. Removal of the templates gave us two isomeric imprinted polymers, (49) and (50), differing only in the position of the binding groups. Rebinding of the trihydroxysteroids (51) and (52), either to their corresponding imprint (matched) or the isomeric imprint (unmatched), followed by reaction with acetyl chloride, gave a series of acetylated products, once they were freed from the polymers. It was found that much higher ratios (up to 23:1) of the 24-acetyl product was seen in the "matched" case, a control polymer (imprinted with ethylene glycol) showed a much poorer uptake and resulted in almost exclusive acetylation at the 3-position (see Table 2), indicating in this case that what little material was bound had reacted with the polymer at the 24-position.

MIPs as Microreactors

In a remarkable demonstration of the ability of the imprinted site to direct chemical transformations, Wulff and Vietmeier[41,42] showed that enatioselective amino acid synthesis could be carried out in a polymer prepared using two distinct covalent imprinting strategies, namely a Schiff's base and a boronate ester group (Fig. 12). In this scheme, the template monomer (53) was used to prepare the l-DOPA imprinted site. Removal of the template reveals the aldehyde and boronic acid residues within the imprint site. Reaction with glycine (55), followed by treatment with base (lithium diisopropylamide, LDA) generated the enolate ion of the glycine Schiff's base. A 2,3-dihydroxybenzyl derivative (56) can then be captured as the corresponding boronate ester. This is followed by condensation between the enolate and the benzylic carbon with loss of the leaving group X. Removal of the product amino acid (54) leaves the site free for a further synthetic cycle. In the same imprint sites, the authors also demonstrated the formation of nickel enolate complex of the glycine, followed by condensation of acetaldehyde, coordinated to the electron deficient boron atom, leading to the condensation products threonine and allo-threonine (not shown). An enantiomeric excess of 36% was seen in the product of this reaction.

Casting in an Imprinted Site—Anti-Idiotypic Imprints

In a conceptually different approach, Mosbach et al[43,44] have proposed the use of the imprinted site as a sort of molecular jigsaw puzzle, in what they call the anti-idiotypic approach

Table 2. Imprinted polymers as protecting groups: yield of 3- and 24-monoacetates

Polymer and Substrate[a]	Bound, μmol	Unmodified, %	Mono-Acetates, %	24-:3-Acetate Ratio
(49) and (51), (matched)	29.0	36	64	10.5:1
(50) and (52), (matched)	26.1	35	65	23.1:1
(49) and (52), (unmatched)	25.5	49	51	5.4:1
(49) and control	8.3	87	13	<1:100

a. See Figure 11. Table adapted from reference 40.

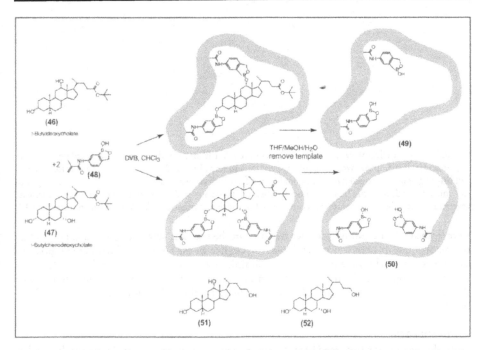

Figure 11. MIPs as protecting groups. Covalent imprinting of (46) and (47) with 3-methacrylamido-boronophthalide (48) results in two isomeric sites (49) and (50) within the respective imprinted polymers. Binding of the trihydroxysteroids (51) and (52) followed by treatment with acetyl chloride results in preferential acetylation of the 24-position only if the triol structure is "matched" to the imprint site. Adapted from reference 40.

(Fig. 13). In the first example of this type, the molecule (57), an inhibitor of the enzyme kallikrein, was imprinted using (2-trifluoromethyl)acrylic acid and DVB. The template (57) is the condensation product of the dichlorotriazine-derivative (58) and the amine (59), if however the triazine is bound to the polymer site and a number of similar amines (59) – (62) are mixed with the partly filled site, those that react within the site will produce products (57), (63) – (65) resembling the template and are likely candidates for new inhibitors. No products

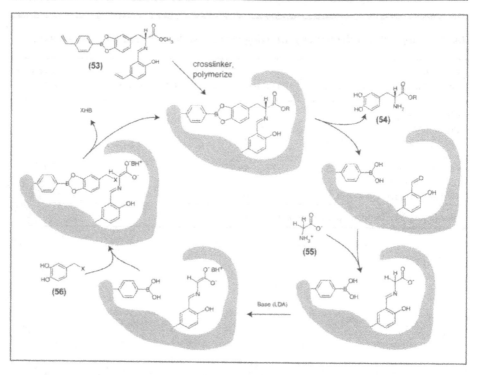

Figure 12. Enantioselective synthesis of l-DOPA in a covalently imprinted polymer. The template monomer (53) was imprinted, using two modes of covalent attachment. Removal of the template (54) is followed by binding of glycine to the aldehyde functionality as a Schiff's base, which is deprotonated to the corresponding enolate. Binding of the benzyl halide derivative (56) occurs such that condensation with the enolate regenerates the original template structure ready for another synthetic cycle. Adapted from reference 42.

were formed when a control polymer was used in the reaction, also (62) produced no product on the MIP due to steric hindrance; it was too large to fit the jigsaw. Of the other compounds, (64) proved to be almost as good as (57) as inhibiting the enzyme. In a second example of this approach, using a slightly different inhibitor as template,[44] the authors also demonstrated that the same approach could be applied to the enzyme active site itself, this was referred to as "direct molding".

Conclusions

In this chapter we have seen how the concept of a transition state analogue can be used to design a template to prepare catalytic imprinted polymers. The use of the "bait and switch" approach and alternative covalent template strategies have shown us how functional groups which can assist in the catalytic process can be assembled within the imprint. We have also seen that imprinted sites can be very effective in directing reactions when used in a noncatalytic manner.

It has not been possible in the space available to discuss some other aspects of the imprinting literature related to this subject, for example the use of imprinted polymers to influence the course of a biocatalytic transformation,[45] how an imprinting approach can be used to modify the activity of an enzyme[46] or how transition metal catalysts can be used in imprinted materials.[47] The interested reader is directed to a number of excellent recent reviews,[48-51] as well as the research papers cited above.

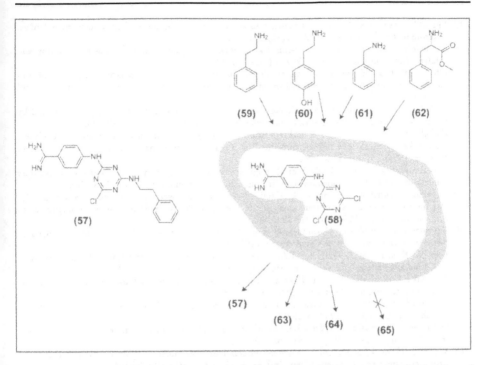

Figure 13. Molecular jigsaw puzzle. The enzyme inhibitor (57) is used to prepare an imprint. Reaction of (58) with a range of amines (59), (60), (61) and (62) will only give a product if both reactants can fit in the imprint site. The range of compounds formed are new candidates for inhibitors of the enzyme for which (58) is know to be an inhibitor. Adapted from reference 43.

Acknowledgements

The work of our group in this area has been supported financially by the UK Biotechnology and Biological Sciences Research Council.

References

1. Svenson J, Nicholls IA. On the thermal and chemical stability of molecularly imprinted polymers. Anal Chim Acta 2001; 435(1):19-24.
2. Tramonato A, Janda KD, Lerner RA. Catalytic antibodies. Science 1986; 234(4783):1566-1570.
3. Schultz PG. Catalytic antibodies. Acc Chem Res 1989; 22(8):287-294.
4. Lerner RA, Benkovic SJ, Schultz PG. At the crossroads of chemistry and immunology – catalytic antibodies. Science 1991; 252(5006):659-667.
5. Schultz PG, Lerner RA. Antibody catalysis of difficult chemical transformations. Acc Chem Res 1993; 26(8):391-395.
6. Tanaka F. Catalytic antibodies as designer proteases and esterases. Chem Rev 2002; 102(12):4885-4906.
7. Jacobs J, Schultz PG, Sugasawara R et al. Catalytic antibodies. J Am Chem Soc 1987; 109(7):2174-2176.
8. Jackson DY, Jacobs JY, Sugasawara R et al. An antibody-catalyzed Claisen rearrangement. J Am Chem Soc 1988; 110(14):4841-4842.
9. Braisted AC, Schultz PG. An antibody-catalyzed bimolecular Diels-Alder reaction. J Am Chem Soc 1990; 112(20):7430-7431.
10. Hedstrom L. Serine protease mechanism and specificity. Chem Rev 2002; 102(12):4501-4523.
11. Beach JV, Shea KJ. Designed catalysts - a synthetic network polymer that catalyzes the dehydrofluorination of 4-fluoro-4-(p-nitrophenyl)butan-2-one. J Am Chem Soc 1994; 11(1):6379-380.
12. Müller R, Andersson LI, Mosbach K. Molecularly imprinted polymers facilitating a beta-elimination reaction. Makromol Chem Rapid Commun 1993; 14(10):637-641.

13. Liu XC, Mosbach K. Catalysis of benzisoxazole isomerization by molecularly imprinted polymers. Macromol Rapid Commun 1998; 19(12):671-674.
14. Leonhardt A, Mosbach K. Enzyme-mimicking polymers exhibiting specific substrate binding and catalytic functions. Reac Polym 1987; 6(2-3):285-290.
15. Ohkubo K, Urata Y, Hirota S et al. Homogeneous and heterogeneous esterolytic catalyzes of imidazole- containing polymers prepared by molecular imprinting of a transition- state analog. J Mol Cat 1994; 87(1):L21-L24.
16. Ohkubo K, Urata Y, Hirota S et al. Homogeneous esterolytic catalysis of a polymer prepared by molecular imprinting of a transition-state analog. J Mol Cat 1994; 93(2):189-193.
17. Ohkubo K, Urata Y, Honda Y et al. Preparation and catalytic property of l-histidyl group-introduced, cross-linked poly(ethylene imine)s imprinted by a transition-state analog of an esterolysis reaction. Polymer 1994; 35(24):5372-5374.
18. Ohkubo K, Funakoshi Y, Urata Y et al. High esterolytic activity of a novel water-soluble polymer catalyst imprinted by a transition-state analog. Chem Commun 1995; (20):2143-2144.
19. Ohkubo K, Funakoshi Y, Sagawa T. Catalytic activity of a novel water-soluble cross-linked polymer imprinted by a transition-state analogue for the stereoselective hydrolysis of enantiomeric amino acid esters. Polymer 1996; 37(17):3993-3995.
20. Kawanami Y, Yunoki T, Nakamura A et al. Imprinted polymer catalysts for the hydrolysis of p-nitrophenyl acetate. J Mol Cat A 1999; 145(1-2):107-110.
21. Lele BS, Kulkarni MG, Mashelkar RA. Molecularly imprinted polymer mimics of chymotrypsin - 1. Cooperative effects and substrate specificity. Reac Func Polym 1999; 39(1):37-52.
22. Toorisaka E, Yoshida M, Uezu K et al. Artificial biocatalyst prepared by the surface molecular imprinting technique. Chem Lett 1999; (5):387-388.
23. Sellergren B, Shea KJ. Enantioselective ester hydrolysis catalyzed by imprinted polymers. Tetrahedron-Asymmetry 1994; 5(8):1403-1406.
24. Sellergren B, Karmalkar RN, Shea KJ. Enantioselective ester hydrolysis catalyzed by imprinted polymers. 2. J Org Chem 2000; 65(13):4009-4027.
25. Wulff G, Gross T, Schönfeld R. Enzyme models based on molecularly imprinted polymers with strong esterase activity. Angew Chem Intl Ed Engl 1997; 36(18):1962-1964.
26. Kim JM, Ahn KD, Strikovsky AG et al. Polymer catalysts by molecular imprinting: A labile covalent bonding approach. Bull Kor Chem Soc 2001; 22(7):689-692.
27. Kim JM, Ahn KD, Wulff G. Cholesterol esterase activity of a molecularly imprinted polymer. Macromol Chem Phys 2001; 202(7):1105-1108.
28. Yu JH, Huang QB, Ma DJ et al. Hydrolysis of carboxylate ester catalyzed by a new artificial abzyme based on molecularly imprinted polymer. Prog Nat Sci 2001; 11(7):516-519.
29. Toorisaka E, Uezu K, Goto M et al. A molecularly imprinted polymer that shows enzymatic activity. Biochem Eng J 2003; 14(2):85-91.
30. Karmalkar RN, Kulkarni MG, Mashelkar RA. Molecularly imprinted hydrogels exhibit chymotrypsin-like activity. Macromolecules 1996; 29(4):1366-1368.
31. Morihara K. Recognition over footprint cavities. ACS Symp Ser 1998; 703:300-313.
32. Wulff G, Knorr K. Stoichiometric noncovalent interaction in molecular imprinting. Bioseparation 2002; 10(6):257-276.
33. Wulff G, Schönfeld R. Polymerizable amidines - Adhesion mediators and binding sites for molecular imprinting. Adv Mater 1998; 10(12):957-959.
34. Strikovsky AG, Kasper D, Grun M et al. Catalytic molecularly imprinted polymers using conventional bulk polymerization or suspension polymerization: Selective hydrolysis of diphenyl carbonate and diphenyl carbamate. J Am Chem Soc 2000; 122(26):6295-6296.
35. Strikovsky A, Hradil J, Wulff G. Catalytically active, molecularly imprinted polymers in bead form. Reac Func Polym 2003; 54(1-3):49-61.
36. Hammond GS. J Am Chem Soc 1955; 77(2):334-338.
37. Matsui J, Nicholls IA, Karube I et al. Carbon-carbon bond formation using substrate selective catalytic polymers prepared by molecular imprinting: An artificial class II aldolase. J Org Chem 1996; 615(16):414-5417.
38. Hilvert D, Hill KW, Nared KD et al. Antibody catalysis of a Diels-Alder reaction. J Am Chem Soc 1989; 111(26):9261-9262.
38. Liu XC, Mosbach K. Studies towards a tailor-made catalyst for the Diels-Alder reaction using the technique of molecular imprinting. Macromol Rapid Commun 1997; 18(7):609-615.
39. Byström SE, Börje A, Akermark B. Selective reduction of steroid 3-ketones and 17-ketones using LiAlH4 activated template polymers. J Am Chem Soc 1993; 115(5):2081-2083.
40. Alexander C, Smith CR, Whitcombe MJ et al. Imprinted polymers as protecting groups for regioselective modification of polyfunctional substrates. J Am Chem Soc 1999; 121(28):6640-6651.

41. Wulff G, Vietmeier J. Enzyme-analogue built polymers .25. Synthesis of macroporous copolymers from alpha-amino-acid based vinyl compounds. Makromol Chem 1989; 190(7):1717-1726.
42. Wulff G, Vietmeier J. Enzyme-analogue built polymers .26. Enantioselective synthesis of amino-acids using polymers possessing chiral cavities obtained by an imprinting procedure with template molecules. Makromol Chem 1989; 190(7):1727-1735.
43. Mosbach K, Yu YH, Andersch J et al. Generation of new enzyme inhibitors using imprinted binding sites: The anti-idiotypic approach, a step toward the next generation of molecular imprinting. J Am Chem Soc 2001; 123(49):12420-12421.
44. Yu YH, Ye L, Haupt K et al. Formation of a class of enzyme inhibitors (drugs), including a chiral compound, by using imprinted polymers or biomolecules as molecular-scale reaction vessels. Angew Chem Intl Ed 2002; 41(23):4459-4463.
45. Ye L, Ramström O, Ansell RJ et al. Use of molecularly imprinted polymers in a biotransformation process. Biotechnol Bioeng 1999; 64:650-655.
46. Ståhl M, Månsson MO, Mosbach K. The synthesis of a d-amino-acid ester in an organic media with alpha-chymotrypsin modified by a bio-imprinting procedure. Biotech Lett 1990; 12:161-166.
47. Cammidge AN, Baines NJ, Bellingham RK. Synthesis of heterogeneous palladium catalyst assemblies by molecular imprinting. Chem Commun 2001; (24):2588-2589.
48. Whitcombe MJ, Alexander C, Vulfson EN. Imprinted polymers: Versatile new tools in synthesis. Synlett 2000; (6):911-923.
49. Ramström O, Mosbach K. Synthesis and catalysis by molecularly imprinted materials. Curr Opinion Chem 1999; 3(6):759-764.
50. Wulff G. Enzyme-like catalysis by molecularly imprinted polymers. Chem Rev 2002; 102(1):1-27.
51. Alexander C, Davidson L, Hayes W. Imprinted polymers: Artificial molecular recognition materials with applications in synthesis and catalysis. Tet 2003; 59(12):2025-2057.

Solid-Phase Extraction on Molecularly Imprinted Polymers:

Requirements, Achievements and Future Work

Lars I. Andersson

Abstract

Molecular imprint based solid-phase extraction is increasingly being used for selective extraction of biological and environmental samples. Interest in imprinted polymers is derived from the high selectivities and affinities achievable, and the fact that by the imprinting process these properties may be qualitatively and quantitatively predetermined for a particular analyte, or a class of structural analogues. Hence, imprinted polymers potentially offer a higher level of sample cleanup than that obtained using conventional extraction materials which has been demonstrated for several systems. This review will discuss recent literature, benefits and limitations of using imprinted polymers in solid-phase extraction applications, as well as method development of imprint-based extraction protocols.

Introduction

The last several years have seen an increasing research activity into molecular-imprint based solid-phase extraction (MISPE). This includes not only research into novel molecularly imprinted polymers, MIPs, and their application to methodology development, but also an increasing number of studies into the use of MIPs for determination of drugs and pollutants in biological and environmental samples. Various formats of solid-phase extraction (SPE) is currently a routine sample preparation technique employed in numerous environmental and bioanalytical applications.[1-5] Separation on most current SPE sorbents is based on physico-chemical retention on the functionalised surface and the SPE column retains not only the target analyte(s) but also other matrix components. Therefore, a considerable amount of method development work is often spent on optimising the complete analytical method. More selective SPE materials, such as immunosorbents[6-7] and imprinted polymers,[8-11] rely on affinity interactions and potentially offer a higher degree of sample clean-up than that achieved using conventional type SPE sorbents. Characteristic for both types of affinity materials are their high ligand selectivity and affinity, where selectivity can be predetermined for a particular analyte by, respectively the choice of antigen used for antibody generation and the choice of template used for MIP preparation.

Since imprinted polymers are a novel type of sorbent, there is a need for better understanding of how to employ robust method development strategies. For instance, most MIP syntheses are organic solvent based, and studies on imprint rebinding are often conducted using organic solvents as the incubation medium, where establishment of conditions for strong and selective rebinding is understood. The same level of understanding is not yet available for aqueous

Molecular Imprinting of Polymers, edited by Sergey Piletsky and Anthony Turner.
©2006 Landes Bioscience.

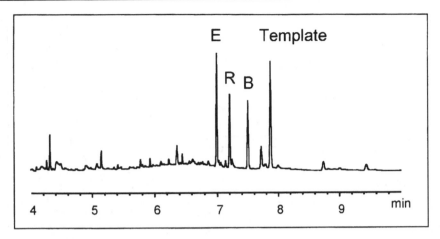

Figure 1. Gas chromatographic trace following MISPE of 500 nmol/L ethycaine (E) and 300 nmol/L of each of ropivacaine (R) and bupivacaine (B) from human plasma using a pentycaine-MIP. Note the presence of a pentycaine peak due to template bleeding. Structures are shown in Figure 2.

rebinding, such as in the presence of biofluids. Furthermore, MIPs are synthesised in the presence of a high concentration of template where trace amounts of the imprint species may remain in the resultant MIP and may later leak during use, so called template bleeding. For trace and ultra-trace analysis, potential influence of template bleeding on assay accuracy must be taken into account. A MIP is best characterised as being a mixed-mode separation material, which in addition to the imprinted affinity sites contains both polar and lipophilic surface functionality. Therefore, optimisation of a MISPE method should be based on an understanding how the strength and nature of imprint-analyte and polymer surface-analyte interactions, respectively, vary with the type of solvent or buffer employed. This review discusses the potential scope and some pitfalls of using MIPs for solid-phase extraction as well as some fundamental aspects of the molecular imprinting technology for such applications.

Preparation of Imprinted SPE Sorbents

A MIP is synthesised through polymerisation of functional and cross-linking monomers in the presence of a high concentration of template. Despite exhaustive washing, trace amounts of the imprint species may remain in the resultant MIP and may later bleed during use[12-18] (Fig. 1). Near-quantitative removal of the imprint species is critical for a MISPE application in trace analysis, where even a small amount of bleeding may greatly affect the assay result. A more thorough extraction yields a MIP where more of the high-affinity sites are free, leading to a material with greater ability to bind analyte from highly diluted samples and less prone to bleed template molecules at use. A comprehensive study into the influence of various post-polymerisation treatments, such as thermal annealing, microwave assisted extraction, Soxhlet extraction and supercritical fluid desorption, on the level of bleeding concluded that none of the treatments eliminated template bleeding completely.[19] While microwave assisted extraction using trifluoroacetic acid or formic acid was found to be the most efficient extraction technique, also polymer degradation and loss of selectivity were observed. Soxhlet extraction using pure methanol or acetic acid in ethanol or methanol is frequently used. Other protocols, which have proved useful, include batch or column mode extractions using chlorinated solvents with strong ability to swell the MIP, and solvents with strong elution power, such as aqueous methanol or ethanol, containing acid or base, as well as alternating acid and base washings.[16] Template bleeding is less critical for many chromatographic and other continuous-flow applications, where the MIP is washed continuously by the mobile phase, and on-line SPE applications suffer less from this problem.

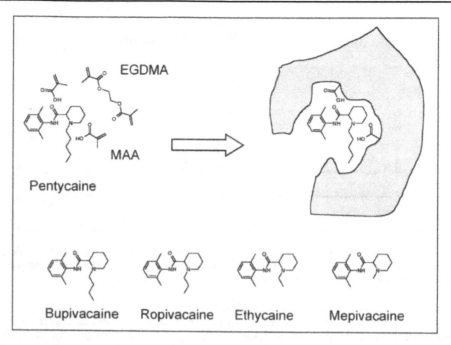

Figure 2. Molecular imprinting of pentycaine using methacrylic acid as the functional monomer and ethylene glycol dimethacrylate as the cross-linking monomer. The resultant imprints recognizes close structural analogues, such as bupivacaine, ropivacaine, ethycaine and mepivacaine, with N-alkyl chains slightly different to that of the template.

The obvious choice of imprint species is to use the target analyte as the template and this approach is employed in the vast majority of molecular imprinting studies. Due to the template bleeding problem discussed above this is, however, not feasible in all situations. Instead a structural analogue of the analyte(s) of interest can be used for the MIP preparation. The alternative template should be selected such that it possesses structural features in common with the analyte and gives rise to imprints that have the ability to bind the target analyte(s) (Fig. 2). A wealth of data is already available on template structure-imprint selectivity relationships, which often will aid the selection of a suitable structural analogue. For trace analysis MISPE, in particular, the alternative-template species should be considered a viable alternative. Should template bleeding occur, the subsequent analytical separation will resolve the template from the analyte(s) and quantification will still be accurate (Fig. 1). This approach was first demonstrated by the preparation of a MIP for extraction of sameridine using a close structural analogue.[12] Another example is the use of dibutylmelamine as a "dummy template" for the preparation of a MIP, which recognizes triazine structures.[20] In the liquid chromatography mode the MIP retained atrazine and related triazines in a group selective manner, whereas structurally unrelated agrochemicals were not bound and eluted with the solvent front. In a subsequent study the MIP was used for selective SPE of atrazine from a mixture of herbicides.[21] Other examples of the alternative template approach are the use of a pentycaine-MIP for extraction of bupivacaine,[16,22] a naproxen-MIP for ibuprofen,[17] a clenbuterol-MIP for brombuterol,[23] a ditolylphosphate-MIP for diphenylphosphate,[24] and a hyoscyamine-MIP for scopolamine.[25]

Whether the alternative template approach is used or not, each MISPE method development must at some stage include a confirmation that template bleeding does not interfere with the assay and gives rise to poor accuracy and precision. Whereas this is very important for off-line extraction protocols using fresh material for each extraction, for on-line SPE protocols,

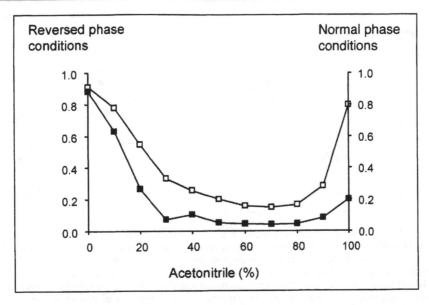

Figure 3. Binding of bupivacaine to a MAA-co-EGDMA-MIP made against bupivacaine (open squares) and a nonimprinted MAA-co-EGDMA polymer (filled squares) in water-acetonitrile mixtures. Under reversed-phase conditions hydrophobic interactions are strong and bupivacaine binds to a large extent via nonspecific adsorption to the hydrophobic polymer surface. Under normal phase conditions electrostatic interactions and hydrogen bonds are strong and bupivacaine binds mainly via selective binding in the imprints.

where the MIP column is constantly washed with mobile phase, template bleeding may not cause any problem.

Development of a MISPE Method

For SPE applications a MIP is best characterised as being a mixed-mode separation material, which in addition to the imprinted affinity sites contains both polar and lipophilic surface functionality. Typically, a MIP is made of a cross-linking monomer, such as ethylene glycol dimethacrylate or trimethylolpropane trimethacrylate, which renders the MIP hydrophobic, and a functional monomer, such as methacrylic acid or vinylpryidine, which contributes weak ion exchange and hydrogen bonding carboxylic acid and pyridine groups, respectively. Under reversed-phase conditions, i.e., water-rich eluents, nonspecific physicochemical retention is due mainly to hydrophobic interactions. Whereas under normal-phase conditions, i.e., organic solvent eluents, nonspecific physicochemical retention is due mainly to polar interactions (Fig. 3). For the analyte the observed retention on a MIP column is the sum of selective and nonspecific retention modes through binding in imprints and physicochemical interaction with polymer surface, respectively. For other components of the sample, the observed retention is due to nonspecific retention modes. If the nonspecific retention mechanisms dominate, the analyte will be retained mainly through the same retention mechanisms as the other sample components and any selectivity shown by the imprints may remain undetected. Hence, efficient MISPE method development should be based on an understanding how the strength and nature of imprint-analyte and polymer surface-analyte interactions, respectively, vary with the type of solvent or buffer employed. A generic off-line extraction protocol is shown in Figure 4. Optimisation of the sample loading conditions and of the wash and elution steps will be discussed in following paragraphs.

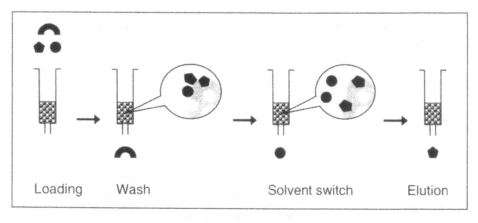

Figure 4. A generic off-line extraction protocol. Following extraction of an aqueous sample the analyte is retained bound selectively in imprints as well as adsorbed to polymer surface through nonspecific hydrophobic interactions. While polar sample components are removed by an aqueous wash step, lipophilic compounds remain adsorbed to the polymer surface. A solvent switch, for instance to acetonitrile or dichlormethane, leads to redistribution of nonspecifically adsorbed analyte to imprinted sites and removal of other nonspecifically adsorbed sample components. Finally, eluention is effected using either a polar organic solvent, such as acetonitrile or methanol, or water, in each case containing acid, such as acetic acid, formic acid or trifluoroacetic acid, or base, such as triethylamine.

Most MIP syntheses are organic solvent based and subsequent studies on imprint rebinding are often conducted using organic solvents as the incubation medium. On theoretical grounds it may be argued optimal to use the same solvent for rebinding as was used for MIP synthesis.[26] While in some instances the use of matched solvents result in best selectivity for the template over close structural analogues,[27] such a practice will be almost impracticable in most real situations which concerns extraction of aqueous environmental or biological samples. Due to the hydrophobic nature of the polymer, extraction of aqueous samples often results in moderately and highly lipophilic compounds being nonspecifically adsorbed to the MIP (Fig. 4). This hydrophobically driven adsorption can be reduced by addition of an organic modifier,[22,28] such as ethanol, methanol or acetonitrile, or a detergent to the sample. The upper limit of the organic modifier content is, however, in part dependent on the type of sample, as protein precipitation may occur for plasma samples. Detergents tested and found useful include Tween 20, Triton X-100 and Brij 35.[22] Also, buffer pH may influence the extent of nonspecific adsorption. An increase with increased pH is seen for adsorption of basic compounds to MAA-type polymers[28,29] and a decrease with increased pH for adsorption of acidic compounds to VPy-type polymers.[30] Nonspecific adsorption may also be reduced by the use of small MIP columns, thereby reducing the polymer surface area available for hydrophobic adsorption. As most applications deal with trace analysis, binding capacity does not seem to be a problem, and column sizes down to 15 mg of MIP have been used.[16]

Following extraction of aqueous samples analyte is retained both bound selectively in imprints and adsorbed to polymer surface through nonspecific hydrophobic interactions (Fig. 4). A wash step using an organic solvent, such as dichloromethane or acetonitrile, improves MIP selectivity and removes all other adsorbed sample components. This solvent switch changes the retention conditions to the normal-phase mode, which leads to redistribution of the analyte to imprint sites and washing off of nonrelated structures (Fig. 4). In apolar solvents the selective imprint-analyte binding is due mainly to hydrogen bonding and electrostatic interactions, which are strong under these conditions, whereas nonspecific hydrophobic adsorption is weak in the same solvent. For environmental analysis the strong hydrophobic, nonspecific adsorption can be employed for capturing the analyte from a large volume of water, which is passed through the column. A subsequent solvent switch assures a selective MISPE method. This protocol was first introduced for extraction of simazine[31] and later used for extraction of chlorotriazines,[32] chlorinated phenoxyacids,[33] 4-nitrophenol[34,35] and bisphenol A[36] from environmental water samples.

Due to the often, strong affinity between imprint and analyte, difficulties in effecting quantitative elution of the analyte have been encountered for some systems. This is most pronounced for extraction of compounds with an amino functionality on methacrylic acid type MIPs. Eluents used in these instances consists typically of acetonitrile or methanol containing acetic acid, trifluoroacetic acid or triethylamine, sometimes in high percentages. For neutral compounds, weak acids and weak bases, however, complete elution may occur simply by treatment with polar solvents or mixtures of polar solvents and water.

Solid-Phase Extraction Applications

Various off-line SPE techniques, not the least those in 96-well format arrays for parallel extraction of large sample batches, are the more popular approaches with respect to the number of samples processed in routine sample preconcentration. Likewise, the majority of studies into MISPE have used cartridges or columns off-line from the downstream analytical separation. Previously, preMISPE transfer of analyte to an organic solvent prior to a MIP extraction protocol using optimal conditions was a common approach. The current trend uses extraction protocols, which are based on direct loading of the aqueous sample, a water-to-solvent switch on-column prior to selective elution using a solvent containing acid or base (Fig 4). As discussed above the purpose is to first quantitatively trap the analyte from the aqueous sample and then change the solvent to one in which the imprints bind the analyte in a highly selective manner, and in which nonspecific MIP-analyte adsorption is weak or absent. This approach has been studied in detail for extraction of clenbuterol from urine,[37] bupivacaine[16] and phenytoin[38] from plasma, chlorotriazines[32] and phenoxy acids[33] from environmental water and quercetin from red wine.[39]

Several on-line systems have been demonstrated. These include both systems where the MIP column is placed after a trapping column, which captures the analyte from the sample for subsequent transfer to the MIP column using an organic solvent, and those where the sample is injected directly on the MIP column. Both systems use the water-to-solvent switch approach discussed above. An example of the first type is a RAM-MIP-LC-MS system for determination of nine triazines in river water samples.[40] Restricted access materials (RAM) combine size exclusion and adsorption chromatography.[41] The material has a hydrophilic outer surface, which permits high molecular weight humic substances and large proteins to flow though the column without retention. Small molecules, which can enter the pores, are retained on the hydrophobic inner surface. The water sample was injected on the RAM column, which reduced the concentration of matrix components. A solvent switch to acetonitrile transferred the analytes into the MIP column, which selectively retained the triazines whereas residual matrix molecules were not retained and separated completely. The cleaned and enriched extract was subsequently eluted with methanol-water-acetic acid to a C18 column and analysed by LC-MS. A similar system was developed for determination of tramadol in human serum.[42] An example of the latter type where the sample is injected directly on the MIP column is the selective on-line MISPE of nitrophenol from spiked river water samples.[34,35] Following acidification to pH 2.5, the sample was applied to the MIP-column. A solvent switch to dichloromethane removed nonspecifically bound compounds, including other phenolic structures, and strengthened the selective imprint-nitrophenol binding. Finally, the analyte was eluted and transferred to the analytical column by acetonitrile containing 1% acetic acid.

A separation system consisting of a MIP with restricted access properties in-line with a conventional C18-column has been used for direct injection of serum and determination of ibuprofen and naproxen.[17] The MIP material was prepared by an initial multistep swelling and thermal polymerisation protocol using 4-vinylpyridine as the functional monomer, followed by coating of the external surface of the polymer particles with an external hydrophilic layer by a second polymerisation of a mixture of glycerol monomethacrylate and glycerol dimethacrylate. Plasma samples were injected directly on the restricted access-MIP column and proteinaceous components washed away. Then, a mixture of phosphate buffer pH 7.3 and 25% acetonitrile eluted the analyte and transfer it to the analytical reversed phase column. Template bleeding prevented accurate determination of the drug, a problem that could be overcome by the use of a restricted access-MIP prepared against naproxen for determination of ibuprofen. By this approach ibuprofen was determined in a pharmacokinetic study in rat plasma with good precision and accuracy, and the column could be used for up to 500 injections.

Provided the extraction is sufficiently selective, the downstream analytical separation can be omitted and the analyte eluted directly to the detector for quantitation. The most well-studied system uses a MIP micro-column and direct in-line UV-detection. The protocol, which is termed MISPE with differential pulsed elution, was used to determine theophylline in human serum.[43-45] Following extraction of the serum sample with chloroform, an aliquot of the organic layer was injected into a theophylline-selective MIP micro-column using chloroform as the mobile phase. An intermediate wash step using a pulse of acetonitrile removed nonspecifically adsorbed interferents, and a pulse of methanol desorbed quantitatively the bound theophylline for in-line UV determination. More polar substances, such as nicotine, were more strongly bound to the respective imprints and acetonitrile could be used as the mobile phase.[46] In this instance, the sample was injected dissolved in methanol, the column was washed with a pulse of methanol and the analyte eluted with 1% TFA in water.

Conclusion and Future Work

Already, a number of highly selective preconcentrations of biological and environmental samples have been reported, where several studies have made direct comparisons with conventional extraction materials and demonstrated superior cleanup using the MIP material.[16,32-35] Compared with immunoaffinity columns MIPs have the advantage of superior stability over a wide range of buffer pH, solvent, temperature and pressure conditions. This provides great flexibility in finding best experimental conditions for good sample cleanup. Since semi-irreversibly trapped template molecules are inherent to the imprinting process, template bleeding must be addressed in each method development. Improved imprinting chemistries and more efficient extraction protocols to reduce template bleeding are warranted. While imprinting of an analyte analogue circumvents the problem rather than solves it, presently this approach may in many instances be vital to successful use of MISPE in trace analysis. Given the very clean extracts often obtained, MISPE with direct detection of the analyte following elution is appealing as it eliminates the need for an analytical column. In many instances, this would simplify the overall separation system and increase speed of analysis. Often, imprints have very high affinity for the analyte, which gives rise to slow dissociation kinetics, and a present limitation may be the large elution volumes often required. Notwithstanding, these challenges are addressable and molecular-imprint based solid phase extraction will likely develop into a viable alternative for environmental and bio-sample analysis.

References

1. In: Poole CF, Wilson ID, eds. Special issue on solid-phase extraction. J Chromatogr A 2000:885.
2. Hennion M-C. Solid-phase extraction: Method development, sorbents, and coupling with liquid chromatography. J Chromatogr A 1999; 856:3-54.
3. Martinez D, Cugat MJ, Borull F et al. Solid-phase extraction coupling to capillary electrophoresis with emphasis on environmental analysis. J Chromatogr A 2000; 902:65-89.
4. Masqué N, Marcé RM, Borrull F. New polymeric and other types of sorbents for solid-phase extraction of polar organic micropollutants from environmental water. Trends Anal Chem 1998; 17:384-394.
5. Ferrer I, Barceló D. Validation of new solid-phase extraction materials for the selective enrichment of organic contaminants from environmental samples. Trends Anal Chem 1999; 18:180-192.

6. Pichon V, Bouzige M, Miege C et al. Immunosorbents: Natural molecular recognition elements for sample preparation of comlex environmental matrices. Trends Anal Chem 1999; 18:219-235.
7. Stevenson D, Immuno-affinity solid-phase extraction. J Chromatogr B 2000; 745:39-48.
8. In: Sellergren B, ed. Molecularly imprinted polymers. Man-made mimics of antibodies and their applications in analytical chemistry. Elsevier, Amsterdam: The Netherlands, 2001.
9. In: Bartsch RA, Maeda M, eds. Molecular and ionic recognition with imprinted polymers. ACS Symposium Series 703. Washington DC, USA: American Chemical Society, 1998
10. Wulff G, Molecular imprinting in cross-linked materials with the aid of molecular templates – A way towards artificial antibodies. Angew Chem Int Ed Engl 1995; 34:1812-1832.
11. Mosbach K, Ramström O. The emerging technique of molecular imprinting and its future impact on biotechnology. Bio/Technology 1996; 14:163-170.
12. Andersson LI, Paprica A, Arvidsson T. A highly selective solid phase extraction sorbent for preconcentration of sameridine made by molecular imprinting. Chromatographia 1997; 46:57-62.
13. Rashid BA, Briggs RJ, Hay JN et al. Preliminary evaluation of a molecular imprinted polymer for solid-phase extraction of tamoxifen. Anal Commun 1997; 34:303-305.
14. Venn RF, Goody RJ. Synthesis and properties of molecular imprints of darifenacin: The potential of molecular imprinting for bioanalysis. Chromatographia 1999; 50:407-414.
15. Berggren C, Bayoudh S, Sherrington D et al. Use of molecularly imprinted solid-phase extraction for the selectivce clean-up of clenbuterol from calf urine. J Chromatogr A 2000; 889:105-110.
16. Andersson LI. Efficient sample preconcentration of bupivacaine from human plasma by solid-phase extraction on molecularly imprinted polymers. Analyst 2000; 125:1515-1517.
17. Haginaka J, Sanbe H. Uniform-sized molecularly imprinted polymers for 2-arylpropionic acid derivatives selectively modified with hydrophilic external layer and their applications to direct serum injection analysis. Anal Chem 2000; 72:5206-5210.
18. Crescenzi C, Bayoudh S, Cormack PAG et al. Determination of clenbuterol in bovine liver by combining matrix solid-phase dispersion and molecularly imprinted solid-phase extraction followed by liquid chromatography/electrospray ion trap multiple-stage mass spectrometry. Anal Chem 2001; 73:2171-2177.
19. Ellwanger A, Berggren C, Bayoudh S et al. Evaluation of methods aimed at complete removal of template from molecularly imprinted polymers. Analyst 2001; 126:784-792.
20. Matsui J, Fujiwara K, Takeuchi T. Atrazine-selective polymers prepared by molecular imprinting of trialkylmelamines as dummy template species of atrazine. Anal Chem 2000; 72:1810-1813.
21. Matsui J, Fujiwara K, Ugata S et al. Solid-phase extraction with a dibutylmelamine-imprinted polymer as triazine herbicide-selective sorbent. J Chromatogr A 2000; 889:25-31.
22. Andersson LI, Abdel-Rehim M, Nicklasson L et al. Towards molecular-imprint based SPE of local anaestethics. Chromatographia 2002; 55:S-65-S-69.
23. Koster EHM, Crescenzi C, Den Hoedt W et al. Fibers coated with molecularly imprinted polymers for solid-phase microextraction. Anal Chem 2001; 73:3140-3145.
24. Möller K, Nilsson U, Crescenzi C et al. Synthesis and evaluation of molecularly imprinted polymers for extracting hydrolysis products of organophosphate flame retardants. J Chromatogr A 2001; 938:121-130.
25. Theodoridis G, Kantifes A, Manesiotis P. Tsoukali-Papadopoulou H, Preparation of a molecularly imprinted polymer for the solid-phase extraction of scopolamine with hyoscyamine as a dummy template molecule. J Chromatogr A 2003; 987:103-109.
26. Sellergren B, The noncovalent approach to molecular imprinting. In: Sellergren B, ed. Molecularly imprinted polymers. Man-made mimics of antibodies and their applications in analytical chemistry. Elsevier, Amsterdam, The Netherlands, 2001:113-184.
27. Spivak D, Gilmore MA, Shea KJ. Evaluation of binding and origins of specificity of 9-ethyladenine imprinted polymers. J Am Chem Soc 1997; 119:4388-4393.
28. Karlsson J, Andersson LI, Nicholls IA. Probing the molecular basis for ligand-selective recognition in molecularly imprinted polymers selective for the local anaesthetic bupivacaine. Anal Chim Acta 2001; 435:57-64.
29. Andersson LI. Application of molecular imprinting to the development of aqueous buffer and organic solvent based radioligand binding assays for S-propranolol. Anal Chem 1996; 68:111-115.
30. Haupt K, Dzgoev A, Mosbach K. Assay system for the herbicide 2,4-dichlorophenoxyacetic acid using a molecularly imprinted polymer as an artficial recognition element. Anal Chem 1998; 70:628-631.
31. Matsui J, Okada M, Tsuruoka M et al. Solid-phase extraction of a triazine herbicide using a molecularly imprinted synthetic receptor. Anal Commun 1997; 34:85-87.

32. Ferrer I, Lanza F, Tolokan A et al. Selective trace enrichment of chlorotriazine pesticides from natural waters and sediment samples using terbutylazine molecularly imprinted polymers. Anal Chem 2000; 72:3934-3941.
33. Baggiani C, Giovannoli C, Anfossi L et al. Molecularly imprinted solid-phase extraction sorbent for the cleanup of chlorinated phenoxyacids from aqueous samples. J Chromatogr A 2001; 938:35-44.
34. Masqué N, Marce RM, Borrull F et al. Synthesis and evaluation of a molecularly imprinted polymer for selective on-line solid-phase extraction of 4-nitrophenol from environmental water. Anal Chem 2000; 72:4122-4126.
35. Caro E, Masque N, Marcé RM et al. Noncovalent and semi-covalent molecularly imprinted polymers for selective on-line solid-phase extraction of 4-nitrophenol from water samples. J Chromatogr A 2002; 963:169-178.
36. Kubo T, Hosoya K, Watabe Y et al. On-column concentration of bisphenol A with one-step removal of humic acids in water. J Chromatogr A 2003; 987:389-394.
37. Blomgren A, Berggren C, Holmberg A et al. Extraction of clenbuterol from calf urine using a molecularly imprinted polymer followed by quantitation by high-performance liquid chromatography with UV detection. J Chromatogr A 2002; 975:157-164.
38. Bereczki A, Tolokan A, Horvai G et al. Determination of phenytoin in plasma by molecularly imprinted solid-phase extraction. J Chromatogr A 2001; 930:31-38.
39. Molinelli A, Weiss R, Mizaikoff B. Advanced solid phase extraction using molecularly imprinted polymers for the determination of quercetin in red wine. J Agric Food Chem 2002; 50:1804-1808.
40. Koeber R, Fleischer C, Lanza F et al. Evaluation od a multidimensional solid-phase extraction platform for highly selective on-line cleanup and high-throughput LC-MS analysis of triazines in river water samples using molecularly imprinted polymers. Anal Chem 2001; 73:2437-2444.
41. Boos K-S, Grimm C-H. High-performance liquid chromatography integrated solid-phase extraction in bioanalysis using restricted access precolumn packings. Trends Anal Chem 1999; 18:175-180.
42. Boos K-S, Fleischer CT. Multidimensional on-line solid-phase extraction (SPE) using restricted access materials (RAM) in combination with molecularly imprinted polymers (MIP). Fresenius J Anal Chem 2001; 371:16-20.
43. Mullett WM, Lai EPC. Determination of theophylline in serum by molecularly imprinted solid-phase extraction with pulsed elution. Anal Chem 1998; 70:3636-3641.
44. Mullett WM, Lai EPC. Molecularly imprinted solid phase extraction micro-column with differential pulsed elution for theophylline determination. Microchem J 1999; 61:143-155.
45. Mullett WM, Lai EPC. Rapid determination of theophylline in serum by selective extraction using a heated molecularly imprinted polymer micro-column with differential pulsed elution. J Pharm Biomed Anal. 1999; 21:835-843.
46. Mullett WM, Lai EPC, Sellergren B. Determination of nicotine in tobacco by molecularly imprinted solid phase extraction with differential pulsed elution. Anal Commun 1999; 36:217-220.

CHAPTER 11

Imprinted Polymers in Capillary Electrophoresis and Capillary Electrochromatography

Alessandra Bossi, Pier Giorgio Righetti and Staffan Nilsson

Abstract

The use of molecularly imprinted polymers (MIPs) as sorbents in capillary electrophoresis (CE) and capillary electrochromatography (CEC) is an attractive way to combine the high selectivity offered by MIPs with the high separation efficiency (10^6 theoretical plates) and short time of analysis (a few minutes) typical of capillary electrophoresis. An overview of the methods proposed for derivatising the capillary column with MIP-stationary phases is given: from bulk polymerization of MIP directly in the capillary to the most recent micro- and nano-spheres of MIPs for filling the capillary. Examples of applications of imprinting technology applied to capillary electrophoresis are indicated and some future developments are discussed.

Introduction

Capillary electrophoresis (CE) is acknowledged as a powerful analytical technique, nowadays largely employed in clinical monitoring, diagnostics, forensic science, environmental analysis, quality control in food and beverages, pharmaceutical industry.[1] Inherent advantages that contributed significantly to the large dissemination of CE techniques are the high selectivity, the high efficiency, the short time of analysis, the low consumption of analytes and chemicals and the full automation.

CE offers a broad choice of separation modes (Table 1). Particular interest is in affinity capillary electrophoresis (ACE) methods, in which sorbents with specific recognition properties are used. ACE allows the achievement of very high selectivity, thus meeting the needs of e.g., environmental control, where qualitative and quantitative analysis are preferably conducted on rough samples, or fulfilling the requirements of pharmaceutical industry dealing with chiral discrimination.

Affinity separation methods in CE were firstly developed by using bio-components as selector.[2-5] However, the problems of grafting biological molecules onto support matrices, the stability of such affinity-biomaterials to the field strength and to temperature gradients, as well as technical problems of bubble formation or replacement of the bio-affinity material in the column limited the expansion of ACE.

Achieving predetermined selectivity with the technology of molecular imprinting appeared a promising way to impart the desired selection properties to the sorbent. Therefore, the combination of MIP and CE started being explored from 1994 as an approach full of potentials. The separation of analytes with MIPs is classified as capillary electrochromatography (CEC).

Molecular Imprinting of Polymers, edited by Sergey Piletsky and Anthony Turner.
©2006 Landes Bioscience.

Table 1. CE: methodologies and applications

Methodology	Mechanism and Applications
Capillary zone electrophoresis (CZE)	Separation based on the difference of mobility of the analytes. Peptide mapping[42] Conformational studies of protein folding[43]
Micellar electrokinetic chromatography (MEKC)	Partition between a micellar system and a mobile phase. Determination of biogenic amines[44] Separation and determination of nalidixic acid and its metabolites in serum and urine[45]
Capillary electrochromatography (CEC)	Partition between two phases: a stationary phase, like a packed particulate inside the column, or a polymeric phase attached to the capillary walls and a mobile phase, i.e., the background electrolyte. Chiral discrimination[46]
Affinity capillary electrophoresis (ACE)	Specific interaction between the analyte and a biocomponent (soluble or fixed to a matrix). Determination of binding constants of ligands to receptors[5]
Isoelectric focusing in CE (cIEF)	A gradient of pH is established in the capillary column and proteins and peptides are separated on the basis of their isoelectric point. Analysis of protein phosphorylation by cIEF-electrospray ionisation- mass spectrometry[47]
CE in sieving liquid polymers	Based on the retardation in the migration due to the sieve effect of the polymeric phase that fills the capillary. Nucleic acid sequencing[48]

Figure 1 reports a chart of the research on MIPs in CE: the number of original papers on imprinted polymers combined with capillary electrochromatography (MIP-CEC) published up to November 2002 are plotted per year.

The number of papers published on the subject is quite small. In 1994 MIP-CEC was proposed as 'premiere', catching the attention of researchers. By 1997 an outbreak of MIP-CEC scientific contributions was registered, but the excitement was silenced by the difficulties encountered in transferring directly the state of the art in polymer preparation into the capillary columns and by the problems posed by the exposure of MIPs to high electric field strengths, i.e., bubble formation, charge repulsion, deformation of the recognition sites.

Over the last few years, intense studies on microscale control of the polymerization and on physicochemical characterization of polymeric phases have been conducted. Such studies were mainly motivated by the burgeoning interest in miniaturization, in chips and in microfluidic systems. At the same time, rules for rational design of MIPs have been indicated recently.[6-8] Thus, the knowledge that has been reached under the flourishing of these research interests has allowed a new start in the field of MIP-CEC with a more solid background that might contribute substantially to make MIP-CEC a competitive technology.

In this chapter, an account of the original research papers on MIP-CEC, with evolutions and drawbacks is given.

The Separation in Capillary Electrophoresis and in Capillary Electrochromatography

Electrophoresis is the migration of charged solutes in solvent under the influence of an electric field.[9] Capillary electrophoresis (CE), firstly developed by Virtanen (10) and then

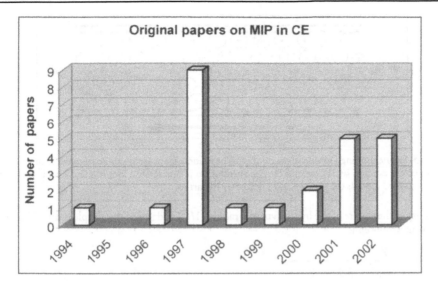

Figure 1. Trend in the research on MIP combined with CEC.

modified to the actual state by Jorgenson and Lukas (11 and 12), is the electrophoresis performed into a capillary tube, as shown schematically in Figure 2. Typical aspects of the technique are the column of capillary dimensions (10-100 μm) and use of high voltage (5-30 kV).

In CE, the separation is governed by the difference in electrophoretic mobilities of the solutes placed under the electric field, which is proportional to the charge/mass ratio of the analyte and depends on the applied field strength, on the pH, on the conductivity of the separation buffer. Although the electrophoretic mobility is usually described with the following equation:

$$\mu = \frac{Z}{6\pi\eta r} \tag{1}$$

where μ is the mobility, Z the net charge, r the radius of the analyte, η the viscosity of the separation medium, recently the equation has been corrected assessing a dependence of the

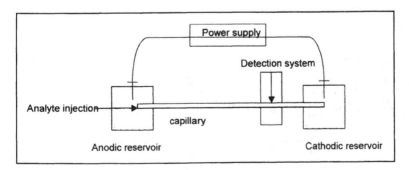

Figure 2. Scheme of the CE apparatus. During the separation, a high voltage is applied across the capillary ends, which are dipped in the electrolyte solution, thus forcing analytes to travel through the column, reaching the detector.

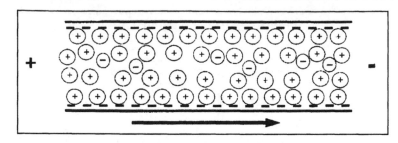

Figure 3. Picture showing a section of the capillary. The silanol groups are highly deprotonated, the negative charge on the capillary walls generates the electroendosmotic flow (EOF). Ions inside the capillary lumen are transported towards the cathode, as indicated by the arrow.

mobility of the square of the hydrodynamic radius ($1/r^2$) and not to the simple radius. The new equation proposed is:

$$\mu = \frac{Z}{6\pi\eta r^2} \times \frac{1}{3.30 \times 10^7 \sqrt{I}} \qquad (2)$$

where I is the ionic strength.[13]

Valuable characteristics of CE are the high selectivity, high efficiency (often theoretical plates as high as 10^6), short time of analysis (few minutes), minute amount of sample (nl) and the low amount of solvents required (μl).

Columns are typically made of silica, thus silanols are exposed at the inner surface of the capillaries. The silanols dissociate with a pK of 6.3 to negative charged species fixed to the capillary walls, thus generating of an electroendosmotic flow (EOF) that drives positively charged solutes towards the cathode, when voltage is applied.[14] The EOF is shown in Figure 3. The entity of the EOF in the silica capillaries is shown in Figure 4.

In capillary electrochromatography (CEC) the EOF is utilised to drive the solutes along the separation column, as first demonstrated by Pretorius.[15] In recent years, electrochromatography refers to the technique that uses electroosmosis (for the most part), instead of pressuredriven flows, to transport the solvent and solutes through a capillary column, hence the name capillary electrochromatography. The separation mechanism is primarily based on differential inter-

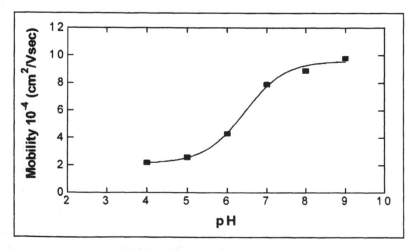

Figure 4. Electroosmotic flow as function of the pH in silica fused columns. Applied voltage 15 kV.

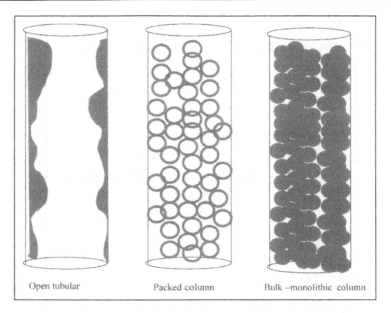

Figure 5. Modified capillary columns for CEC: 1) open tubular, 2) bulk polymerization or monolithic phase, 3) packed columns.

actions (e.g., partitioning) between two phases; if the analyte is charged, electrophoresis will also have a main contribution to the separation. The interest in CEC results from the possibility of performing analytical separations by using electrically driven flows on chromatographic beds. The electric field is applied across the capillary column, as in case of CE, generating a flow of liquid (i.e., the EOF). The EOF carries the solvent and the solutes through the column. The solutes are separated on the basis of their differential interaction between two phases inside the column, typically a stationary and a mobile phase. As shown in Figure 5, capillary columns can be packed with particulate material that contains the stationary phase (packed-CEC), or the stationary phase can be attached to the inner walls of the capillary (open tubular, OT-CEC), or the stationary phase can be polymerized in situ generating a monolithic phase (bulk phase). Basically CEC is a hybrid of CE and HPLC and MIP-CE can be classified as a particular type of CEC.

Column Derivatization Chemistry

Open tubular phases and bulk polymeric phases are most often anchored to the walls of the capillary column with covalent bonds. The modification of the silica surface of the capillaries is obtained by organosilanization, by exploiting the silane-coupling procedures available from high performance liquid chromatography.[16]

Fused silica capillaries are typically reacted with organosilanes to yield a Si-R functionally attached to the support (Fig. 6A). Organosilanes have two different types of reactive groups: the first one, X, couples the Si-OH of the walls and the second group, R, is incorporated in the growing polymer.

In order to improve the efficiency and the reproducibility of the coating procedure pretreatments with alkali are suggested for maximizing the number of free hydroxyl groups (Si-OH) and heat and vacuum treatments are suggested for removing the residual water adsorbed onto the surface of the capillary, which is cause of auto-polymerisation of organosilanes.

The silanization is commonly carried out with tri-functional organosilane agents, with general formula R_1-Si-X_3, as shown in the reaction scheme of Figure 6B, with X triethoxy- or

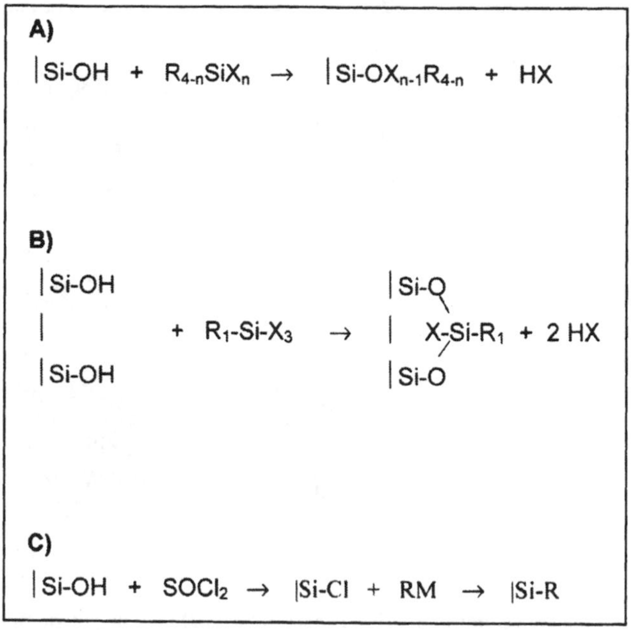

A)

$$|Si\text{-}OH + R_{4\text{-}n}SiX_n \rightarrow |Si\text{-}OX_{n\text{-}1}R_{4\text{-}n} + HX$$

B)

$$
\begin{array}{ccc}
|Si\text{-}OH & & |Si\text{-}O \\
| & + R_1\text{-}Si\text{-}X_3 \rightarrow & | \quad X\text{-}Si\text{-}R_1 + 2\,HX \\
|Si\text{-}OH & & |Si\text{-}O
\end{array}
$$

C)

$$|Si\text{-}OH + SOCl_2 \rightarrow |Si\text{-}Cl + RM \rightarrow |Si\text{-}R$$

Figure 6. Reactions used for the modification of the silica capillaries. A) General scheme of the reaction between an organosilane and the silica wall. R is an alkyl or substituted alkyl group, X is an easily hydrolyzable group such as halide, amine, alkoxy etc., n ranges between 1 and 3, and the vertical line represents the support surface. B) Modification of the silica wall via trifunctional organosilane and formation of a siloxane bond (SI-O-C), X is often a triethoxy- or trimethoxy- group; R is a function with a double bond, which provides anchorage point for the polymer. C) Modification of the silica wall via Grignard and formation of a direct SI-C bond. M is lithium or MgBr and contains a terminal double bond for the anchorage of the polymer to the capillary wall.

trimethoxy-; R is a function with a double bond, which provides covalent anchorage for MIPs or for control (blank) polymers. Such derivatization method originates siloxane bonds (Si-O-Si-C) onto the walls, which in turn are subjected to hydrolysis under alkaline or weak acidic conditions. An alternative approach for the modification of the silica walls of the capillaries makes use of monofunctional reagents in a two-step reaction which leads to the formation of direct Si-C bonds, which is far more stable to hydrolysis than siloxane bonds.[17,18] In such modification route, silanols are first treated with a chlorinated agent (e.g., thionyl-chloride), then a reaction with an alkylating reagent follows (Fig. 6C). Suitable alkylating reagents are Grignard or organolithium compounds.

The Traditional, Bulk Polymer Approach

The first monolithic polymer prepared with an imprinting approach was reported in 1994.[19] A methacrylic acid polymer was prepared in situ, using a dispersion-precipitation polymerization, in which the monomers are soluble but not the polymer.[20] The polymer consisted of micron-sized agglomerates, or sub-micron particles, with microporous or mesoporous morphology, as shown in Figure 7. The monolithic phase was anchored to the capillary walls through trimethoxysilyl-propyl-methacrylate with a polymerization carried out for 24 hours in porogen solvent (cyclohexanol:dodecanol or isopropanol). Templates were: pentamidine, benzamidine, L-phenylalanine-anilide. The monolithic polymer seemed to last several weeks, thus displaying a fairly high stability, but no enantioselection was observed (the monolithic polymer was unable to discriminate between L and D-phenylalanine). The lack of enatiodiscrimination could

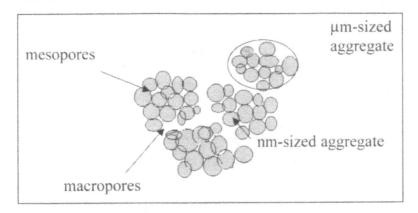

Figure 7. Structure of a macroporous monolithic polymer obtained via dispersion-precipitation bulk-polymerization. The monolith presents microaggregates of 100-200 nm dimensions and containing micropores (5-15 nm), which are clustered into macroaggregates (micro-sized), containing a system of mesopores (20-50 nm). Good flow-through properties of the polymer are assured by the macropores (50-1000 nm) between the macroaggregates.

be ascribed to a low ratio crosslinkers to monomers employed, chosen to facilitate the passage of the solvent through the capillary, that made the monolith too soft and flexible, thus corrupting the fidelity of the imprinted cavities.

It were Lin and colleagues, who first reported on a MIP-CEC monolith for the successful separation of enantiomers.[21] The capillary was activated via a Grignard reaction. An in situ bulk polymerization of template (L-phenylanaline-anilide), functional monomers (MAA and/ or 2-vinylpiridine) and crosslinker (EGDMA) took place in chloroform by thermal initiation at 60°C and was continued for 24 h.

Bubble formation and shrinkage in the volume of the polymer were frequently observed during the phase transition in the polymerization process and the absorbance of the analyte was suppressed by the polymer high UV absorbance. Consequently, the authors proposed a quite ingenious way for overcoming such problems. In their experimental set-up, reported in Figure 8, the separation column consists in two portions: the first one is MIP-derivatized, the second one is an empty capillary filled with buffer. The two portions are joined together with a Teflon sleeve. The detector is placed 5 mm behind the connection, on the empty capillary. The system is of course valid for avoiding the polymer UV-absorption, but is rather complicated and suffers from vaporization of the solvents at the connection; not surprisingly the authors declare a poor repeatability of the system.

The selectivity of the bulk-polymer column was tested with the discrimination between D and L-phenylalanine, as shown in Figure 9. The enantiomers were baseline separated. The resolution of D, L-phenylalanine was explored as function of the rigidity of the polymer showing an optimum (Rs 1.15) for a 5:1 molar ration crosslinker: monomer, which accounts for a balance between flexibility and rigidity of the polymer. The runs were performed in acidified organic solvent (acetonitrile: water: acetic acid 80:10:10). The field strength plays a crucial role in the separation: optimal field strength was 400 V/cm, while lower resulted in no separation and peak broadening.

Packed Columns

Apart from the in situ polymerization, a widely used method for preparing MIP columns for conventional chromatography is to synthesize a monolithic MIP, then grind the polymer and sieve the particles for obtaining homogeneous particulate, which is used to pack the columns. Lin et al[22] prepared MIPs using L-phenylalanine and its anilide derivative as templates.

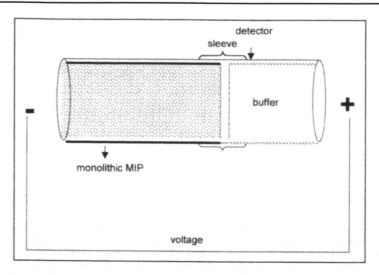

Figure 8. Scheme of the capillary column derived from Lin et al.[21] In the first part of a capillary a bulk, monolitihic MIP was polymerized. An empty portion of the capillary was connected to the monolithic part via teflon sleeves. The empty portion was placed on the detector window. Racemic mixtures of aminoacids were successfully separated on the present MIP-CEC.

The bulk polymer was ground and sieved to particles with diameter of <10 μm and packed in the capillary column for CEC, by using a slurry method. A short plug of polyacrylamide gel served as a retaining frit for holding the particles in the column.

The synthesis of bulk polymers is relatively straightforward, but the packing of the columns needs retaining frits, which are difficult to fabricate (nowadays frits are normally made of silicate) and often contribute to bubble formation within the column. Another drawback of the bulk grinding is the irregularity of the shape of the sieved particles that limits the efficiency of the column.

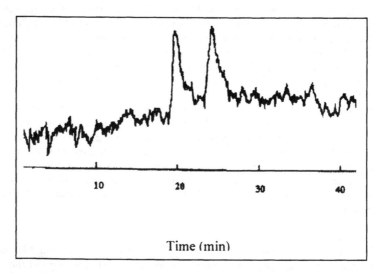

Figure 9. A typical electropherogram obtained injecting a racemic mixtures of phenylalanine in the MIP-CEC column showed in Figure 14. Running conditions were: acetonitrile: water: acetic acid 80:10:10 (v/v), field strength 400 V/cm. Adapted from Lin et al. [21]

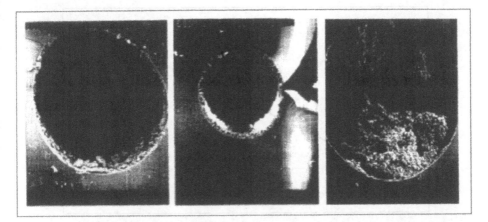

Figure 10. Electron microscopy disclosed information on the morphology of the MIP-monolithic polymers produced by Brueggeman and colleagues: the more efficient polymers were superporous (adapted from ref. 23).

Polymer Technology for MIP-CEC

Brueggeman and colleagues concentrated on polymer technology aspects for MIP-CE.[23] The needs and requirements in morphology of the imprinted polymers for CE separations were studied. Some conditions were found for producing MIPs inside the capillary, preserving the 'three-dimensional' quality of the polymers, so fundamental for the stereoselective interaction with the template and generating porosity, in order to facilitate the association/dissociation equilibrium of the analyte to the polymer.

Capillaries were first activated with the 'classic' 3-methacryloxypropyl-trimethoxy-silane to provide a monolayer of anchorage points on the capillary surface. Then, they were filled with a mixture of template (2-phenylpropionic acid), crosslinkers (DVB, EGDMA), acting also as functional monomers, and a porogen. The effect of hexane, THF, toluene, acetonitrile, chloroform, DMF, DMSO were investigated. Capillaries were sealed and let react at 65°C for 48 hours. In late experiments *trans*-3-(3-pyridyl)-acrylic acid was introduced as interactive functional monomer. The morphology of all the polymer prepared was systematic investigated by electron microscopy (see Fig. 10).

As stated in the paper of Brueggeman: "the protocol for producing a thick but not too thick polymer was a matter of empirical recipes". Nevertheless, few valid guidelines for the preparation of efficient MIPs in CE can be derived from the experiments:

1. the thickness of the coating is linearly linked to the concentration of crosslinker (e.g., Fig. 11 indicate that 15% crosslinker produces a 2 μm coating);
2. the rigidity of the polymer depends on the concentration of the crosslinker;
3. a highly porous structure is effectively generated by making use of the dispersion polymerization strategy, which is based on a polymerization carried out in a solvent where the monomers are well soluble, while the growing polymer chains are not fully dissolved, yielding polymer coils that collapse and precipitate generating the superporosity.[20]

Superporous MIP and the Hydrodynamic Pressure

The group of Nilsson gave to the MIP-CE technology a turn.[24] The benefits of MIPs in CE, i.e., entailing a determined selectivity to the column for chiral discrimination, were known, but these authors searched for effective solutions for quickly removing unreacted species, replacing the electrolyte in the capillary and flushing the column to get rid of bubbles. In this respect, rigid polymer structures were the best to withstand pressure, while good flow-through properties were required to the polymer for hydrodynamic pumping. Both requirements met in the superporous, monolithic MIP proposed.

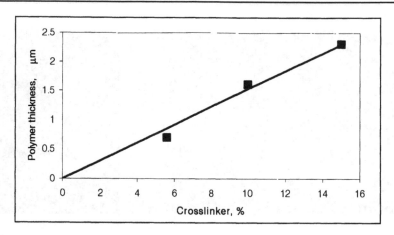

Figure 11. Dependence of the thickness of the coating on the concentration of crosslinker employed (modified from 23).

The recipe for monolithic columns copolymerizes MAA with TRIM 10:1 mol/L and template (metoprolol or propranolol) in toluene on silanized columns. Interestingly, the authors make use of a photoinitiated polymerization, by photodecomposition of AIBN upon exposure to UV light (350 nm) for 80 min. Photoinitiation allowed a more precise control of the polymerization. Moreover, the polymer was prepared at -20°C, as low temperature favors fidelity in the imprinting.[25] Upon scanning electron micrograph (Fig. 12) the monolithic polymers showed aggregates of micrometer size globular particles surrounded by 1-20 μm wide interconnected superpores, which permitted bulk flow throughout the capillary length. The small size of the globular units, 0.5-1 μm, provides good diffusion properties and thus rapid access of the sample to the imprinted sites in the globules. Enantiomeric separations were obtained with Rs > 1, as shown in Figure 13. Worth to note are the extremely appealing separation times, i.e., within few minutes.

MIP Nanoparticles

The latest type of MIP-phase introduced consists of micron-sized nano-particles, shown in (Fig. 14), obtained via a precipitation-polymerization procedure similar to those used for the superporous polymers. In the polymerization of nano-particles, the monomer-crosslinker solution is highly diluted, so that each nucleation center does not enter in contact with other nucleation centers, thus inducing the formation of spherical particles, that reach a certain dimension and then precipitate.[26] MIP nano-particles are particularly convenient to use in partial filling technique, where scattering and absorbance can be avoided. In partial filling the particles are injected in the capillary as a plug in front of the sample, the mobility of the particle is opposite to the direction of the EOF. The mobility of the sample is in the same direction of the EOF. When the sample is injected, it migrates with the EOF, passes the nano-particles and reaches the detector prior the plug of nano-particles.[27] The nano-particles have the advantage of being easily replaced after each run and therefore are effective to avoid problems of column-ageing and poor results reproducibility. Another advantage is in principle that by mixing in the CE column MIP microparticles made for the recognition of different templates, it should be possible to obtain the simultaneous separation of multiple analytes in a single run.

Advantages and Disadvantages of MIP-CEC Separations

MIP-CEC offers in ideal case: exquisite selectivity, high number of theoretical plates, fast time of analysis, high resolution. Moreover, the electrical current applied to freshly polymerized

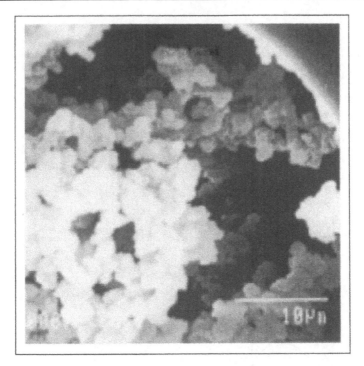

Figure 12. Electron scanning micrograph of the superporous MIP-phase proposed by Nilsson et al (modified from 24).

MIP-CEC columns is more effective in removing the template than the pressure in chromatography.[28]

Limitations in MIP-CEC are substantially the same encountered in the chromatographic use of imprinted polymers, thus principally separations suffers from severe tailoring of the template peak. Factors responsible for the tailoring are slow interaction kinetic between the template and the binding site [29] and the heterogeneous nature of the binding sites with respect of geometry and accessibility. Typically a nonlinear isotherm of adsorption describes the binding of the template to the MIP.[30] In practice tailing can be ameliorated to some extent by conducting the separations at high temperatures[24] and by using gradient elution. Tailoring problems hinder in particular separations carried out with packed columns, when polymers are made with the traditional bulk-polymerization approach, followed by grinding and microcolumn packing, because the shape of the particles is highly irregular.

Applications

In general MIP-CEC is used for separating small molecules, the specific interest being in drug separation. The task of MIP-CEC is chiral separation.[30] Table 2 gives a list of chiral compounds separated in MIP-CEC.

An inherent feature of the MIPs is that some cross-selectivity can occur between the template and compounds whose structures are closely related. The template will always be retained the most in the MIP and the specificity can be tuned to some degree during the recognition and by changing the cross-linking degree of the polymer.

The cross-selectivity is interesting as the MIP cavity act as an artificial receptor: a known drug is used as template to create the MIP-artificial receptor, then libraries of similar compounds can be screened on the MIP-CEC to find the compounds with similar or more

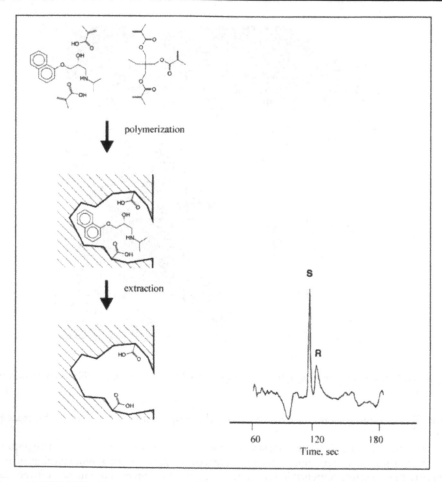

Figure 13. MIP-CEC with superporous monolithic polymers. The MIP was prepared in toluene by pho-
toinduced polymerization with (R)-propranolol as template (0.030 mol/L), MAA as functional monomers
(0.024 mol/L) and TRIM as crosslinker (0.024 mol/L). Template and non reacted monomers were efficiently removed by hydrodynamic pumping with acetonitrile. Running buffer was acetonitrile/acetate pH
3.0 (80:20); racemic mixtures of 100 μM propranolol were injected electrokinetically and separated at 30
kV applied voltage (875 V/cm). The enantiomers were baseline resolved with a Rs of 1.27.

favorable interaction characteristics. The concept was proven by a small library of structurally
similar tricyclic antidepressant drugs that was successfully separated onto MIP-CEC.[32]

Conclusions and Future Perspective

MIP-CEC is still under development. Research in the field demonstrated the feasibility of
polymerizing MIPs with specific recognition properties for CEC separations. Different techniques are available for preparing the MIPs: bulk polymerization of monolith followed by
grinding and packing capillaries, on-column polymerization of porous monoliths and the more
recent polymerization of nano-particles which are next packed or loaded into the capillary
column. MIP-CE allows high-resolution separations of analytes and of particular interest is the
application of MIP-CE to enantioseparation. Among the advantages of MIP-CE is the extremely low amount of template molecule required for the preparation of the polymer, which
makes the technique interesting for the separation of analytes which are purified in minute

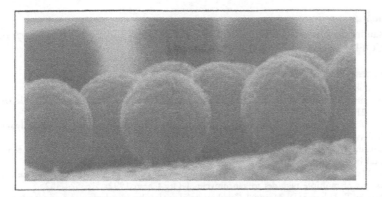

Figure 14. Scanning electron micrograph of MIP nanoparticles.

quantities from e.g., cells or tissues. MIP-CE is suitable also for the separation of expensive analytes, requiring minute amount of sample both for the preparation of the imprinted polymer and for the analysis. Still, typically the analyte used as template is separated with severe tailing in the peak on the MIP-CE.

The future of MIP-CE surely includes and benefits from the MIP nano-particles: being the microparticles replaced after each run, they offer the possibility of operating each time with 'fresh' MIP sorbents, moreover nano-particles can be used in partial filling techniques.

Future efforts would be directed towards multiple imprints for the preparation of oligo-selective or pluri-selective sorbents. Such an interesting possibility might be set up particularly with nanoparticle based MIPs, mixing different templated nanoparticles. Finally, most of the MIP-CE work is anticipative for downsizing the technology to the nanoscale. Chip technology with MIP sorbents would offer analytical chemistry a new powerful analytical tool and the possibility of parallel screening on different sorbents.

Table 2. Chiral separations reported in MIP-CE

Analytes	MIP Type
Beta-Adrenergic Agonists:	
Metoprolol, propranolol,	Superporous monolytic polymer[24]
atenolol propranolol	MIP-microparticles[33]
	Open-tubular column[34]
Aminoacids	
(phe, tyr, Phegly, trp, ser)	Bulk polymer ground into particles immobilised
	in the capillary using a polyacrylamide gel[21]
	Bulk polymer[35]
Aminoacid Derivatives:	
Dansyl-Phenylalanine	Open-tubular polymer[36]
Phenylalanine anilide	Silica coated with MIP, packed column[37]
Local Anesthetics:	
Ropivacaine, bupivacaine, mepivacaine	Superporous monolytic polymer[38]
Salbutamol	MIP microparticles[39,40]
Ephedrine	MIP microparticles[39,40]
2-phenylpropionic acid	Macroporous monolithic polymer[23]
Caffeine	Monolithic polymer[41]

Acknowledgements

Alessandra Bossi is grateful to the Ministry of Education and Research for supporting this paper (COFIN 2001; COFIN 2003).

References

1. Electrophoresis 2002; 23:3789-4052.
2. Guijt-van Duijn RM et al. Recent advances in affinity capillary electrophoresis. Electrophoresis 2000; 21:3905-18.
3. Baba Y et al. Specific base recognition of oligodeoxynucleotides using polyacrylamide poly(9-vyniladenine) conjugated gel. Anal Chem 1992; 64:1920-1925.
4. Birnbaum N, Nilsson S. Protein-based capillary affinity gel-electrophoresis for the separation of optical isomers. Anal Chem 1992; 64:2872-2874.
5. Chu YH, Whitesides GM. Affinity capillary electrophoresis can simultaneously measure binding constants of multiple peptides to vancomycin. J Org Chem 1992; 57:3524-3525.
6. Takeuchi T, Fukuma D, Matsui J Combinatorial molecular imprinting: An approach to synthetic polymer receptors. Anal Chem 1999; 71:285-290.
7. Piletsky SA et al. Recognition of ephedrine enantiomers by molecularly imprinted polymers designed using a computational approach Analyst 2001; 126:1826-1830.
8. Lanza F, Sellergren B. Method for synthesis and screening of large groups of molecularly imprinted polymers Anal Chem 1999; 71:2092-2096.
9. Tiselius AWK. Trans Farad Soc 1937; 33:524.
10. Virtanen R. Zone electrophoresis in a narrow-bore tube employing potentiometric detection. Theoretical and experimental study. Acta Polytech Scand Chem Incl Metall Ser 1974; 123:67.
11. Jorgenson JW, Lukacs KD. Zone electrophoresis in open tubular glass capillaries. Anal Chem 1981; 53:1298.
12. Jorgenson JW, Lukacs KD. Capillary zone electrophoresis. Science 1983; 222:266.
13. Cross RF, Wong MG. Electrophoretic mobilities and migrating analytes: Part 1: Relationships. J Cap Elec and Microchip Tech 2002; 7:119-124.
14. Bello MS, Capelli L, Righetti PG. Dependence of the electroosmotic mobility on the applied electric field and its reproducibility in capillary electrophoresis. J Chromatogr A 1994; 684:311-322.
15. Pretorius V, Hopkins BJ, Schieke JD. Electroosmosis: A new concept for high-speed liquid chromatography. J Chromatogr A 1974; 99:23-30.
16. In: Righetti PG, ed. Capillary Electrophoresis in Analytical Biotechnology. Boca Raton: CRC Press, 1996.
17. Simò-Alfonso E et al. Novel acrylamido monomers with higher hydrophilicity and improved hydrolytic stability. I: Synthetic route and product characterization. Electrophoresis 1996; 17:723-731.
18. Simò-Alfonso et al. Novel acrylamido monomers with higher hydrophilicity and improved hydrolytic stability. II: Properties of N-acryloyl amino propanol. Electrophoresis 1996; 17:732-737.
19. Nilsson NKG, Lindell O et al. Sellergren Imprinted polymers as antibody mimics and new affinity gels for selective separations in capillary electrophoresis. J Chromatogr A 1994; 680:57-61.
20. Sellergren B. Imprinted dispersion polymers: A new class of easily accessible affinity stationary phases. J Chromatogr A 1994; 673:133-141.
21. Lin JM et al. Molecularly imprinted polymer as chiral selector for enantioseparation of amino acids by capillary gel electrophoresis. Chromatographia 1996; 43:585-591.
22. Lin JM. Enantioseparation of d,l phenylalanine by molecularly imprinted polymer particles filled capillary electrochromatography. J Chromatogr Rel Technol 1997; 20:1489-1506.
23. Brueggemann O et al. Comparison of polymer coatings of capillary electrophoresis with respect to their applicability to molecular imprinting and electrochromatography. J Chromatogr A 1997; 781:43-53.
24. Schweitz L, Andersson LI, Nilsson S. Capillary electrochromatography with predetermined selectivity obtained through molecular imprinting. Anal Chem 1997; 69:1179-1183.
25. O'Shannessy DJ, Ekberg B, Mosbach K. Molecular imprinting of amino acid derivatives at low temperature (0°C) using photolytic homolysis of azobisnitriles. Anal Biochem 1989; 177:144-149.
26. Ye L, Cormack PAG, Mosbach K. Molecularly imprinted monodisperse microspheres for competitive radioassay. Anal Commun 1999; 36:35-37.
27. Spegel P, Schweitz L, Nilsson S. Molecularly imprinted microparticles for capillary electrochromatography: Studies on microparticle synthesis and electrolyte composition. Electrophoresis 2001; 22:3833-3841.
28. Lin et al. Capillary electrochromatographic separation of amino acid enantiomers with molecularly imprinted polymers as chiral recognition agents. Fresenius J Anal Chem 1997; 357:130-132.

29. 'O Brien et al. Mechanistic aspects of chiral discrimination on a molecular imprinted polymer phase. J Liq Chrom Rel Technol 1999; 22:283.
30. Sellergren B, Shea K. Origin of peak asymmetry and the effect of temperature on solute retention in enantiomers separations on imprinted chiral stationary phases. J Chromatogr A 1995; 690:29.
31. Gubitz G, Schmid MG. Recent progress in chiral separation principles in capillary electrophoresis. Electrophoresis 2000; 21:4112-4135.
32. Vallano ZT, Remcho VT. Proceedings of the 21st International Symposium on Capillary chromatography and electrophoresis. Park City, UT, USA: 1999.
33. Schweitz L, Spegel P, Nilsson S. Molecularly imprinted microparticles for capillary electrochromatographic enantiomer separation of propranolol. Analyst 2000; 125:1899-1901.
34. Schweitz L. Molecularly imprinted polymer coatings for open-tubular capillary electrochromatography prepared by surface initiation. Anal Chem 2002; 74:1192-1196.
35. Lin JM et al. Capillary electrochromatographic separation of amino acid enantiomers using on-column prepared molecularly imprinted polymer. J Pharmaceut Biomed Anal 1997; 15:1351-1358.
36. Tan ZJ, Remcho VT. Molecular imprint polymers as highly selective stationary phases for open tubular liquid chromatography and capillary electrophoresis. Electrophoresis 1998; 19:2055-2060.
37. Quaglia M et al. Surface initiated molecularly imprinted polymer films: A new approach in chiral capillary electrochromatography. Analyst 2001; 126:1495-1498.
38. Schweitz L, Andersson LI, Nilsson S. Capillary electrochromatography with molecular imprint-based selectivity for enantiomer separation of local anesthetics. J Chromatogr A 1997; 792:401-409.
39. de Boer T et al. Proceeding of the 1st workshop on molecularly imprinted polymers. Cardiff, UK: 2000.
40. de Boer T et al. Spherical molecularly imprinted polymer particles: A promising tool for molecular recognition in capillary electrokinetic separations. Electrophoresis 2002; 23:1296-1300.
41. Yan LS et al. Molecularly imprinted polymer monoliths prepared in capillaries by photoinitiated in situ polymerization for the screening of caffeine. Chem J Chin Univ 2001; 22:2008-2010.
42. Righetti PG et al. Capillary electrophoresis of peptides and proteins in acidic, isoelectric buffers: recent developments. J Biochem Biophys Methods 1999; 40:1-15.
43. Verzola B, Fogolari F, Righetti PG. Monitoring folding/unfolding transitions of proteins by capillary zone electrophoresis: Measurement of deltaG and its variation along the pH scale. Electrophoresis 2001; 22:3728-373.
44. Kovacs A, Simon-Sarkadi L, Ganzler K. Determination of biogenic amines by capillary electrophoresis. J Chromatogr A 1999; 836:305-313.
45. Perez-Ruiz T et al. Separation and simultaneous determination of nalidixic acid, hydroxynalidixic acid and carboxynalidixic acid in serum and urine by micellar electrokinetic capillary chromatography. J Chromatogr B Biomed Sci Appl 1999; 724:319-324.
46. Gübitz G, Schmidt MG. Chiral separation by chromatographic and electromigration techniques. A review. Biopharm Drug Dispos 2001; 22:291-336.
47. Wei J et al. High resolution analysis of protein phosphorylation using capillary isoelectric focusing –electrospray ionisation– mass spectrometry. Electrophoresis 1998; 19:2356-2360.
48. Righetti PG, Gelfi C. Capillary electrophoresis of DNA for molecular diagnostics. Electrophoresis 1997; 18:1709-1714.

Molecularly Imprinted Polymers in Drug Screening

Chris Allender

Introduction

Molecular imprinted polymers (MIPs) are no longer new materials. Three decades have passed since the early Mosbach and Wulff studies[1,2] and the technology is rapidly coming of age. However just what lies ahead for molecular imprinting is far from clear. A search of the literature reveals that researchers have applied molecular imprinting strategies to almost every conceivable problem requiring a molecular recognition solution. From sensors to SPE (solid phase extraction), from column chromatography to catalysis, MIPs have been applied with varying degrees of success.[3-8] One area of clear value, and one with a set of uniquely challenging and applicable problems, is drug discovery[9] and in particular the process of primary drug screening.

Within the pharmaceutical industry the current drug discovery philosophy is to prepare increasingly massive libraries of potential drug candidates and to then screen the whole population against a number of 'drug targets'. However, despite this approach resulting in huge increases in the number of individual primary screening events, the number of new drugs actually reaching the market has fallen. This trend is of considerable concern to the industry. There is constant pressure on researchers to increase throughput and to improve reliability. As a result high-throughput drug screening is perceived as an area amenable to new technologies and open to new ideas.[10]

The Drug Discovery Process

In general terms the drug discovery process can be divided into a number of sections:[11]
1. Synthesis or isolation of a lead compound (natural product or synthetic route)
2. Primary screening in vitro
3. Secondary screening, confirmation of target binding in native tissue in vivo or ex vivo
4. Pharmacokinetic study: absorption, distribution, metabolism and excretion (ADME) and drug stability
5. Pharmacodynamic in vivo validation of lead efficacy
6. Toxicology investigation into potential toxicity
7. Patient based clinical trials

A potential drug candidate can be eliminated from this process at any point and, highly significantly, the costs to a company of a failed candidate, in terms of both time and resources, increases at an almost exponential rate the further a candidate progresses. It is therefore hugely important to the pharmaceutical industry that compounds that are destined to be fail, are eliminated from the process at an early stage.

Molecular Imprinting of Polymers, edited by Sergey Piletsky and Anthony Turner.
©2006 Landes Bioscience.

In the 1970s and 1980s the rate limiting step in this process was the synthesis or isolation of new chemical entities. Increasingly this is changing and currently the slowest step is primary screening. The core reason for this change in emphasis has been the emergence of parallel or combinatorial synthesis.

The Rise of Combinatorial Chemistry and High-Throughput Screening

Historically, the synthesis of new drug candidates relied on application of the principles of rational drug design.[12,13] This involved the use of traditional medicinal chemistry to design and synthesis a molecule which would be extensively studied and logically modified through an iterative process that would ultimately give rise to a 'lead' compound. This process is commonly referred to as the study of structure activity relationships (SARs) and quantitative structure activity relationships (QSARs). The success of this process relied on the skills and intuitive powers of a medicinal chemist to prepare a relatively small number of molecules. This process can be described as 'series' synthesis.

In recent years a new approach has emerged and has matured so that currently it dominates the thinking of the major pharmaceutical companies. The process of combinatorial synthesis can be perceived as the flip-side of the rational drug design coin. It involves the parallel synthesis of a large library of compounds which is screened, either in part or in its entirety, for drug-like activity against available drug targets or suitable indicators of activity. This latter process is referred to as high-throughput screening.

Combinatorial libraries are created by combining a number of chemical building blocks in large number of different way. To illustrate the power of this approach consider a linear assembly of ten different building blocks, the number of different linear compounds that could be prepared by combining the building blocks in different ways is 10^{10}. Between 1991 and 1999 975 libraries were reported with the largest of these containing greater than a million compounds. However throughout the nineties, and despite huge efforts, lead compound attrition rates remained high and little time was cut from the R&D pipeline. During the nineties R&D expenditure doubled whilst the number of new chemical entities halved.[14,15]

So why has the attrition rate been so high and why has so little time been shaved of the drug development pipeline? There are a number of key issues:

1. combinatorial libraries contain many 'nondrug like' compounds
2. libraries lack diversity
3. inability to effectively screen the huge numbers of compounds produced against an ever-increasing number of drug targets

Combinatorial Libraries Contain Many 'Non-Drug-Like' Compounds

One commonly used system for predicting 'drug-like character' is the Lipinski 'rule of five'.[16,17] This predicts that poor adsorption and permeability of potential drug candidates will occur if:

i. the molecule contains more than five hydrogen bond donors
ii. the molecular weight is more than 500
iii. the logP is greater than 5
iv. the molecule contains more than 10 hydrogen-bond acceptors

80%-90% of current drugs fall within the limits proposed by Lipinski whilst many combinatorial libraries contain a significant proportion of compounds that fall outside.

Combinatorial Libraries Lack Diversity

The issue of diversity within libraries is increasingly of concern to industry. The nature of combinatorial chemistry results in libraries of compounds all related to a central scaffold. Additionally, practical issues that limit the range of synthetic strategies, further reduce the degree of diversity possible within a particular library.

The Inability to Screen Huge Numbers of Compounds against an Increasing Number of Targets

The issue of ineffective screening is complex. The need for reliable and reproducible drug screening protocols, with the potential for high-throughput automation, has resulted in a number of extremely elegant solutions. However, the demands on high-throughput screening continue to increase as the number of new chemical entities and potential drug targets continues to escalate. Currently ~500 drug targets are exploited in drug discovery but it is estimated that this number represent only 10% of the total number of targets that will arise from genomic studies. This statistic has major implications on the future of high-throughput drug screening.[14,18]

Drug Screening

In its simplest terms, a drug-screening test comprises a target for ligand binding and a reporter system. Currently, around 60% of drug screening processes rely on enzymatic targets and approximately 80% use UV/VIS/FLU detection technologies in the reporter system.

The Targets

In a large majority of cases the target for specific drug action is either a protein or a nucleic acids.[19-21]

Proteins

Protein drug targets can divided into three groups:
- Membrane bound receptor proteins
- Intracellular receptor proteins
- Enzymes

Membrane Bounds Receptor Proteins
G-Protein Coupled Receptors (GPCRs)

The GPCRs are the largest family of cell surface receptors and characteristically comprises of seven domains. They operate by transmitting signals to intracellular targets via the action of guanine nucleotide-binding proteins (G proteins): G-proteins comprise of three subunits α, β and γ. The receptor is closely associated with the cell membrane and winds back and forth across the bi-layer. The ligand binding site can lie extra-cellularly or within the cell membrane. When the ligand interacts with the receptor it induces conformational changes in the protein which result in intracellular binding of G-protein. This binding step destabilizes G-protein resulting in it being split into two subunit parts; $\alpha\gamma$ and β, which are then released from the receptor. The α subunit (there are many classes of G-protein and α subunit) has a number of different targets which can result in a cascade of effects (Fig. 1).

The G-protein coupled receptor family contains some of the most important drug targets including the histamine, α-adrenergic, β-adrenergic, and dopaminergic receptor types.

Kinase-Linked Receptors

Kinase-linked receptors differ from G-protein receptor in that they activate enzymes directly and do not require a G-protein intermediate. They are trans-membrane proteins with an extra-cellular ligand binding domain (N terminal), a single helical hydrophobic membrane region and an intracellular catalytic domain (C terminal) i.e., the ligand binding site and the catalytic site occupied opposite ends of the same molecule. Many members of this family undergo ligand-induced dimersiation as the first step in activation. Important examples of this type of receptor are the insulin receptor and the growth hormone receptor (Fig. 2).

Ion Channel Receptors

These (trans)membrane proteins are ligand gated ion channels. Cationic and anionic ion channels can select between different ions and in general their activation leads to the depolarization of the membrane. Well characterised and important examples include the nicotinic acetylcholine (nACh) receptor and the γ-aminobutyric acid glutamate receptor (GABA$_A$) (Fig. 3).

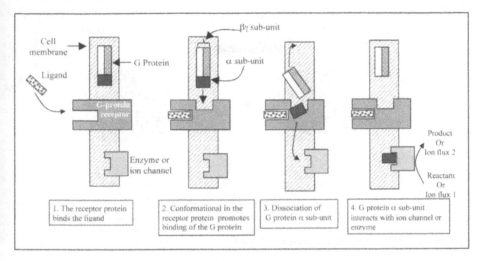

Figure 1. Mode of action of G-protein coupled receptor.

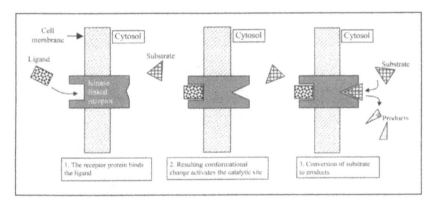

Figure 2. Mode of action of kinase linked receptor.

Intracellular Receptors

Certain ligands can have longer-term effects on cellular activity by effecting gene expression e.g., sex hormones. These ligands interact with intracellular receptors that exist in an inactive state, as 'free' receptor protein, within the cytosol or nucleus. The receptor-ligand complex then has a direct affect on gene expression. Important examples of this class of receptor are the steroidal receptors e.g., estrogen receptor and androgen receptor (Fig. 4).

Enzymes

Enzymes control all essential metabolic and anabolic processes in the body. It is therefore not surprising that many have been utilized as targets for drug action. Drugs can be used to attenuate or even amplify enzyme activity through a number of mechanisms:

    i. Competitive inhibitors: where the inhibitor competes with the substrate for the active site and can be subsequently displaced by the substrate

    ii. Noncompetitive inhibitors: brought about by the irreversible binding of the inhibitor to the active site of an enzyme

    iii. Noncompetitive, reversible inhibitors or allosteric inhibitors: such inhibitors do not bind to the active site but bind reversibly to a secondary regulatory site.

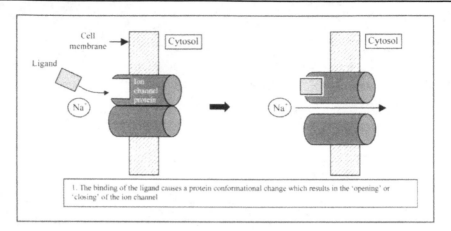

Figure 3. Mode of action of a ligand gated ion channel.

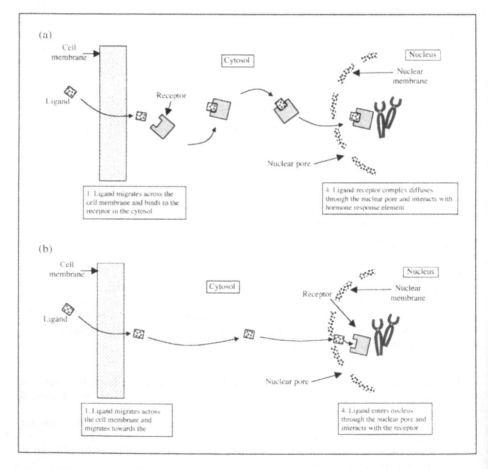

Figure 4. Mode of action of intracellular receptor (a) intracellular ligand-receptor binding (b) intranuclear ligand-receptor binding.

Table 1. Current drug targets

Target	Number of Drugs (n = 483)
GPCRs	217
Enzymes	135
Hormones and factors	53
Unknown	34
Ion channels	24
Nuclear receptors	10
DNA	10

Adapted from reference 22.

Nucleic Acids

Drugs that are targeted at the nucleic acids bring about pharmacological effect by changing cellular protein concentrations (enzyme or receptor) by affecting protein synthesis. This is an efficient mechanism through which to elicit drug action. However initiating a specific response can be an issue.

Deoxyribonucleic Acid (DNA)

The mechanism of drug action when DNA is targeted is transcription (that is the reading of the genetic code and its transfer to ribonucleic acid (RNA)) or replication (the duplication of the genetic material that occurs before cell division). Typically, drugs which target DNA can be catagorised into one of three groups:

1. intercalating agents
2. alkylating agents
3. chain cleaving agents

Intercalating agents act by slipping between base pairs causing disruption to the tertiary DNA structure. This results in 'lethal' errors in transcription or replication and subsequent cell death. This class of drugs includes the antimalarial quinine and the antibiotic and anticancer drug actinomycin D. Alkylating agents give rise to a similar effect by forming covalent attachments to either one of the bases or to the sugar-phosphate backbone. This leads to inhibition of transcription or replication due to the formation of covalent cross-links between the DNA strands or by disrupting the docking of transcriptional or replication enzymes. Cisplatin acts in this way and is used in anticancer strategies. Other drugs are capable of actually cleaving the DNA chain. One example of this type is bleomycin, a large glycoprotein anticancer drug, which causes chain cleavage and subsequent impedance of the repair mechanisms.

Ribose Nucleic Acid (RNA)

Targeting RNA has a number of advantages over targeting DNA or protein. By selectively targeting sequence specific messenger RNAs (mRNAs), protein synthesis could be attenuated in a highly controlled manner. In practice this is remains a difficult problem and RNA targeting drugs are limited mainly to a number of antibiotics. These include the aminoglycosides which act by inhibiting bacterial gene translation (transfer of genetic information from DNA to RNA prior to protein synthesis).

80% of current drugs have a protein target and of these 45% target GPCRs (Table 1).[22]

The major issue for screening is how do you practically go about screen millions of compounds against a range of potential protein and nucleic acid targets? This problem is currently growing as genomics and proteomics continue to identify new drug targets. As an example: the first draft of the human genome led to the identification of 35,000 human genes. 750 of these genes were GPCRs. It is thought that around 400 of these genes code for potential GPCR drug targets and only 30 of these are targeted by the current drugs.[23] This has major implications for the future of drug targeting and drug screening.

Screening the Targets

Broadly speaking primary screening approaches can be subdivided into a number of areas.
1. Virtual or in silico screening
2. Isolated target assays in vitro
3. Whole cell assays in vitro

In silico screening relies on computer prediction of ligand—target fit and the derivation of calculate physicochemical indicators of drug-like character, whilst the in vitro approaches aim to demonstrate target—ligand affinity via a reporter mechanism. The reporter systems range from simple heterogeneous radiolabelled-linked assays to modern reporter gene mechanisms. In general the target is nearly always recombinant human receptor or enzyme protein. There is a trend towards the use of whole cell systems in which a ligand-binding event leads to up-regulation of a transduction cascade which results in a change in expression of a reporter gene. Although the use of whole cells in drug screening adds complexity to the screening process, their use in primary screening effectively brings forward pharmacokinetic and toxicological evaluation.[24]

Molecular Imprinting and Drug Screening

The use of noncovalent molecularly imprinted polymers as synthetic mimics of biological receptor proteins was first reported by Ramstrom et al in 1994.[25] The concept was simple. Biological activity relies on highly specific interactions between a ligand and a target. This process relies on complementary chemical functionality and molecular shape. It was reasoned that when a biologically active molecule or agonist was molecularly imprinted, the imprint site would, in some way, be analogous to the biological target. On this premise it was proposed that molecules demonstrating cross-reactive binding to a molecular imprint of a biologically active molecule would themselves be potentially biologically active. The affinity of a molecule for a molecular imprint could be used as an indicator of biological activity and that MIPs could be used to select for potentially interesting molecules from large and complex libraries of compounds (Fig. 5). In the context of drug discovery, MIPs could be used in drug screening protocols instead of biological macromolecules.

Ramstrom et al's peptide receptor mimic was prepared by molecularly imprinting a methacrylic acid-coethylene glycol dimethacrylate copolymer (poly(EGMA-coMAA)) with a dipeptide (N-Ac-L-Phe-L-Trp-OMe).[25,26] This polymer was evaluated in terms of its ability to chromatographically differentiate between the stereoisomers of the template molecule. The data in Table 2 suggests that the MIP had a high degree of specificity for the template.

A subsequent publication from the Mosbach group built on the concept of molecular imprinted biological mimicry and proposed that mimics of the opioid receptor could be prepared by molecularly imprinting morphine and the endogenous neuropeptide leu-enkephalin (poly(EGMA-coMAA)). Andersson et al reported MIPs with high template affinities and similar cross-reactivity profiles to antibodies.[27] The selectivity of the morphine MIP compared favorably with antibodies both in water and in acetonitrile (Table 3). However, the leu-enkephalin MIP, whilst showing excellent selectivity in acetonitrile, was significantly less specific than antibodies when evaluated in water (Table 4).

This study was comprehensive and systematic and provided significant evidence that MIPs could be engineered that possessed binding properties analogous to those of biological systems.

A related study aimed to prepare α_2-adrenoreceptor mimics by imprinting yohimbine (poly(EGMA-coMAA)): a rauwolfia alkaloid and antagonist of the α_2 adrenoreceptor.[28] When evaluated in acetonitrile/acetic acid this polymer was shown to have a dissociation constant (K_d) for the template of 6×10^{-8}M. This compares very favorably with the reported K_d of the endogenous α_2-adrenoreceptor for yohimbine of 8.0×10^{-9}M. However, when similar studies were carried out in an aqueous environment the K_d increased to 1.2×10^{-7}M. The selectivity of

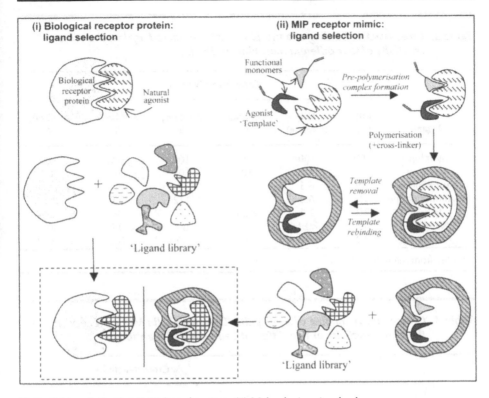

Figure 5. Ligand selection (i) Biological receptor (ii) Molecular imprinted polymer.

Table 2. Chromatographic retention factors (k') and separation factors (α) for stereoisomers of N-Ac-Phe-Trp-OMe on a N-Ac-L-Phe-L-Trp-OMe imprinted HPLC column

Methacrylic acid   Ethyleneglycol dimethacrylate

| Stereoisomers | | | | |
1	2	k'_1	k'_2	α
DD	DL	0.36	6.40	17.8
LL	LD	0.44	6.20	14.2
DL	DD	1.06	5.51	5.21
LL	LD	0.45	0.98	2.20
LD	DD	0.38	1.03	2.75
LL	DL	0.38	0.38	1.00

Adapted from reference 25.

Table 3. *Cross-reactive binding of a morphine MIP compared against the cross-reactivity of four different morphine antibodies*

Ligand	MIP (aq)	MIP (toluene)	Antibody 1	Antibody 2	Antibody 3	Antibody 4
Morphine	100	100	100	100	100	100
Codeine	25	4.7	18	104	36	<0.1
Normorphine	9.9	8.3	-	-	-	-
Hydromorphone	15	6.0	-	112	9.8	-
Heroin	8.3	2.3	<0.5	-	-	-
Naloxone	0.4	<0.1	-	0.1	0.7	<0.1
Naltrexone	0.3	<0.1	-	<<0.1	0.2	<<0.1

Adapted from reference 27.

Table 4. *Cross-reactive binding of a morphine Leu-enkephalin MIP compared against the cross-reactivity of two different Leu-enkephalin antibodies*

	MIP (aq)	MIP (MeCN)	Antibody 1	Antibody 2
Leu-enkephalin (H-Tyr-Gly-Gly-Phe-Leu-OH)	100	100	100	100
Met-enkephalin (H-Tyr-Gly-Gly-Phe-Met-OH)	68	101	122	1.4
H-Tyr-D-Ala-Gly-Phe-Leu-OH	86	<<0.1	13	36
H-Tyr-D-Ala-Gly-Phe-D-Leu-OH	55	<<0.1	<1	0.036
α-Endorphin	47	-	-	-
Gly-Gly-Phe-Leu	5.2	-	<1	0.011
Morphine	5.2	<<0.1	-	<<0.1

MeCN = Acetonitrile. Adapted from reference 27.

the yohimbine imprinted receptor mimic was assessed chromatographically and in equilibrium binding studies against corynanthine (a diastereoisomer of yohombine) (Table 5). Predictably the selectivity of the MIP for the two diastereoisomers was significantly enhanced when the porogen used in the MIP preparation was chloroform rather than the more polar methanol (Table 6). It was surprising, however, that only the yohimbine imprinted polymer discriminated between the two stereoisomers.

A further significant contribution in this area was published by Ramstrom et al.[29] This paper proposed that a β-adrenergic receptor mimic could also be prepared by imprinting a 1,1,1-Trimethylolpropane trimethacrylate-co-methacrylic acid copolymer with the nonendogenous adrenergic agonists ephedrine and pseudoephedrine. The polymers' ability to discriminate between a series of related stereoisomers (Tables 7 and 8) was evaluated by HPLC (Tables 9 and 10).

Table 5. Separation factors (α) for yohimbine and corynanthine on a number of molecularly imprinted HPLC stationary phases

	Yohimbine MIP 1	Corynanthine MIP 1	Control Polymer 1	Yohimbine MIP 2	Corynanthine MIP 2	Control Polymer 2
α	1.20	1.01	0.97	2.27	0.67	0.96

MIP1 prepared in methanol; MIP2 prepared in chloroform. Adapted from reference 28.

Table 6. High affinity and low affinity dissociation constants for yohimbine MIPs prepared in both methanol and chloroform and assayed in acetonitrile / acetic acid (CH_3CN / CH_3COOH) and an aqueous buffer

Yohimbine MIP	Ligand	Mobile Phase	K_d High Affinity Sites (μM)	K_d Low Affinity Sites (μM)
	Yohimbine	CH_3CN / CH_3COOH	47	5400
MIP1	Corynanthine	CH_3CN / CH_3COOH	330	2500
	Yohimbine	(aq) buffer	2.3	150
	Corynanthine	(aq) buffer	25	640
	Yohimbine	CH_3CN / CH_3COOH	0.06	4.8
MIP2	Corynanthine	CH_3CN / CH_3COOH	37	1300
	Yohimbine	(aq) buffer	0.12	62
	Corynanthine	(aq) buffer	5.6	170

MIP1 prepared in methanol; MIP2 prepared in chloroform. Adapted from reference 28.

Both polymers were shown to possess very high specificity for their respective templates and showed little stereochemical cross-reactivity (Table 9). Interestingly both polymers showed some enantio-selectivity for the endogenous agonist adrenaline although this was significantly less than for the template enantiomers. Additionally, and highly significantly, both MIPs were shown to be able to discriminate between the enantiomers of a number of synthetic β-adrenergic antagonists (Table 10).

Another interesting example of this type was a testosterone receptor mimic reported by Cheong at al.[30] This study uses the steroid testosterone as a template to prepare a high affinity imprinted polymer. The aim of this work was to evaluate the specificity of the testosterone imprint for a range of related compounds. Testosterone and related steroids are particularly good targets. They are rigid, conformationally restrained and possesses defined yet complex stereochemistry. Testosterone has two polar functional groups which can act as points of

Table 7. Structures of the stereoisomers of various β-adrenoreceptor ligands

1,1,1-Trimethylolpropane trimethacrylate (TRIM)

	R₁	R₂	R₃	R₄	R₅	R₆
(1S,2R)- Ephedrine	OH	H	CH₃	H	H	H
(1R,2S)- Ephedrine	H	OH	H	CH₃	H	H
(1S,2S)- Pseudoephedrine	OH	H	H	CH₃	H	H
(1R,2R)-Pseudoephedrine	H	OH	CH₃	H	H	H
(S)- Halostachine	OH	H	H	H	H	H
(R)- Halostachine	H	OH	H	H	H	H
(S)- Adrenaline	OH	H	H	H	OH	OH
(R)- Adrenaline	H	OH	H	H	OH	OH

Adapted from reference 29.

Table 8. Structures of various β-adrenoreceptor antagonists

	R1	R2
Propranolol		
Metoprolol		
Atenolol		
Timolol		

Adapted from reference 29.

Table 9. *Retention factors (K') and separation factors (α) for a number of stereoisomers of ephedrine and pseudoephidrine on a (S,R) ephedrine and a (S,S) pseudoephidrine MIPs*

Ligand	(S,R) Ephedrine MIP			(S,S) Pseudoephedrine MIP		
	K'_1	K'_2	α	K'_1	K'_2	α
Ephedrine	2.59 (R,S)	8.84 (S,R)	3.42	1.62 (R,S)	1.62 (S,.R)	1
Pseudoephedrine	2.01 (R,R)	2.29 (S,S)	1.14	2.58 (R,R)	8.22 (S,S)	3.19

Adapted from reference 29.

Table 10. *Retention factors (K') and separation factors (α) for a number of the β-adrenoreceptor agonists and antagonists on a (S,R) ephedrine and a (S,S) pseudoephidrine MIPs*

Ligand	(S,R) Ephedrine MIP			(S,S) Pseudoephedrine MIP		
	K'_1	K'_2	α	K'_1	K'_2	α
Halostachine	3.79 (R)	7.30 (S)	1.92	3.51 (R)	7.44 (S)	2.12
(R,S) Adrenaline	16.2 (R)	25.9 (S)	1.60	16.0 (R)	28.1 (S)	1.76
Propranolol	2.67 (S)	3.50 (R)	1.31	3.22 (S)	4.76 (R)	1.48
Metoprolol	2.35 (S)	3.02 (R)	1.29	2.08 (S)	3.14 (R)	1.50
Atenolol	11.6 (S)	13.5 (R)	1.15	12.3 (S)	15.9 (R)	1.29
Timolol	1.27 (S)	1.27 (R)	1.0	1.12 (S)	1.34 (R)	1.20

Adapted from reference 29.

interaction during the imprinting process. The steroids are a close-knit family of molecules based on a conserved, chiral, steroidal backbone (Fig. 6). They tend to have good solubility in apolar solvents and can contain a number of polar groups. Changes in configuration of the carbon atoms give rise to *cis* and *trans* type fused ring boundaries which have major effects on the three dimensional structure of the molecule. Additionally, the A ring (Fig. 6) can be either be aliphatic or aromatic. Again this has a profound effect on the overall 3D structure of the molecule.

By rationally and systematically probing MIP binding affinity and specificity, with a number of appropriately selected steroidal family members, a three dimensional picture of the imprinted site can be developed. Using a chromatographic approach, Cheong et al studied the effect of modification of the testosterone structure by introducing an aromatic A ring and by changing the α, β unsaturated ketone at the 3 position to a phenolic hydroxyl (this modification also means that there can be no methyl substitute at the 10 position). The effect of modifying the substituting group at the 17 position was also investigated (Fig. 7 and Table 11). In addition a degree of polymer optimization was achieved through varying polymerization temperature, cross-linker, functional monomer and template to functional monomer ratio.

They concluded that the 17-hydroxyl groups were dominant in determining the affinity of the ligand for the polymer and also that the highest separation factors were achieved with the rather high functional monomer: template ratio of 1:12. Again, the selectivity of the

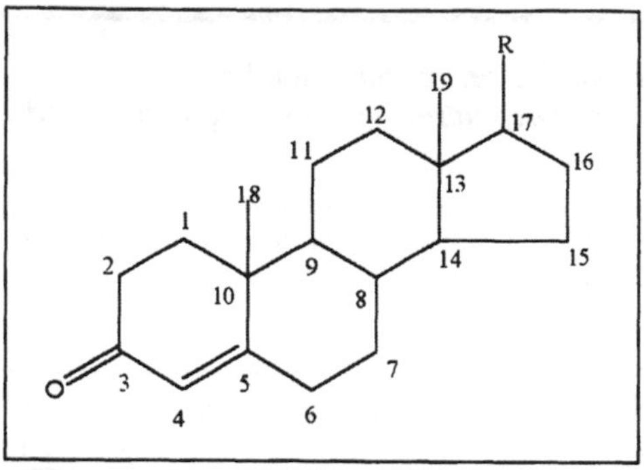

Figure 6. The steroidal backbone.

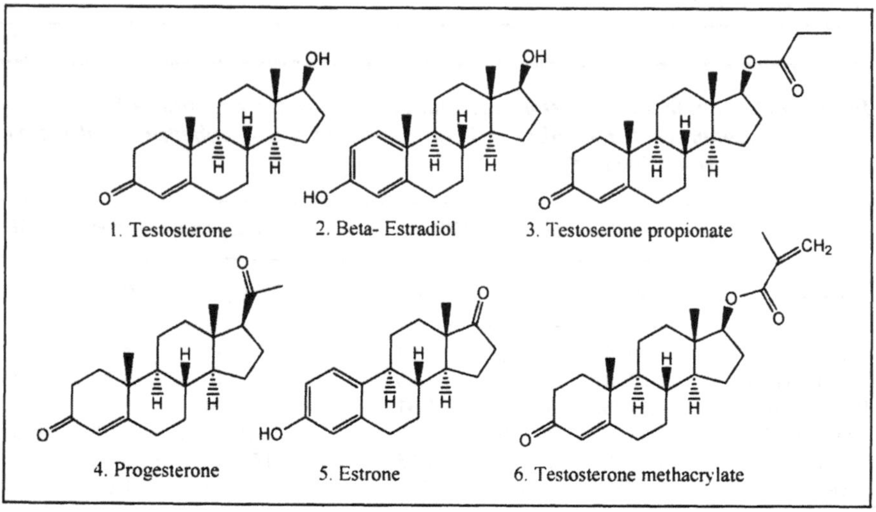

1. Testosterone   2. Beta- Estradiol   3. Testoserone propionate

4. Progesterone   5. Estrone   6. Testosterone methacrylate

Figure 7. Steroidal structures.[30]

testosterone MIP was excellent. Perhaps significantly it should be noted that the mobile phase was acetonitrile.

Berglund et al described the preparation of an α_2-adrenoreceptor mimic by imprinting the α_2-adrenoreceptor antagonist yohimbine (poly(EGMA-coMAA))[31] whilst Ramstom et al used the same approach to prepare two steroid receptor mimics by imprinting 11-a-hydroxyprogesterone and corticosterone (poly(EGMA-coMAA))[32]. In both of these cases, the aim of the researchers was to use the receptor mimics to directly screen combinatorial libraries. The α_2-adrenoreceptor mimic (yohimbine imprinted polymer) was used to screen a yohimbine selected phage display hexapeptide library whilst a commercially available steroid library was the target for the steroidal receptor mimics (11-a-hydroxyprogesterone and corticosterone imprinted polymers).

The results from the screening of the phage display peptide library demonstrated that the affinity of the yohimbine selected library for the yohimbine MIP was three-fold greater than that for the primary (nonselected) library. Of the 90 characterized phage clones in the selected library eight showed high affinity for the yohimbine imprinted polymer. The remaining clones all demonstrated low affinity. The researches took their findings one stage further and elucidated the amino acid sequence of eight of the low affinity peptide clones and five of the high affinity peptide clones. There results showed that the low affinity hexapeptides were composed of hydrophobic amino acid residues whilst the high affinity hexapeptides were composed largely of positively charged residues. Significantly four of the five high affinity hexapeptide expressing

Table 11. Chromatographic parameter for a range of steroidal molecules on three noncovalent testosterone MIPs (P1 – P3)(poly(EGMA-co-MAA))

MIP	Template: Monomer	Steroid*	K'_{imp}	α_{imp}	K'_{non}	α_{non}	I	Sa
P1	1:4	1	1.39	1	0.795	1	1.75	1
		2	1.13	1.24	0.928	0.857	1.21	1.44
		3	0.398	3.50	0.331	2.40	1.20	1.46
		4	0.530	2.63	0.464	1.71	1.14	1.53
		5	0.464	3.00	0.398	2.00	1.17	1.50
P2	1:8	1	5.10	1	1.26	1	4.05	1
		2	1.52	3.35	1.19	1.06	1.28	3.16
		3	0.597	8.55	0.464	2.72	1.28	3.16
		4	0.795	6.42	0.597	2.11	1.33	3.04
		5	0.530	9.63	0.464	2.72	1.14	3.55
P3	1:12	1	6.56	1	1.59	1	4.12	1
		2	1.92	3.42	1.26	1.26	1.52	2.71
		3	0.729	9.00	0.464	3.43	1.57	2.63
		4	1.06	6.19	0.663	2.40	1.60	2.58
		5	0.597	11.0	0.398	4.00	1.50	2.75

K'= retention factor; α= separation factors relative to testosterone; I= imprinting factor ($K'_{MI P}$ / $K'_{control}$); *Key for steroid structures Figure 1; S= selectivity factor (I_{ligand} / $I_{template}$). Adapted from reference 30.

clones had identical amino acid sequences. Initially, this data appears very exciting, however when the researchers investigated the effect further they observed that the addition of high concentrations of yohimbine had little effect on the binding of the selected library to the yohimbine imprinted polymer. Although it is possible that the concentration of yohimbine used in the experiment (0.11 μmol/ml) was too low to induce competition, the authors doubt that this was the case. It was proposed that it was more probable that the phage library had not selected for the imprinted site through a mechanism of 'best fit' but had selected for a "common regular structure" within the polymer matrix. Although the findings of this study are ultimately inconclusive, the principle of phage selection, using an imprinted material, is supported and represents an early example of the exciting interface that exists between molecular imprinted materials and biological systems.

The steroidal receptor mimics, 11-a-hydroxyprogesterone and corticosterone imprinted polymers, were evaluated chromatographically. Each polymer was used to screen a small combinatorial steroid library (Table 12) of twelve closely related steroids (differing only at positions 1, 11, and 17). The chromatographic data from this study strongly suggested that high affinity imprinted sites had been prepared for both of the templates. The data also suggested that both imprinted polymers possessed high selectivity for their respective templates but perhaps little affinity or selectivity, compared with the nonimprinted control polymer, for the rest of the library. Although the evidence is by no means conclusive it does suggest that the steroidal receptor mimics may be too selective and that better differentiation between cross-reactants would be achieved if a less specific polymer was used. Obviously this has major implications for drug-screening where a biological receptor mimic must possess a cross-reactivity profile akin to the natural target.

In two separate studies chromatographic phases were prepared that were selective for estrogenic molecules. Ye et al[33] described the preparation of four imprinted polymers: three imprinted with estrogenic steroids [11α hydroxyprogesterone and 11 deoxycortisol (A rings contain an α,β- unsaturated ketone) and 17β estradiol (A ring is aromatic)] and one with the

Table 12. Key to steroid structures

	R	Other Groups
11α-Hydroxyprogesterone	COCH₃	11 α-OH
11β-Hydroxyprogesterone	COCH₃	11 β-OH
17α- Hydroxyprogesterone	COCH₃	17 α-OH
Progesterone	COCH₃	
4-Androsten-3,17-dione	=O	
1,4-Androstadiene-3,17-dione	=O	$C_1=C_2$
Corticosterone	COCH₂OH	11 β-OH
Cortexone	COCH₂OH	
11-Deoxycortisol	COCH₂OH	17 α-OH
Cortisone	COCH₂OH	11 =O; 17 α-OH
Cortisone 21-acetate	COCH₂OAc	11 =O; 17 α-OH
Cortisol 21-acetate	COCH₂OAc	11 β_OH; 17 α-OH

Adapted from reference 32.

synthetic estrogen dienestrol, whilst Tarbin et al[34] imprinted polymers with two nonsteroidal estrogenic compounds, diethylstilbestrol and hexestrol, and one with 17β-estradiol (Fig. 8).

In general the results from both studies are aligned. The major observation being that, under chromatographic conditions, the steroidal imprinted polymers were highly selective for

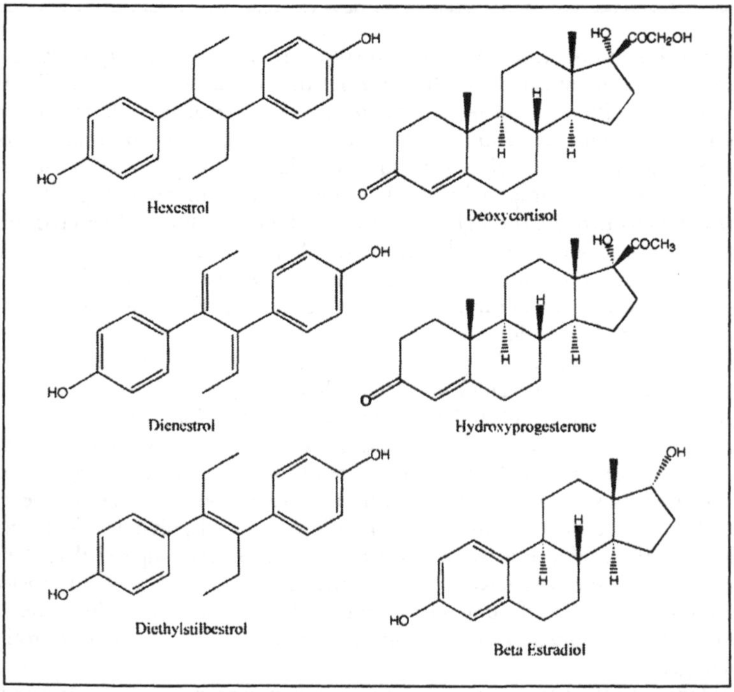

Figure 8. Estrogens and synthetic estrogen structures.

their template and showed only limited cross-reactivity for other estrogenic compounds. For both studies the estrogenic compounds studied fell into one of three groups:

1. Steroidal, aromatic A ring
2. Steroidal, nonaromatic A ring
3. Nonsteroidal

Cross-reactivity appears to occur between molecules within a group to a greater extent than between groups. Also, in the Ye study, the general level of cross-reactivity for the steroidal imprinted polymers was lower than for the dienestrol imprinted polymer. Significantly both studies were able to discriminate between 17α estradiol and 17β estradiol.

Molecularly Imprinted Receptor Mimics and Drug Screening

In general, industry has viewed molecular imprinting, and receptor mimicry in particular, with a degree of skepticism. So what would be the advantages and disadvantages of synthetic receptor mimics compared to biological systems in drug screening?

A purely synthetic drug screening system would have a number of significant advantages over a biological system. These would include lower costs, simpler protocols, improved reproducibility, longer shelf life and greater stability. Most significantly, since MIPs are prepared from robust synthetic materials, they can be formatted in a number of ways and incorporated into a range of systems and devices.[35-37] The disadvantages include:

- Low confidence in the ability of a molecular imprints to mimic a biological target
- Drug screening is moving away from simple affinity systems
- Template selection

Low Confidence in the Ability of a Molecular Imprints to Mimic a Biological Target

A molecularly imprinted primary drug screen would 'select' a potential drug candidate purely on the basis of affinity and not activity, pharmacokinetics or toxicology. This is a major issue. A number of the examples described in Section 3, rely purely on chromatographic retention parameters, usually obtained in organic solvents, as the basis for candidate selection. Considering that MIPs are commonly prepared in organic solvents, it is perhaps unsurprising that little analogy has been perceived between biology and molecular imprinting. Indeed it can reasonably be argued that ligand binding within an imprinted site in an organic solvent, has little relevance to drug screening.

Drug Screening Is Moving away from Simple Affinity Systems

It should be reemphasized that high levels of activity or affinity are only part of the story. Ideally, primary and secondary drug screens would reveal compounds that not only demonstrated activity but also possessed desirable pharmacokinetic and toxicological properties. In practice this has resulted in a move towards more comprehensive primary and secondary screening, in particular 'whole-cell', and away from simple affinity based models. This further erodes the potential of MIPs for application in primary drug screening.

Template Selection

MIP receptor mimics are prepared by imprinting a biologically active molecule. However, for a particular drug target a number of agonists and antagonists will usually be available. So which one should be imprinted? Furthermore, it is possible, considering their high levels of specificity observed,[25-34,38] that a MIP prepared in this way would only bind molecules that are very closely related to the template. In drug screening this could potentially result in nontemplate related drug candidates being 'missed'. In an industry where false positives are a nuisance but a false negative could mean missing out on the next 'block buster' drug, this represents an unacceptable level of risk.

Concluding Remarks

The problems associated with the use of MIPs in primary drug screening are significant. However, what is apparent is MIPs are able of specifically rebinding their template molecule and will also rebind template-related molecules. The evidence from many studies described in the literature is that for known agonists and antagonists the binding profiles of the MIP receptor mimics largely reflect those observed in biological systems. So is there another role for molecularly imprinted materials in drug discovery? Potentially molecularly imprinted screens, capable of selecting for related compounds, could find application in the characterisation, fractionation and focusing of large combinatorial libraries, alternatively, they may have a role in tailoring the synthesis of candidate libraries.[39] To summarise, there is currently insufficient evidence to conclude that reliable biological receptor mimics can be prepared by molecular imprinting. However, this is not the end of the story, and it is certainly not inconceivable that a fully validated comprehensive study, comparing the binding profiles of a molecular imprinted mimic and the biological target, could turn the current situation on its head.

References

1. Wulff G, Sarhan A, Zabrocki K. Enzyme-analogue built polymers and their use for the resolution of racemates. Tetrahedron Letters 1973; 4329-4332.
2. Arshady R, Mosbach K. Synthesis of substrate-selective polymers by host-guest polymerization. Macromolecular Chemistry and Physics-Makromolekulare Chemie 1981; 182:687-692.
3. Wulff G. Enzyme-like catalysis by molecularly imprinted polymers. Chem Rev 2002; 102(1):1-27
4. Ye L, Mosbach K. Molecularly imprinted materials: Towards the next generation. Molecularly Imprinted Materials-Sensors and Other Devices 2002; 723:51-59.
5. Spégel P, Schweitz L, Nilsson S. Molecularly imprinted polymers. Anal Bioanal Chem 2002; 372:37-38.
6. Nicholls IA, Rosengren JP. Molecular imprinting of surfaces. Bioseparation 2002; 10:301-305.
7. Haupt K. Creating a good impression. Nat Biotechnol 2002; 20:884-885.
8. Piletsky SA., Turner APF. Electrochemical sensors based on molecularly imprinted polymers. Electroanalysis 2002; 14:317-323.
9. Lai E. New Developments Towards the use of molecularly imprinted polymers in drug discovery. Business Briefings 2002; 92-95.
10. Wolcke J, Ullman D. Miniaturised HTS technologies -uHTS. Drug Discov Today 2001; 6(12):637-646.
11. Patrick GL. An introduction to medicinal chemistry. 2nd ed Oxford, UK: Oxford University Press, 2001.
12. King FD. (Ed) Medicinal chemistry principles and practice. 2nd ed. Cambridge, UK: Royal Society of Chemistry, 2002.
13. Thomas G. Medicinal chemistry: An introduction. UK: John Wiley & Sons, Chichester, 2000.
14. Ausman D. Creating the high-throughput mind-set. Modern Drug Discov 2001; 19-23.
15. Ausman D. Screening's age of insecurity. Modern Drug Discov 2001; 33-39.
16. Lipinski CA. Computational alerts for potential absorption problems: Profiles of clinically tested drugs. Tools for Oral Absorption. Part Two. Predicting Human Absorption. BIOTEC, PDD symposium, AAPS. Miami, FL: 1995.
17. Lipinski CA, Lombardo F, Dominy BW et al. Experimental and computational approaches to estimate solubility and permeability in drug discovery and development settings. Advanced Drug Delivery Reviews 2001; 46:3-26.
18. Ausman D. Screening's age of insecurity. Modern Drug Discovery May 2001; 33-39.
19. Waller DG, Renwick AG, Hillier K. Medical pharmacology and therapeutics. London, UK: Harcourt publishers Ltd., 2001.
20. Rang HP, Dale MM, Ritter J. Pharmacology. 3rd ed. Churchill Livingstone, Edinburgh, UK: 1995.
21. Cooper GM. The cell, a molecular approach. 2nd ed. Washington DC: ASM Press, 2000.
22. Drews J. Drug discovery: A historical perspective. Science 2000; 287:1960-1964.
23. Wise A, Gearing K, Rees S. Target validation of G-protein coupled receptors. DDT 2002; 7(4):2002.
24. In: Milligan G, ed. Signal transduction:A practical approach. Oxford, UK: Oxford University Press, 1999.
25. Ramström O, Nicholls IA, Mosbach K. Synthetic peptide receptor mimics - highly stereoselective recognition in noncovalent molecularly imprinted polymers Tetrahedron-Asymmetry.1994; 5:649-656.

26. Nicholls IA, Ramström O, Mosbach K. Insights into the role of the hydrogen-bond and hydrophobic effect on recognition in molecularly imprinted polymer synthetic peptide receptor mimics. J Chromatography A 1995; 691:349-353.
27. Andersson LI, Müller R, Vlatakis G et al. Mimics of the binding-sites of opioid receptors obtained by molecular imprinting of enkephalin and morphine. Proc Natl Acad Sci USA 1995; 92:4788-4792.
28. Berglund J, Nicholls IA, Lindbladh C et al. Recognition in molecularly imprinted polymer alpha(2)-adrenoreceptor mimics. Bioorg Med Chem Lett 1996; 6:2237-2242.
29. Ramström O, Yu C, Mosbach K. Chiral recognition in adrenergic receptor binding mimics prepared by molecular imprinting. J Mol Recognit 1996; 9:691-696.
30. Cheong SH, McNiven S, Rachkov AE et al. Testosterone receptor binding mimic constructed using molecular imprinting. Macromolecules 1997; 30:1317-1322.
31. Berglund J, Lindbladh C, Nicholls IA et al. Selection of phage display combinatorial library peptides with affinity for a yohimbine imprinted methacrylate polymer. Anal Commun 1998; 35:3-7.
32. Ramström O, Ye L, Krook M et al. Screening of a combinatorial steroid library using molecularly imprinted polymers. Anal Commun 1998; 35:9-11.
33. Ye L, Yu YH, Mosbach K. Towards the development of molecularly imprinted artificial receptors for the screening of estrogenic chemicals. Analyst 2001; 126:760-765.
34. Tarbin JA, Sharman M. Development of molecularly imprinted phase for the selective retention of stilbene-type estrogenic compounds. Analytica Chimica Acta 2001; 433:71-79.
35. Schweitz L, Andersson LI, Nilsson S. Molecular imprinting for chiral separations and drug screening purposes using monolithic stationary phases in CEC. Chromatographia 1999; 49:S93-S94.
36. Stefan RI, van Staden JKF, Aboul-Enein HY. Design and use of electrochemical sensors in enantioselective high throughput screening of drugs. A minireview. Comb Chem High Throughput Screen 2000; 3:445-454.
37. Piletsky SA, Piletska EV, Chen BN et al. Chemical grafting of molecularly imprinted homopolymers to the surface of microplates. Application of artificial adrenergic receptor in enzyme-linked assay for beta agonist determination. Anall Chem 2000; 72:4381-4385.
38. Bowman MAE, Allender CJ, Brain KR et al. A high-throughput screening technique employing molecularly imprinted polymers as biomimetic selectors, In: Reid E, Hill HM, ed. Drug-development assay approaches including molecular imprinting and biomarkers. New York: Springer-Verlag, 1998:37-43.
39. Mosbach K, Yu YH, Andersch J et al. Generation of new enzyme inhibitors using imprinted binding sites: The anti-idiotypic approach a step toward the next generation of molecular imprinting. J Am Chem Soc 2001; 123:12420-12421.

CHAPTER 13

MIPs in Biotechnology, Perspective and Reality

David A. Spivak

Abstract

O ver the last five decades, molecularly imprinted polymers (MIPs) have been important as both models and analytical tools for biotechnology. More recently, direct applications as drugs, biosensors, or bioassay materials are increasing the utility of MIPs in bio-related fields. This review will discuss some of the exciting new applications of MIPs in the biological sciences, as well as the basic concepts that make this possible.

Introduction

Since their inception, molecularly imprinted polymers (MIPs) have served biotechnology and perspectives on biotechnology. In the late 1940s, Linus Pauling and Frank Dickey discussed the origins of antibody recognition, based on an induced fit mechanism to explain the wide variety of molecules that antibodies can bind.[1] Inspired by these discussions, Dickey demonstrated induced "specific adsorption" was possible by imprinting silicate materials, and thus developed one of the first experimental models of antibody recognition.[2] These experiments provided didactic perspective on the biotechnology of antibodies and clarified the reality of the imprinting concept.

The modern age of molecular imprinting was ushered in by Wulff,[3] Shea,[4] and Mosbach;[5] who continued to advance the specific binding aspects of MIP materials in addition to pioneering efforts toward catalytic MIPs. Thus, MIPs can serve either of two types of biological models; first, MIPs created for binding and molecular recognition serve as antibody mimics or "plastic antibodies".[5] Second, MIPs created for catalysis serve as models for enzymes, and could similarly be referred to as "plastic enzymes".[7] The ability to mimic important properties of these, and other biological molecules (e.g., receptors), is the primary application of MIPs for biotechnology. This chapter reviews some key examples of how MIPs can be used in place of biomolecules in biotechnology, and even improve the performance of these applications. The organization of topics in this review begins with some of the technical advances of MIPs for biology, and continues with traditional applications of MIPs in biotechnology.

Bioactive Pharmaceuticals

Breaking new ground in recent years, MIPs have been investigated as drugs that lower cholesterol levels by sequestering and removing target compounds from the human gastrointestinal system.[8,9] The strategy is based on an established approach for treating high cholesterol levels and related diseases, where ion-exchange polymers are utilized as drugs for lowering bile acid in the gastrointestinal system (Scheme 1).[10] The polymers ingested are not absorbed into the bloodstream, and pass into the gastrointestinal system where they bind and sequester bile

Molecular Imprinting of Polymers, edited by Sergey Piletsky and Anthony Turner.
©2006 Landes Bioscience.

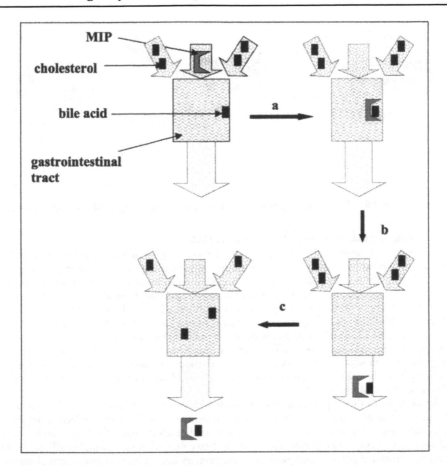

Scheme 1. Schematic representation of MIP modulated sequestration and removal of bile acids leading to lowering of cholesterol levels.

acids that are subsequently removed. Cholesterol in the body is then converted to bile acids to replace those lost, resulting in an overall lowering of cholesterol levels. To increase potency and selectivity of the polymers used, the imprinting method was applied to similar polyammonium materials using cholesterol as the template.[9] In vitro studies showed enhanced binding of cholesterol to imprinted polymers versus nonimprinted control polymers. In vivo studies were carried out in animals which also showed enhanced potency over control polymers.

Another potential pharmaceutical application of MIPs as controlled release and transdermal devices for pharmaceutical delivery has been investigated by Allender and coworkers.[11] The main problem in development of a MIP transdermal/controlled release device was the interference of water with the affinity and selectivity properties of MIP materials. To solve this problem, reduction in the water content surrounding the MIPs was achieved by embedding the MIP and drug in a secondary polymer matrix used commercially for nonpolar transdermal adhesives. Devices were prepared by adding MIP particles incorporating the drug propranolol to the adhesive; which was dried, cut to size, and pressed onto the center of a 4 cm² silicone membrane. The membrane was mounted in a Franz type diffusion cell, which was submerged in a continuously stirred water bath at physiological temperature. Samples taken over 24 hours revealed a lower flux of propranolol into the receptor phase, versus control membranes made with nonimprinted polymer. This modulation of drug permeation may have potential for controlling the flux and delivery profile of drug delivery devices.

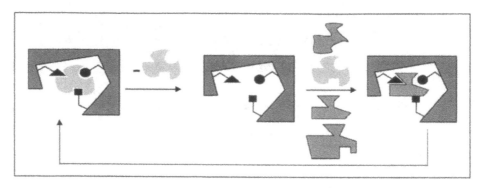

Scheme 2. Method for affinity screening of receptor-binding molecules using an MIP artificial receptor

Screening Combinatorial Drug Libraries

The essence of molecular imprinting is that it provides a general method for forming artificial receptors toward and using a target compound. This concept can be used in a strategy to screen libraries of drug compounds where the actual receptor is not available or known, but the structure of a lead compound that binds the natural receptor has been identified. In this case, an MIP can made using the lead compound as a template, which will create an artificial receptor that will bind the lead compound in a fashion similar to the real receptor, i.e., "drug-lead casting" (Scheme 2). In this way, an artificial receptor can be formed (the "cast") which can substitute for the real receptor in affinity assays. Further screening can be accomplished by using eluents with stronger and stronger elutropic strength. Remaining compounds can finally be eluted from the column and their structure analyzed. This process can be repeated until a suitable inhibitor can be found.

An example of this application was demonstrated by Mosbach, Nicholls and coworkers, who prepared an MIP that was an \alpha\-2-adrenoreceptor mimic by the molecular imprinting of yohimbine.[12] The MIP receptor-mimic was used to select high-affinity pepeptides from a phage display hexapeptide library. The selected library showed three-fold higher affinity overall for the imprinted polymer compared with the primary library. Furthermore, eight of ninety characterized phage clones from the selected library showed high affinity for the polymer. In this study, a direct correlation was seen between affinity and the number of positive charges on the hexapeptide.

High throughput analyses of inhibitor compounds are also possible using MIPs. Traditionally, the exploration for new receptor binding molecules (e.g., enzyme inhibitors or neurotransmitters) involves the systematic substitution of one functional group (i.e., an isostere) for another. These traditional or "rational" methods synthesize target compounds one at a time, and consequently assay the inhibitory properties one at a time. New methods for combinatorial synthesis of compounds have allowed the generation of large numbers of libraries of different isosteres simultaneously. Correspondingly, methods have been developed to assay these libraries simultaneously, commonly referred to as screening. One important method for screening binding properties is to use the targeted receptor for affinity chromatography techniques. If the library is eluted on a column with immobilized receptor, the library members with the strongest affinity will adhere to the column while the compounds with lower affinity are eluted from the column. For example, Remcho and coworkers have demonstrated the potential utility of MIP-based chromatographic sorbents for affinity screening of a library of structurally similar tricyclic antidepressant drugs and related compounds.[13] An MIP was elicited using one of the antidepressants, nortriptyline (NOR), library was screened using an HPLC format. The results of the study revealed that library species which possess the major structural features of the template, specifically the ring structure and pendant secondary amine, were best recognized by the MIP, while the most structurally dissimilar compounds exhibited the least selective interaction.

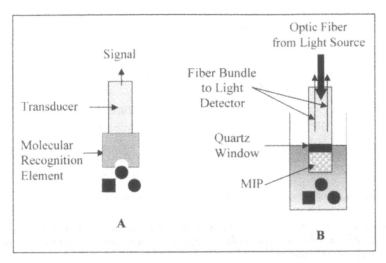

Figure 1. A) Generic format for recognition-based sensor. B) Diagram of a fluoresence optical sensor utilizing MIP recognition elements (adapted from reference 14).

Bio-(Mimetic)-Sensors

Biosensors are defined as sensors that utilize a biological molecule to carry out one or more of the following three requirements for sensors (Fig. 1):

1. Detection (e.g., binding) of a target analyte
2. Transduction of the binding event to a signal generation event
3. Signal generation corresponding to the binding event

Biological molecules used for sensor applications are usually antibodies or enzymes which can provide the initial binding event. However, these sensor devices do not have storage or operational stability, because antibodies and enzymes are easily denatured due to heat, organic solvent, pressure, excessive salts, and other denaturants. Therefore, MIPs provide an attractive alternative for biosensors (or bio-mimetic sensor) since they are more stable under these conditions. Furthermore, the MIPs can be used for detection of target analytes, and in some cases serve as the transduction and signaling event. In general, an MIP sensor should have the detection and transduction elements within close proximity; otherwise, conducting these events separately would be considered an assay. A fine early example of an MIP-based sensor was demonstrated by Kriz and coworkers, who developed a fluorescence-based optical fiber probe packed with MIP particles, diagram B in Figure 1.[14] In this example, a polymer was imprinted by traditional methods using the fluorescent template molecule, dansyl-L-phenylalanine. The polymer particles were held in place on the quartz window with a nylon net, which was attached to the fiber optic bundle for transduction (and excitation) of the fluorescent signal generated to the detector. Using this sensor, it was possible to follow concentration dependence of dansyl-L-phenylalanine solutions. Furthermore, the fiber optic device was able to show enantioselective discrimination for the L form versus dansyl-D-phenylalanine.

Another strategy for formation of a MIP sensor material employs a fluorescent monomer for signal generation from the polymer itself, which does not require the analyte be fluorescent for signal generation. This general approach to fluorescent MIP sensor materials has been demonstrated recently by Mosbach and coworkers with imprinted polymers capable of proximity scintillation (Scheme 3).[15] In this strategy, an organic scintillator (i.e., a fluor) is incorporated into the imprinted polymer matrix along with functional monomers and crosslinkers (and template). In toluene, when the imprinted polymer selectively binds a tritium-labeled template, a nearby organic scintillator is stimulated to give a fluorescent signal. A more recent example of this strategy by Lei and coworkers has eliminated the need to carry out this method

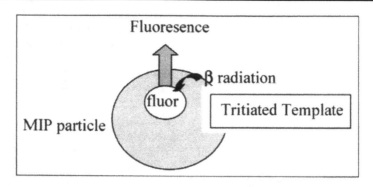

Scheme 3. Mechanism for proximity scintillation induced fluorescence in MIPs.

in aromatic solvents.[16] Many other methods for sensor apparatus and applications using MIP materials have been published, and readers interested in more examples are directed to recent review articles on MIP sensors.[5,17,18]

Biocatalysis

In order to create an antibody-like MIP artificial receptor that can bind to a target molecule, polymers are imprinted toward the actual molecule. However, in order to create an enzyme-like catalytic MIP, the strategy is more complicated. Catalytic MIPs are often made by imprinting a stable analog of a reaction's transition state, following similar methods utilized to elicit catalytic antibodies.[19] According to transition state theory put forth by Linus Pauling, receptors capable of binding intermediate transition states of a reaction will lower their overall energy of activation, and thus speed up the rate of the reaction. A typical example is the hydrolysis of an ester illustrated in Figure 2.

The transition state of the hydrolysis reaction forms a tetrahedral intermediate, with a negatively charged oxy-anion available for electrostatic binding interactions. Thus an MIP that will bind the transition state will catalyze the hydrolysis reaction. Because transition state analogs are ephemeral and unstable, a transition state analog is used as the template for imprinting, such as the phosphate compound shown in Figure 2. This strategy was used by Mosbach and Robinson,[20] who used the phosphonate compound in Figure 2 as the template to form MIPs that hydrolyze p-nitrophenol acetate (the reaction shown in Fig. 2) 1.6 fold faster than a nonimprinted control polymer. More complicated systems developed by Sellergren and Shea enabled enantioselective ester hydrolysis by MIPs.[21]

A recent biotechnological advance has been the use of MIPs cast to a transition state analog, in order to catalyze the formation of biological inhibitors in a fashion similar to that employed for combinatorial library screening. The technique, referred to as "anti-idiotypic imprinting" has been demonstrated by Mosbach and coworkers and illustrated in Scheme 4.[22] First, an MIP was cast around an enzyme inhibitor template, followed by removal of the enzyme inhibitor to leave a binding and catalytic site that is anticipated to resemble many of the features of the actual enzyme active site. Then, reactive building blocks are mixed with the MIP, which catalyzes the coupling reaction of reactive partners that bind the MIP best. This method has also been directly carried out on an enzyme by both the groups of Mosbach[23] and Sharpless.[24] Referred to as "direct molding", the building blocks are mixed with the enzyme which catalyzes the coupling of reactive partners that bind the enzyme active site best. The examples provided here show both traditional and novel application of catalytic MIPs for biotechnological applications; a recent review by Wulff provides a very thorough treatment of MIP catalysis.[25]

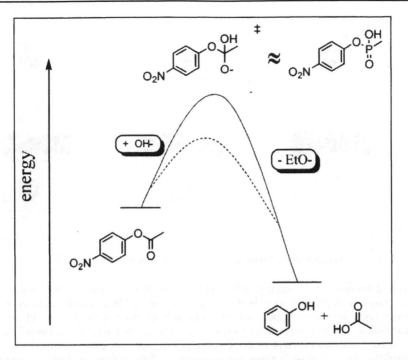

Figure 2. Energy diagram for catalyzed and uncatalyzed saponification of esters.

Bioimprinting

The molecular imprinting method has been used as a technology to improve the performance of enzymes or create them from other proteins. The method is referred to as bioimprinting, where the starting material is a protein instead of organic monomers. There are several methods reported for biohimprinting proteins. The first approach was reported by Alexander Klibanov who dissolved a protein in a concentrated aqueous solution of an organic template and subsequently freeze-dried the mixture.[26] The template was washed out using ethanol, and the resultant protein assayed for improved binding versus nonimprinted protein. This method was first tested using the protein bovine serum albumin (BSA) with para-hydroxybenzoic acid; after which imprinted BSA showed 9-fold enhanced binding versus nonimprinted protein. In this case, rebinding experiments must be carried out in solvents that will not solvate the protein and consequently allow relaxation back toward its native structure. Once the protein is exposed to water, the hydrated protein chains reassemble randomly and the templated binding site structure is lost.

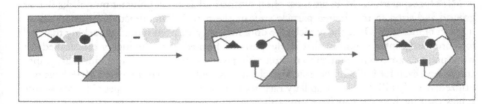

Scheme 4. Outline of the "anti-idiotypic imprinting" method.

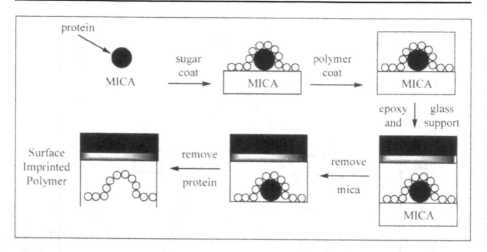

Scheme 5. Surface imprinting method utilized for proteins (adapted from reference 28).

A second approach in the bioimprinting field is to lyophilize a protein in the presence of a template molecule. A premier example of this was demonstrated by Dordick and coworkers.[27] In this approach, the enzyme subtilisin Carlsberg was lyophilized in the presence of the template thymidine. The rate of reaction of thymidine with vinylbutyrate was enhanced 50-fold versus the same reaction in the presence of nonimprinted enzyme. Using this method, it was postulated that small changes in the microenvironment of the active site of the enzyme were tailored specifically to the molecular structure of the template.

A different type of "bioimprinting" involves the imprinting of large biomolecules, such as entire proteins. Because of their large size, proteins primarily become entrapped in the imprint polymer matrix. One method to circumvent the encapsulation problem is to imprint the surfaces of polymers, thereby allowing the mass transfer of proteins to and from the imprinted sites. An example of this was demonstrated by Ratner and coworkers, who adsorbed a target protein to a mica surface (Scheme 5).[28] Next, the surface adsorbed protein is coated with a disaccharide that serves as the "functional monomer" via hydrogen bonding interactions with its hydroxy groups. The sugar coating is held in place by a layer of hexafluoropropylene, and the entire matrix epoxied to a glass support. The mica layer is peeled off, followed by solvent removal of the protein to leave nano-cavities with the imprinting effect. The future of "bioimprinting" will most likely be for materials that recognize biomolecules rather than imprinting biomolecules themselves, since the imprinted biomolecules still suffer from the same stability disadvantages as unmodified biomolecules.

Bioseparations and Bioassays

One of the first biotechnological applications, and still one of the most important, is the use of MIPs for separations. MIPs are most often synthesized as either polymer monoliths that are ground and sized to the desired particle size, or the particles are directly fabricated using a number of methods. Once the particles are obtained, they are predisposed as packing materials for chromatographic columns; that is, the particles formed from the highly crosslinked network polymer are robust enough to maintain shape and performance under chromatographic conditions, even for HPLC. There are four chromatographic formats in which MIPs have been utilized; namely HPLC, SPE, Capillary Electrophoresis, and TLC. The types of bioactive molecules used in these formats have primarily been small molecules of interest with molecular weights approximately less than 1200.[29] This is due to either slow or limited mass transfer of larger substrates into and out of the imprinted polymers, or entrapment of larger molecules within the polymer matrix during polymerization. Early reports by Wulff and Mosbach developed HPLC techniques for chiral separations molecules, one of the most challenging applications in separation science. For example, early work by the group of Wulff involved separation of enantiomeric and diastereomeric carbohyhdrate compounds.[30,31] The key to these separations was the use of vinyl phenylboronic acid as a functional monomer for binding targeted carbohydrate derivatives (e.g., Phenyl-\alpha\-D-mannopyranoside), which were positioned within a divinyl benzene matrix. Later it was determined that ethyleneglycol dimethacrylate (EGDMA) was the best crosslinker available for forming the matrix of MIPs.

Mosbach and coworkers devised easier methods for creating MIPs for chiral separations using noncovalent interactions between the template and functional monomers, eliminating any time consuming synthetic steps.[32] Using L-phenylalanine anilide as the template, MIPs were made by polymerizing the template with a mixture of monomers, methacrylic acid (MAA), and EGDMA. The MIPs were capable of enantiomeric resolution of the phenylalanine anilide enantiomers; and to this day, this monomer mixture has become the standard of MIP procedures. Using this monomer formulation, Mosbach and coworkers developed a highly successful ligand-binding assay for the drugs theophylline and diazepam, using a format similar to immuno-assays which they called a "molecularly imprinted sorbent assay" or MIA.[33] Using a radiolabeled ligand assay, the researchers were able to accurately measure theophylline levels in human serum. A molecularly imprinted sorbent assay using diazepam imprinted polymers was also investigated, and found to similar cross-reactivities as an antibody-based immunosorbent assay. More recently, Mosbach and coworkers have developed a competitive binding assay analogous to an enzyme-linked immunosorbent assay (ELISA).[34] A polymer was imprinted with the template 2,4-dichlorophenoxyacetic acid using a precipitation polymerization technique that produced molecularly imprinted microspheres. The polymer particles were "linked" to the enzyme tobacco peroxidase, which allowed for both colorimetric and chemiluminescent detection strategies. The polymer particles selectively bound the template in aqueous solution, with subsequent colorimetric or chemiluminescence generated by the tobacco peroxidase. The concentration of analyte was determined using a calibration curve, successfully demonstrating an enzyme-linked molecularly imprinted sorbent assay (ELMIA).

Conclusions: Present and Future Role of MIPs in Biotechnology

MIPs will continue to find roles in biotechnology research and development, both now and in the future. MIPs are currently finding broad use as solid phase extraction media for clean-up and preparation of biological as well as environmental samples. Similarly, there are several applications of MIPs to HPLC analysis of chiral pharmaceuticals and other bioactive molecules. Bioassays using MIPs may compete in the near future with antibody-based assays; where time, temperature, and solvent stable MIP polymer materials would be preferred over the less robust antibody-immobilized materials. Similar applications in the future of MIPs may be the utilization of these materials as the biomolecule or cell recognition components microanalytical devices, i.e., "lab-on-a-chip" analytical formats. The ability to tailor MIPs to create substrate specific catalysts coupled with the stability of MIPs may make these industrial useful, even with moderate rates of catalysis. MIPs have tremendous potential for applications as biosensors, an increasing need in the field of biology. Last, applications to drug delivery devices and even directly as pharmaceuticals are exciting prospects for biotechnological advances for MIPs.

References

1. Spivak DA, Dickey F. Personal communication. Dickey FH. Preparation of specific adsorbents. Proc Natl Acad Sci USA 1949; 35:227-229.
2. Wulff G. Polymeric Reagents and Catalysts. In: Ford T, ed. ACS Symposium Series 308. Washington: Am Chem Soc 1986:186-230.
3. Shea, Kenneth J. Molecular imprinting of synthetic network polymers: The de novo synthesis of macromolecular binding and catalytic sites. Trends in Polymer Sci 1994; 2:166-173.
4. Ekberg B, Mosbach K. Molecular imprinting: A technique for producing specific separation materials. Trends in Biotech 1989; 7:92-96.

5. Haupt K, Mosbach K. Plastic antibodies: Developments and applications. Trends in Biotech 1998; 16:468-75.
6. Wulff G, Sarhan A. Models of the receptor sites of enzymes. Studies in Organic Chemistry. Amsterdam 1982; 10:106-118.
7. Sellergren B, Wieschemeyer J, Boos KS et al. Imprinted polymers for selective adsorption of cholesterol from gastrointestinal fluids. Chem Mater 1998; 10:4037-4046.
8. Huval CC, Bailey MJ, Braunlin WH et al. Novel cholesterol lowering polymeric drugs obtained by molecular imprinting. Macromolecules 2001; 34:1548-1550.
9. Rosenbaum DP, Petersen JS, Ducharme S et al. Absorption, distribution and excretion of GT31-104, a novel bile acid sequestrant, in rats and dogs after acute and subchronic administration. J Pharm Sci 1997; 86:591-595.
10. Allender CJ, Richardson C, Woodhouse B et al. Pharmaceutical applications for molecularly imprinted polymers. Int J Pharmaceutics 2000; 195:39-43.
11. Berglund J, Lindbladh C, Mosbach K et al. Selection of phage display combinatorial library peptides with affinity for a yohimbine imprinted methacrylate polymer. Anal Comm 1998; 35:3-7.
12. Vallano PT, Remcho VT. Affinity screening by packed capillary high-performance liquid chromatography using molecular imprinted sorbents. I. Demonstration of feasibility. J Chrom A 2000; 888:23-34.
13. Kriz D, Ramstrom O, Mosbach K. Molecular imprinting. New possibilities for sensor technology Anal Chem 1997; 69:345A-349A.
14. Ye L, Mosbach K. Polymers recognizing biomolecules based on a combination of molecular imprinting and proximity scintillation: A new sensor concept. J Am Chem Soc 2001; 123:2901-2902.
15. Ye L, Surugiu I, Haupt K. Scintillation proximity assay using molecularly imprinted microspheres. Anal Chem 2002; 74:959-64.
16. Yano K, Karube I. Molecularly imprinted polymers for biosensor applications. Trends in Anal Chem 1999; 18:199-204.
17. Haupt K, Mosbach, K. Molecularly imprinted polymers and their use in biomimetic sensors. Chem Rev 2000; 100:2495-2504.
18. Lerner RA, Benkovic SJ, Schultz PG. Science 1991; 252:659-657.
19 Robinson DK, Mosbach K. Molecular imprinting of a transition state analog leads to a polymer exhibiting esterolytic activity. J Chem Soc Chem Comm 1989; 969-970.
20. Sellergren B, Karmalkar RN, Shea KJ. Enantioselective ester hydrolysis catalyzed by imprinted polymers 2. J Org Chem 2000; 65:4009-4027.
21. Mosbach K, Yu Y, Andersch J et al. Generation of new enzyme inhibitors using imprinted binding sites: The anti-idiotypic approach, a step toward the next generation of molecular imprinting. J Am Chem Soc 2001; 123:12420-12421.
22. Yu Y, Ye L, Haupt K et al. Formation of a class of enzyme inhibitors (drugs), including a chiral compound, by using imprinted polymers or biomolecules as molecular-scale reaction vessels. Angew Chem Int Ed 2002; 41:4460-4462.
23. Lewis WG, Green LG, Grynszpan F et al. Click chemistry in situ: Acetylcholinesterase as a reaction vessel for the selective assembly of a femtomolar inhibitor from an array of building blocks. Angew Chem Int Ed 2002; 41:1053-1057.
24. Wulff G. Enzyme-like catalysis by molecularly imprinted polymers. Chem Rev 2002; 102:1-27.
25. Braco L, Dabulis K, Klibanov AM. Production of abiotic receptors by molecular imprinting of proteins. Proc Natl Acad Sci USA 1990; 87:274-277.
26. Rich JO, Dordick JS. Controlling subtilisin activity and selectivity in organic media by imprinting with nucleophilic substrates. J Am Chem Soc 1997; 119:3245-3252.
27. Shi H, Tsai W-B, Garrison MD et al. Template-imprinted nanostructured surfaces for protein recognition. Nature 1999; 398:593-597.
28. Spivak DA, Shea KJ. Investigation into the scope and limitations of molecular imprinting with dna molecules. Anal Chim Acta 2001; 435:65-74.
29. Wulff G, Sarhan A, Zabrocki K. Enzyme-analogue built polymers and their use for the resolution of racemates. Tetrahedron Lett 1973; 44:4329-4332.
30. Sarhan A, Wulff G. Enzyme-analogue Built Polymers, 13. On the introduction of amino- and boronic acid groups into chiral polymer cavities. Makromol Chem 1982; 183:85-92.
31. Andersson L, Sellergren B, Mosbach K. Imprinting of amino acid derivatives in macroporous polymers. Tetrahedron Lett 1984; 25:5211-14.
32. Vlatakis G, Andersson LI, Mueller R et al. Drug assay using antibody mimics made by molecular imprinting. Nature 1993; 361:645-7.
33. Surugiu, Ioana Ye, Lei Yilmaz et al. An enzyme-linked molecularly imprinted sorbent assay. Analyst 2000; 125:13-16.

CHAPTER 14

Business Models for the Commercialisation of MIPs

Peter Leverkus

Abstract

A high priority for today's researcher is the need to extract commercial value from a new technology – and MIPs (molecularly imprinted polymers) are no exception to the rule. It is essential to understand that a technology is only of value when used in a specific application, in a market segment, by a customer. With a relatively new technology such as MIPs, customers need to be taken through a sequence of creating Awareness, Interest, Desire and Action in order to gain their commitment to using the technology. To move through this sequence, MIPs need to be marketed effectively to overcome the technical shortcomings which have previously hindered their widespread commercialisation. The optimum business model for the exploitation of MIPs will build customers' confidence in the technology, the options including:

- Contract research and consultancy
- Licensing the technology
- Selling the intellectual property
- Manufacturing MIP material
- Manufacturing MIP based components or devices

The model to be adopted will be decided by the research team's attitude to risk and the availability of funding. A "soft start" model enables a MIP business to be created with modest funding, moving from a contract research and consultancy model to become a manufacturer of MIP material or products. Such an approach would create confidence in the technology and ensure that MIPs have a bright commercial future as a platform technology.

Introduction

How do you create value from a technology which, while proven, has yet to find widespread application? It's particularly tough when the technology has been around for several years and is familiar to a relatively large proportion of the scientific community. Scepticism and doubt can rule, even though the technology may eventually pave the way for substantial improvements in the cost and performance of end products. In this chapter we will address this challenge, consider the options available to developers of Molecularly Imprinted Polymer (MIP) technology and suggest a route forward for the commercial exploitation of MIPs.

Why Commercialise?

Why is the commercialisation of a technology such a big issue? Indeed, what do we mean by "commercialisation"? The starting point has to be the financial driver, the need to earn a return on the investment which has been made to date in R&D. Most academic researchers these days

Molecular Imprinting of Polymers, edited by Sergey Piletsky and Anthony Turner.
©2006 Landes Bioscience.

realise full well that they cannot undertake publicly or privately funded research without delivering outcomes of demonstrable value. Equally, private sector researchers in all industries are finding their budgets under increasing pressure, as corporations seek to improve their bottom line profits by minimising costs – of which research is just one element.

This means that it is vital for researchers to deliver outcomes which can, in some way, earn money. If the intellectual property emerging from the research can be protected, especially in the form of patents, then immediately the researcher has a bargaining tool which has some value. But what comes next? What should the researcher and his colleagues do to create the value that we all seek?

Issues in Commercialising Technologies

It's all too easy for the scientific researcher to regard a full set of impressive experimental results as the end game. Whilst MIPs display exciting characteristics of specificity and selectivity, this alone is not enough. We need to think how we take this particular phenomenon and apply it through the hierarchy of applications, markets and customers.

A technology is only of value when it is used in an application, such as chiral separation or chemical sensing. In most cases a single technology can be used in a large number of applications, and the greater the number of applications the greater the potential value of the technology. This is where the concept of the "platform technology" arises, since it underpins a wide range of applications. Lasers are just one example, finding application in everything from CD players to eye surgery to telecommunications. Could MIPs become such a platform technology?

From applications we move to markets. A market, and its constituent segments, represents a grouping of users of the application with certain characteristics in common. For example, buyers of CDs all have an interest in music and will buy CDs through certain established channels, such as high street shops, mail order or over the internet. Within the wider music buying market, segments exist with more specific needs and purchasing patterns. These segments can be defined by age, type of music, purchase channel used, and so on. In the world of MIPs, market segments may include the "big pharma" drug manufacturers, manufacturers of separation columns or industrial sensor manufacturers.

And then we come to customers. These are the people—like you and me—who specify, choose and purchase the product. To go back up the hierarchy, groupings of customers who purchase products or services in a similar way form market segments. So the Heads of Diagnostics Research in big pharma form a market segment with an interest in purchasing new technologies which will aid their diagnostics work.

In summary, then, the market hierarchy looks like an inverted pyramid, underpinned by the core technology (Fig. 1).

In commercialising a technology, it therefore becomes apparent that there are a number of stages to go through and a number of players to interact with before serious money changes hands.

One simple aide memoire to take you through this process is AIDA:
- Awareness
- Interest
- Desire
- Action

This acronym means that, before any sale of a product or service can take place, the potential customer first has to be aware of it, then has to show an interest in it, needs to develop a desire to purchase, and finally needs to act by completing the deal.

The model is helpful in exploiting the commercial potential of MIPs. Is the research community aware of what MIP technology is and what it offers in various applications? If not, how should one create that awareness? What interest is expressed in MIPs? Do MIPs offer a sufficient advantage in performance to make it worth switching, e.g., a current separation technique from using a natural receptor to a synthetic material such as a MIP?

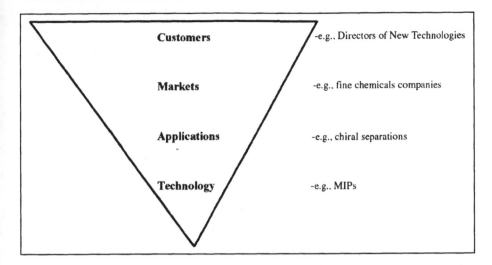

Figure 1. The hierarchy from technology to customer.

How do you create the desire to change the laboratory or production process to one based on MIPs? What types of demonstrations or trials should be carried out to create such a desire? And lastly, how do you ensure that the potential customer acts on this desire? At the end of the day, the key objective is to create value from MIPs by selling a product, system or service, which means that signing the contract is a vital step.

If the AIDA process is to be followed, there are several actions which may be taken at each step to commercialise MIPs:

Awareness

Once a MIP technology is protected by, e.g., filing a patent application, it may be promoted on various technology transfer websites or databases, such as Yet2.com. Papers may be published and patent applications filed, so publicising to the world that one is working on certain aspects of MIPs. A more proactive, focused approach would be to contact individual potential users in order to assess their specific interests in MIPs.

Interest

Developing a potential customer's interest in MIPS is likely to be through the description of some performance advantage. For example, if a specific MIP promises an improvement in selectivity in a chiral separation from an α factor of 1.5 to 5, this may be of sufficient interest to attract the attention of the scientific team. The key point is that any performance advantage offered by MIPs must be sufficient to warrant the company changing from its established, proven technique to one which is inherently of higher risk. The vital question to ask is "Do MIPs offer ten times better performance in this application?". An improvement of just 50%, although substantial, may not be enough to justify the switch to MIPs.

Interest will also be engendered by reading scientific papers, press articles and reviewing patents. In the last 10 years, the number of publications on MIPs has risen from just 15 to around 250 per annum (see Fig. 2 below). This near exponential growth is itself an expression of increased interest in MIPs by the scientific community.

Desire

The key here is to show to the potential user of MIPs that they offer specific benefits to his business. If the rapid development of a new MIP through rational, computational methods enables a new process or drug to be screened or developed faster, this will be of significant

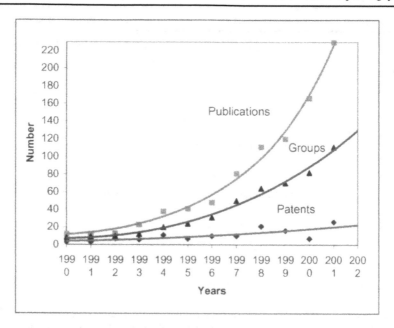

Figure 2. Growth of MIP technology (courtesy of IBST, Cranfield University).

benefit. Provision of a MIP sample to a potential customer permits him to validate published experimental results, so gaining his confidence in the technology. The intention is to stimulate the desire to act!

Action

This is the point where the MIP developer needs to formalise the commercial relationship with the customer. It will require mutual agreement on the potential benefits in order to move ahead and draft, then sign, a contract.

Challenges and Opportunities for MIPs

Whilst the preceding sections have largely dealt with the process of commercialising a new technology, there are several facets of MIPs which require special comment.

In particular, MIPs have been around a long time. One could argue that Dickey's work on silica gels in the 1940s was the first on an affinity technique using a removable template, the principle of MIPs. However the technology has really come into its own as a result of the work by Wulff and by Mosbach, starting in the 1970s. In the last 30 years the number of teams working on MIPs has grown to around 80 worldwide. The question therefore is, why have MIPs not found widespread application in industry, given such an extensive history?

One reason may be that MIPs have displayed certain shortcomings which, until recently, have proved sufficient to prevent their usage. For example, leaching of the template has been known to limit sensitivity in sensors and SPE applications and the preference for non-aqueous solvents has restricted the range of applications. At the same time, existing, competing techniques, such as chromatographic separation or diasteric crystallisation, have improved in performance. This means that MIPs have to catch and overtake a moving target.

The design of MIPs has also markedly improved recently, with the introduction of computational techniques. While previously MIPs were developed empirically over many months, rational design now allows a new MIP to be designed in a few weeks. The consequential benefits of reduced time and lower cost make MIPs far more attractive than previously.

Sceptics may also point to the improved selectivity of the range of chiral separation techniques now available. Yet, whilst biocatalysis can give 100% enantiomeric specificity, chemocatalytic processes usually deliver separation efficiencies in the purity range of 90-98%. In pharmaceutical manufacture, where chiral purity must be 100%, there is therefore a need for further "polishing" of the racemate, potentially using MIPs, to achieve the required enantiomeric purity.

These examples suggest that MIPs' time may now have come. With the extensive amount of R&D work currently underway around the world, the cost-performance package offered by MIPs is becoming increasingly attractive. What is now required is the application of MIPs in the screening, development or manufacture of a high profile drug, which will generate the publicity and credibility that MIPs need.

Which Business Model Is Right for MIPs?

We have seen above that the major hurdle for the successful commercial exploitation of MIP technology is to achieve credibility. This primarily means delivering sufficiently greater performance to justify switching from alternative diagnostic or separation techniques to MIPs. In addition, there is a need for the application under consideration to gain credibility; for example, so that MIPs become the preferred route to chiral separations following chemocatalysis. And thirdly there is the need for the research team, university or company to achieve credibility in the world of MIPs. To put it simply:

- How good is the MIP technology?
- How successful is the application?
- How strong is the team?

There are several ways to gain this credibility and we will explore them briefly here. Traditionally, academic researchers have achieved recognition through publishing scientific papers in peer-reviewed journals. Yet this approach does not generally lead to the creation of significant financial income. Other ways of proving the technology which will generate real value include:

- Contract research and consultancy
- Licensing the technology
- Selling the intellectual property
- Manufacturing MIP material
- Manufacturing MIP based components or devices

We will now look at each of these in turn, to assess their relative merits.

Contract Research and Consultancy

The quickest and lowest risk way to create a track record in MIPs is to undertake contract research assignments for industrial clients (e.g., large pharma companies). Such companies recognise the value of research and are prepared to pay for it. This is particularly the case where the company does not have the technical skills to design or produce MIP materials in-house. So the contract deliverables could range from design of a MIP material, to manufacture of small quantities of the polymer, to supply of trial quantities of packed columns. Another reason for such a client to work with a centre of MIP expertise is the availability of specialist equipment, for example for measuring the surface porosity of MIP beads, use of which will enhance the quality of the research.

A key issue here is ownership of intellectual property (IP). Very often the industrial (funding) partner will claim ownership of any IP emanating from the research, given the finance he has provided. The research team, whether academic or industrial, should ensure that the research contract clearly addresses the issue of ownership of IP, prior to the start of the work. In particular, both parties should be aware of the possibilities offered by sectoral licensing. While the industrial partner may demand exclusive rights to the technology in their core field, there may be scope to negotiate additional terms which allow the inventor to exploit the technology in other fields or sectors. This approach allows a win-win solution, whereby both the industrial partner and the research team gain from the IP generated.

Once the first contract has been successfully completed, the MIP research team is on its way to creating a track record. The only real potential barriers to continued success are the ability to market the team's skills and the possibility of conflicts of interest. For example, it would not be professionally ethical for the team to work on the same MIP development for two competing pharma companies. For academic teams, the demands of teaching and pure research may limit the time available for commercial work.

So is contract research the end game? For some it might be, as it represents a relatively low risk strategy. But the limitation is that of any fees-for-time consultancy – revenue is constrained by the headcount and the time available; for X staff charged out at £Y per hour, the maximum income is £XY per hour. So to create real value by leveraging the group's expertise, different models need to be considered.

Licensing the Technology

The increasing level of activity in patenting aspects of MIP technology suggests that research teams perceive latent value in their work. Licensing the intellectual property to interested parties, preferably by application or sector, represents a straightforward way of deriving value from the intellectual property emerging from research. However, in the case of MIPs, patents are often bound up in a web of knowhow, such that the licence alone may have little value. Only if the licensee is prepared to invest in people and time to develop their own knowhow will the licence be of great value.

In addition, the licensee may not wish to move far from their core expertise. For example, a pharma company may see its role as one of drug discovery, development and marketing and therefore be unwilling to invest in novel processes for purifying active ingredients. This would mean that the company would prefer to buy in the purified material or product, rather than license in a technology such as molecular imprinting.

Where licensing may be of greater appeal is in devices. If MIPs can be used in diagnostic devices or drug delivery systems, there will be scope to license to interested players making such products. An associated royalty deal would hold the promise of future cash inflows in the long term.

The attraction of licensing is of course that it generates cash which can be reinvested in further research. If the organisation's strategy is one of research, development and licensing, this can be a valid business model. However it may not generate the capital value that a manufacturing business could command.

An additional factor is the need to consider who will enforce the patent in the case of a potential infringement by a third party. If an academic institution has licensed its MIP technology to a big pharma company, the company may expect the institution to defend the IP in the courts of law. Yet most academic institutions do not have the financial resources to do this. Therefore the terms of the licence should identify who pays the costs of defending the patent. Of course if the patent is assigned to the company, it would be normal for the new owner of the IP to take on the obligation of defending it.

Selling the Intellectual Property

Research teams working on MIPs may wish to sell their intellectual property for one of several reasons. It is likely that they will create IP which is non-core to their MIP mission and so it may be preferable to sell the rights and generate some cash while the technology is still fresh.

Equally, the team may quit the MIPs arena or adopt a new research focus. Or it may just need cash in the short term. Whatever the reason, selling the IP is a simple way of raising cash quickly, provided that a ready buyer can be found. Yet of course, once sold, the team will need to generate new IP. This scenario suggests that sale or assignment of IP, especially if there is no significant reward, is of short term benefit only.

Manufacturing MIP Material

A natural sequel to the contract research route is to manufacture and sell MIP materials for specified applications. Pharma companies prefer to keep their research objectives and programmes secret, so it is safer for them to specify a given separation or selectivity and purchase material for their own confidential use.

This "design and manufacture" service may be a viable business model, though the quantities of materials sold for research purposes are likely to be small. Only when MIPs are used regularly in production processes will quantities move from grams to kilograms or even tonnes. This larger scale opportunity raises questions over the scalability of the process for making MIPs. Until a relatively large scale manufacturing process is demonstrated satisfactorily, scepticism will be encountered over this issue. Again, it is a question of credibility.

Manufacturing MIP Based Components or Devices

The real value added in manufacturing occurs where a more complex system is produced, especially where, as in the case of MIPs, the raw materials are generally of low cost. Such a system may be, for example, a MIP separation column or a MIP-based biosensor, where a number of materials and components are integrated. In addition, the revenue potential is greatest when these items are disposable.

Both affinity columns and biosensors represent applications of MIPs which are relatively close to market. For this reason, companies in the MIP industry are typically focusing on these opportunities. However the downside is the need to invest in manufacturing hardware, such as column packing equipment and screen printing equipment. This investment then requires a continuing sales effort to win the orders which will keep the manufacturing equipment fully utilised and earning revenues. As in most businesses, success depends on effective marketing and sales operations.

From Track Record to Turnover

When starting any new business, it is vital to have a clear vision of what the business model will be. With a new technology such as MIPs, it is helpful but not essential to have such a vision. In the same way that clients seek credibility in the MIPs offering, the supplier must build confidence based on his track record.

So how does a MIP business succeed and grow, while avoiding excessive financial or technical risks? If the vision is to manufacture, e.g., MIP biosensors in high volumes, it may be possible to raise substantial funding from venture capitalists, for investment in buildings, manufacturing plant, people and working capital, in addition to the funds needed to support R&D and marketing. The cash outflow will be high in the early stages, yet the return will hopefully be even higher as sales accumulate (Fig. 3).

Such an approach is inherently high risk, high return. Whilst the technological risk can be reduced progressively through a staged development programme, the commercial risk remains high until the first sales (and, especially, repeat sales) are made. Thus there is a heavy dependence on highly effective marketing and sales, as well as professional technical development.

An alternative approach is to develop the business more gradually, focusing initially on funding R&D and the marketing of services rather than investment in fixed assets. This "soft start" model would take a new MIP business through the stages of:

1st Contract research and consultancy

2nd Manufacturing MIP material

3rd Manufacturing MIP based components or devices

In this model, the cash exposure is more modest in the early stages, possibly financed by the founders, government grants or business angels (Fig. 4).

The financial rewards may be slightly slower in arriving than in the previous model, but the financial risks are far less. As experience accumulates, so the technological risk is reduced and the IP portfolio strengthened. Simultaneously the business' reputation in the market place is

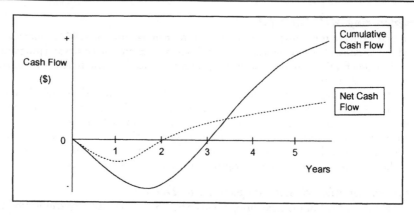

Figure 3. The high risk, high return approach to business creation.

enhanced. With an increasingly sound track record, the business will find it easier to raise the second or third round funding it will need to invest in manufacturing facilities and to expand.

Whichever model is adopted, the fundamental need is to market the business and its capabilities. Remembering the AIDA acronym, there is no point in attempting to commercialise MIPs unless you are prepared to invest in making the market aware of your offering. This means that substantial sums will need to be spent on identifying prospective customers, contacting their Technical Directors, visiting them and supporting such proactive approaches with promotional initiatives such as publishing papers, advertising in appropriate journals and exhibiting at trade fairs. This activity will create the interest in MIPs that you seek, enabling you to generate the desire to purchase your MIP products and services. The action is then for the customer to sign the contract.

This is how you build a successful MIPs business.

The Commercial Future for MIPs

The exponential increase in activity in the world of MIPs suggests that they are shortly to find their time. Whilst there will always be a need for new research in the field, MIPs will only succeed when the market is confident that molecular imprinting is a robust and credible technology. This requires pioneering entrepreneurs to establish businesses, possibly following one of the models outlined above, to convert MIPs from being a scientific novelty into a proven, large scale, platform technology.

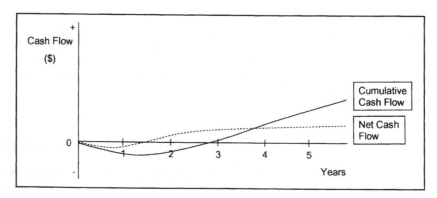

Figure 4. The "soft start" approach to business creation.

CHAPTER 15

A General Survey of Patents in the Field of Molecularly Imprinted Polymers

Jeffrey B. McIntyre[1]

This chapter presents a nonexhaustive survey of the types of subject matter for which patent protection has been sought in the field of molecularly imprinted polymers. First, a brief discussion of patents and their practical significance to corporations and universities conducting research and development in this field is provided. Then, examples of issued patents and published patent applications in this field are generally discussed.

Patents—Generally[2]

Patents are property rights conferred by governments to inventors of novel and unobvious processes or compositions. Patents basically constitute a contractual agreement between inventors and the government granting such rights: in exchange for publicly disclosing their inventions,[3] inventors are granted a short period of exclusivity during which they can exclude others from making, using or selling their inventions in the countries in which they have secured patent protection. That is, patents do not bestow upon inventors the right to practice their inventions. Rather, patents provide inventors with the right to exclude others from using or capitalizing on the inventions. In effect, when a government grants a patent, the government grants a limited monopoly.

The theory behind granting inventors a monopoly and, thus, precluding competition with respect to the patented invention for a brief period of time is that the prospect of a monopoly, albeit only a limited monopoly, provides inventors with sufficient incentive to publicly disclose their inventions. By making their inventions public, inventors add to the knowledge of the scientific community and contribute to the advancement of science and technological development. Without the limited monopoly provided by patents, inventors would not be motivated to publicly disclose their inventions and would secret them away for personal use, thereby impeding the advancement of science.

The practical effect of this monopoly power can be awesome for a patent holder or, conversely, devastating for an infringer. For example, assume two competitors exist in the market for a particular type of analytical device utilizing molecularly imprinted polymers. One company has a patent covering the device or related processes; the other company does not, but has spent several years and millions of dollars researching, developing and marketing its product. If

---

1. The author is a partner in the intellectual property law firm of Oblon, Spivak, McClelland, Maier & Neustadt, P.C., Alexandria, VA, USA.

2. The following discussion of patents is based upon U.S. patent law, although the majority of the discussion also applies to the laws of many other countries.

3. This disclosure must be sufficiently detailed to allow those skilled in the art to which the invention relates to reproduce and to practice the claimed invention without undue experimentation.

Molecular Imprinting of Polymers, edited by Sergey Piletsky and Anthony Turner.
©2006 Landes Bioscience.

the patent holder successfully asserts its patent against the competitor and obtains a ruling that the competitor has infringed its patent, not only would the patent holder be entitled to compensation for the competitor's past infringement, but it should also be entitled to an injunction prohibiting the competitor from continuing to sell its product, effectively rendering all the time, effort and money the competitor spent developing its product useless and potentially leaving the competitor without a commercial product.

Patent infringement can either be literal or under the doctrine of equivalents, and either direct or indirect. Literal infringement exists where each element in the claimed process or composition is present in an accused process or composition. Infringement under the doctrine of equivalents exists where most elements in the claimed process or composition are literally present in the accused product or process and, with respect to the remaining elements of the claimed invention, equivalent elements (that is, elements which are not substantially different from the claimed elements) exist in the accused product or process. Direct infringement exists where the accused infringer makes, sells or uses the accused product or process itself. Indirect infringement exists where the accused infringer does not directly infringe the claimed invention, but rather in some way aids, abets or encourages another to directly infringe the claimed invention.

For example, in the hypothetical above, assume the patent covers a process for making molecularly imprinted polymers using specific monomers. If the competitor uses the claimed monomers to make the polymers itself, this would constitute direct literal infringement; or if the competitor uses a slightly-modified monomer (that is, a monomer which is not substantially different from the claimed monomers) to make the polymer, such activity could constitute infringement under the doctrine of equivalents. On the other hand, if the competitor merely manufactures the claimed monomers, such activity would not infringe the patent which covers only a process for making the polymers. However, if the competitor sells the claimed monomers to customers, advertises that the monomers can be used to make molecularly imprinted polymers, and provides instruction regarding how to make the polymers, this activity would likely constitute indirect literal infringement of the patent.

In view of this background, the types of subject matter for which patent protection has been sought in the field of molecularly imprinted polymers will be now be discussed.

Patents/Patent Applications Related to Molecularly Imprinted Polymers

Patent protection has been sought for several different types of subject matter in the field of molecularly imprinted molecules including the polymers themselves, methods of making the polymers and methods of using the polymers (for example, as sensors, catalysts, separators/purifiers, etc.). This chapter discusses the types of subject matter for which patent protection has been sought;[4] however, it is neither the intent nor the purpose of this chapter to analyze, discuss or opine in any way regarding the validity, scope or enforeceability of any of the patent references discussed herein. Accordingly, to facilitate such discussion, patents/patent applications will be categorized according to the three subject matter categories set forth above and discussed in chronological order.[5]

---

4. The patents/patent applications discussed below were identified by conducting computerized searches seeking patents/patent applications in which variations of the phrase "molecularly imprinted polymers" occurred. For sake of convenience to the author, the vast majority of patent references discussed are U.S. patents. However, it should be understood that most of these patent references have non-U.S. counterparts. That is, corresponding applications were also filed in non-U.S. jurisdictions. For example, U.S. patent 6,255,461 corresponds to Australian patent application no. 2,721,797 as well as to PCT patent application publication no. 97/38015. As explained in footnote 6, filing a PCT patent application permits a patent applicant to pursue worldwide patent coverage, if desired. Thus, the patent references discussed below are for the most part representative of attempts to patent technology related to molecularly imprinted polymers in multiple jurisdictions worldwide.

Polymers

U.S. patent 5,110,833 issued May 5, 1992 to Mosbach discloses preparing synthetic enzymes and synthetic antibodies using transition state analogues and antigen-like compounds as imprint molecules.

U.S. patent 5,372,719 issued December 13, 1994 to Afeyan et al discloses molecularly imaged sorbents which reversibly bind preselcted macromoleclues via spacially matched multipoint interactions between functional groups synthesized on the sorbent surface (such as, for example, charged groups, metal coordinating groups, hydrophobic moities) and those on the macromolecule's surface.

U.S. patent 5,786,428 issued July 28, 1998 to Arnold et al discloses molecularly imprinted polymers for purification and enantiomeric resolution of amino acids and peptides based on optically active amino acids and peptides being capable of selectively chelating with metal ions that are located in complexes with other ligands inside of the imprinted cavities, where the ligands covalently anchor metal complexes in a specific orientation within a polymeric matrix allowing formation of cavities that are selective for enantiomers used in the formation of the metal complex.

U.S. patent 6,217,901 issued April 17, 2001 to Perrott et al discloses "synethetic polymer complements" ranging in size from about 20 to about 1000 nm which are prepared by contacting a template molecule with monomers within a liposome and forming a polymer surrounding the template within the liposome.

U.S. patent 6,255,461 issued July 3, 2001 to Mosbach et al discloses molecularly imprinted polymers which are artificial corticosteroid antibodies.

U.S. patent 6,274,686 issued August 14, 2001 to Mosbach et al discloses molecularly imprinted copolymers containing a polymer having a free amide group which provide for reversible binding of a target molecule.

U.S. patent 6,316,235 issued November 13, 2001 to Mosbach et al discloses molecularly imprinted polymers which contain a recognition site for the imprinted molecule and a magnetically susceptible component. These polymers are used for separation purposes. The magnetically susceptible component can be used to separate (via a magnetic field) polymers which have bound the imprint molecules.

U.S. patent 6,525,154 issued February 25, 2003 to Shea et al discloses molecularly imprinted polymers containing an amino acid sequence having an N-terminal histidine residue as well as methods of making such polymers.

Methods of Making Polymers

U.S. patent 5,310,648 issued May 10, 1994 to Arnold et al discloses a method for producing a molecularly imprinted polymer in which a complex containing chelated metal ion and enzyme is polymerized with crosslinker to imprint the polymer with enzyme and discloses a method for preparing imprinted polymers that subsequently maintain the ability to selectively bind the imprinting chemicals.

U.S. patent 5,587,273 issued December 24, 1996 to Yan et al discloses a method allowing the manufacture of thin films disposed on a substrate such as the surface of a silicon wafer in which a monomer- and imprint molecule-containing solution is placed on a substrate, the solution is evaporated, energy is applied to form a crosslinked polymer, and the imprint molecule is removed.

---

5. It should be understood that such categorization of patents/patent applications is somewhat arbitrary given that most of the patents and patent applications discussed herein can be classified as belonging to more than one of the three identified categories. For example, a patent may disclose a molecularly imprinted polymer, a method of making the polymer and a method of using the polymer, meaning that classification under any of the three categories identified above would be appropriate.

U.S. patent 5,872,198 issued February 16, 1999 to Mosbach et al discloses preparing molecularly imprinted polymer supports via suspension polymerization in which the dispersing phase is a perfluorocarbon liquid containing polyoxyethylene ester groups.

U.S. patent 5,959,050 issued September 28, 1999 to Mosbach et al discloses a method for producing molecularly imprinted polymers via suspension polymerization involving polymerizing at least two distinct acrylic monomers and an imprint molecule in a perfluorocarbon liquid containing a polyoxyethylene ester dispersing phase. Such polymerization can result in molecularly imprinted polymers in spherical form.

U.S. patent 5,994,110 issued November 30, 1999 to Mosbach et al discloses a method for producing molecularly imprinted polymers capable of binding a virus or cell that involves coating the virus or cell with a crosslinkable polymer, crosslinking the monomer, and removing the crosslinked coating from the virus or cell.

U.S. patent 6,057,377 issued May 2, 2000 to Sasaki et al discloses a method for molecularly imprinting the surface of a sol-gel material using a solution containing a sol-gel material, an imprint molecule and a functionalizing siloxane monomer. This method allows preparation of inorganic solid materials such as metal oxide sol gels.

U.S. patent 6,127,154 issued October 3, 2000 to Mosbach et al discloses a site-specific method for producing a molecularly imprinted polymer which is complementary to a target molecule or portion thereof.

U.S. patent 6,310,110 issued October 30, 2001 to Markowitz et al discloses a method for producing molecularly imprinted polymers including forming a surfactant-containing solution where the surfactant assembles to form a supramolecular structure having exposed imprint groups, combining monomer with this surfactant-containing solution, polymerizing the monomer, and removing the supramolecular structure to yield a porous material having molecularly imprinted sites.

U.S. patent 6,379,599 issued April 30, 2002 to Vaidya et al discloses a method for producing molecularly imprinted polymers useful for separating enzymes in which a crosslinked polymer is formed by reacting the enzyme of interest with monomers, crosslinkers and polymerization initiator molecules to form a crosslinked polymer, crushing the polymer so formed, and extracting the enzyme from the polymer.

U.S. patent 6,489,418 issued December 3, 2002 to Mosbach discloses a method for producing anti-idiotypic molecularly imprinted polymers in which an initial molecularly imprinted polymer is formed, the imprinted molecule is removed from the polymer, and then the polymer is mixed with monomers to form an anti-idiotypic polymer in the cavity of the original polymer, where the anti-idiotypic polymer corresponds to the original molecule.

PCT patent application publication no. WO 01/55235[6] published August 2, 2001 to Chen et al discloses a method for producing a molecularly imprinted molecule including producing a virtual library of molecular models of functional monomers having polymerizable portions and binding portions capable of binding a template, providing a molecular model of the template, screening the virtual library with the template model to identify monomers which bind to it, and using this information to create a molecularly printed polymer which binds the template.

PCT patent application publication no. WO 02/29412 published April 11, 2002 to Piletsky et al discloses a process for preparing a selective binding material for a template including preparing a solution containing the template and a carrier fluid, freezing the solution, and at least partially removing the template from the frozen composition.

---

6. PCT ("Patent Cooperation Treaty") makes it easier for inventors to file for patent protection worldwide. If an inventor files a PCT patent application, he/she will be able to prosecute his/her patent application in countries which he/she designates without having to file an original patent application in each country. Thus, filing a PCT application greatly facilitates filing patent applications in multiple countries. PCT patent applications are published 18 months after their priority date.

Methods of Using Polymers

PCT patent application publication no. WO 94/14835 published July 7, 1994 to Mosbach et al discloses a method for using molecularly imprinted polymers to synthesize and/or to selectively remove from solution stereospecific molecules.

U.S. patent 5,461,175 issued October 24, 1995 to Fischer et al discloses a method for separating enantiomers of aryloxipropanolamine derivatives in which the derivatives are contacted with a chiral solid-phase chromatography material which is a molecular imprint of an optically pure enantiomer of the derivative to be separated.

U.S. patent 5,541,342 issued July 30, 1996 to Korhonen et al discloses a method for separating enantiomers of amino acids using molecularly imprinted polymers.

U.S. patent 5,630,978 issued May 20, 1997 to Domb discloses a method for preparing mimics of biologically active compounds such as drugs which retain a desired activity but exhibit improved properties. The disclosed methods include polymerizing functional monomers around a biologically active molecule exhibiting a desired activity, removing the molecule from the polymer; and polymerizing a second class of monomers in the void left by the removed molecule. Reportedly, the prepared molecule will maintain the desired properties similar to that of the template molecule and are more stable because the polymerized monomers provide a stabilizing backbone.

U.S. patent 5,910,286 issued June 8, 1999 to Lipskier discloses a chemical sensor having a layer of molecularly imprinted polymer, where detection occurs via an acoustic wave transducer.

U.S. patent 5,942,444 issued August 24, 1999 to Rittenburg et al discloses a method for using a molecularly imprinted polymer as a marker for product identification to allow determination whether a product is genuine or counterfeit.

U.S. patent 6,068,981 issued May 30, 2000 to Rittenburg et al discloses a method for using molecularly imprinted polymers as markers to enable marking orally ingested or injected products to enable subsequent confirmation and monitoring of the marked product to assist, for example, in ensuring compliance with oral administration regimens of pharmaceuticals (drug monitoring).

U.S. patent 6,177,513 issued January 23, 2001 to Takeuchi et al discloses a method for evaluating an artificial receptor which involves forming a molecularly imprinted polymer using a first template molecule, removing the template molecule, exposing the molecularly imprinted molecule to a second template molecule which may be the same as the first template molecule or different, and then analyzing the polymer based on its binding activity with the second template.

U.S. patent 6,232,783 issued May 15, 2001 to Merrill discloses using molecularly imprinted polymers for detecting contaminants in water.

U.S. patent 6,322,834 issued November 27, 2001 to Leone discloses using molecularly imprinted polymers which recognize at least a portion of the caffeine molecule to decaffeinate an aqueous solution such as a cup of tea or coffee.

U.S. patent 6,458,599 issued October 1, 2002 to Huang discloses a method for separating macromolecules without requiring purified samples of the macromolecule by forming a molecularly imprinted polymer corresponding to a portion of the macromolecule of interest and using such polymer to capture or isolate the macromolecule from a sample.

U.S. patent 6,461,873 issued October 8, 2002 to Catania, et al discloses a caffeine detector which uses a paper strip having molecularly imprinted polymers for caffeine on one side of the strip and molecularly imprinted polymers for substances which could interfere with caffeine quantification such as theobromine on the other side.

Conclusion

Patents confer valuable, exclusive rights to inventors of novel and unobvious processes or compositions. In the field of molecularly imprinted polymers, patent protection has been sought for several different types of subject matter relating to the polymers themselves, methods for making the polymers and methods of using the polymers. As with most technologies, patents relating to molecularly imprinted polymers have evolved from being directed to broader, more general concepts (for example, WO 94/14835 which is directed to using molecularly imprinted polymers in peptide synthesis or separation) to being directed to more specific refinements and/or uses of such polymers (for example, U.S. patent 6,461,873 which is directed to using molecularly imprinted polymers in a particular type of caffeine detector or U.S. patent 6,525,154 which is directed to molecularly imprinted polymers having a specific structure). Mosbach and colleagues have been very active in seeking patent protection in this field. However, based on the number of recently-issued U.S. patents[7] to numerous different entities, it appears that patent activity in this field is increasing, and that this activity is broad-based. Given this increased activity, entities conducting research and development in this field should be mindful of the potential patent-related pitfalls which may await them in the future.

---

7. The majority of U.S. patents discussed above have numbers greater than 6,000,000, meaning that these patents have issued in the past four years (since January 1, 2000).

Index

A

Adsorption 26, 27, 31, 32, 34, 35, 41-46, 48, 67, 81, 101, 102, 107, 143-145, 159, 165, 182
Affinity 64, 66, 67, 69, 70, 81, 85, 87, 90, 91, 96, 100-102, 104, 105, 110, 112, 140, 141, 143, 145, 146, 149, 150, 170, 173, 175-177, 179, 183, 184, 194, 197
AIDA 192, 193, 198
Aldehyde 35, 42-48, 134, 136
Aldol reaction 131
Anti-idiotypic imprinting 186, 187

B

β-elimination 18, 125
Bacteria 23, 50, 55-58, 62
Basic metal oxide surface 41, 44, 48
Beads 1, 3-6, 31, 56, 62, 90, 110, 115, 118, 195
Binding isotherm 101, 102
Binding site 3, 13, 14, 16-19, 21, 23, 65, 69, 74, 92, 96, 97, 100, 101, 105, 106, 112, 114-116, 118, 125, 133, 159, 166, 187
Bioimprinting 12-19, 21-24, 57, 187, 188
Biological 50, 51, 52, 54, 56, 59, 64, 76, 80, 84, 85, 100, 101, 122, 137, 140, 144, 146, 149, 170, 171, 177, 179, 180, 182, 185, 186, 189
Biomimetic 64, 68, 84, 122, 185
Blank 86, 90, 126, 154
Bulk polymerization 149, 153, 155, 160

C

Capillary 95, 112, 149-158, 160, 161, 188
Capillary electrochromatography (CEC) 95, 114, 115, 149-153, 155-160
Capillary electrophoresis (CE) 112, 149-153, 157, 158, 160, 161, 188
Catalysis 12, 14, 19, 21, 27, 28, 32, 35, 41-43, 45, 75, 84, 110, 122, 125, 126, 131, 164, 182, 186, 189
Cationic polymerisation 4
Cell 23, 50-57, 65, 68, 84, 161, 166, 169, 170, 183, 189, 202

Chemical

Chemical sensor 35, 47, 48, 50, 51, 64, 110, 114, 118, 203
Chemical vapor deposition 28, 41, 42
Chromatography 31, 34, 50, 92, 95, 96, 100, 112, 116, 142, 145, 150, 153, 155, 159, 164, 184, 203
Coating 1, 3, 6, 7, 51, 52, 55, 87, 115, 146, 153, 157, 158, 188, 202
Column 1, 7, 55, 70, 96, 99, 102, 104, 105, 109, 110, 112, 113, 140, 141, 143-146, 149-153, 155-161, 164, 171, 184, 188, 192, 195, 197
Combinatorial synthesis 106, 165, 184
Complex 2, 4, 5, 16, 22, 23, 35, 36, 65, 67-69, 72, 73, 83, 84, 88, 97, 108, 115, 129, 131, 132, 134, 166, 167, 170, 173, 197, 201
Computational 66, 106, 107, 118, 193, 194
Core-shell nanoparticle 3
Cross-linking 1, 7, 12, 21-23, 52, 86, 87, 90, 98, 108, 141-143, 159, 202

D

Dendrimer 4
Diels-Alder reaction 124, 125, 132
Differential pulse voltammetry 69
Drug 7, 65, 75, 85, 95, 100, 110, 116, 140, 146, 159, 160, 164-167, 169, 170, 177, 179, 180, 182-184, 189, 192, 193, 195, 196, 203

E

Electrochemical 27, 30, 51, 64, 66, 67, 69-71, 74, 75, 81
Electrode 6, 30, 31, 51, 54, 58, 66-70, 73, 84
Electropolymerization 66
Emulsion 2, 3, 30, 57, 110, 111, 116, 127, 128
Enantiomer 68, 70, 95-97, 99-102, 104-106, 110, 112-118, 155, 160, 173, 189, 201, 203
Enantioseparation 160
Entropy 16, 97, 99
Enzyme 3, 4, 12, 13, 16-19, 22, 23, 26, 31, 50-52, 64-66, 70, 73, 75, 84, 101, 122, 123, 125, 127, 129, 131, 135-137, 166, 167, 169, 170, 182, 184-189, 201, 202

Enzyme mimic 129
Ester hydrolysis 186
Esterification 19
Extraction 68, 83, 95, 101, 110, 140-146, 164, 189

F

Film 1, 6, 53, 55, 57, 58, 66-68, 85-88, 110, 112-115, 117, 118, 201
Fluorescence 3, 67, 70-72, 185, 186
Fluorescent sensor 72
Fluorocarbon 4, 5
Format 1, 3, 5-7, 83, 110, 114, 140, 145, 184, 185, 188, 189
Frequency 54-56, 58, 62, 68, 69
Frontal analysis 101-104, 107
Functional monomer 2, 22, 27, 65-68, 71, 72, 97, 98, 101, 107, 108, 110, 111, 125, 126, 129, 132, 142, 143, 145, 155, 157, 160, 175, 185, 188, 189, 202, 203

G

Gate effect 71, 72, 80, 87, 88, 90, 92
Grafting 6, 59, 67, 87, 112, 114, 149

H

Hydrogel 6, 7, 128
Hydrogen bond 12, 16-19, 21, 53, 60, 72, 98, 105, 110, 115, 117, 129, 143, 144, 165, 188
Hydrophilic 3, 16, 57, 87, 110, 145, 146
Hydrophobic 3, 12, 16, 17, 19, 53, 57, 60, 143-145, 166, 176, 201

I

Immobilization 64, 67
Imprinting 1, 3-7, 12, 13, 17, 18, 22, 23, 26-28, 30-32, 34-36, 41, 50-54, 57-60, 62, 64-66, 68, 72, 73, 80, 81, 86, 88, 90, 91, 95, 97, 101, 102, 107, 108, 110, 112, 115-118, 122, 125, 127-129, 134-136, 140-142, 146, 149, 154, 158, 164, 170, 172, 175-177, 179, 180, 182-184, 186-188, 191, 196, 198, 201, 202
Initiator 6, 98, 112, 114, 202
Inorganic 2, 26, 29, 31, 32, 41, 47, 52, 56, 65, 82-84, 86, 202
Inorganic / organic hybrid material 86

Interaction 1, 3, 4, 6, 12, 13, 16-19, 22, 43, 44, 52-58, 67, 71, 81, 87, 88, 90, 91, 97, 99, 100, 102, 107, 108, 110, 115, 116, 125, 129, 130, 140, 141, 143, 144, 150, 152, 153, 157, 159, 160, 170, 175, 184, 186, 188, 189, 201
Ion pair 12, 16, 115
Ionic strength 16, 66, 105, 152
Isomer 22, 26, 28, 35, 45, 47, 48, 91, 105, 134
Isotherm 101-103, 105, 107, 159

K

Kinetic 30, 43, 72, 73, 95, 102, 123, 125, 146, 159

L

Ligand 2, 3, 12-14, 16, 18, 20, 21, 70, 102, 140, 150, 166-168, 170-175, 177, 179, 189, 201
Light 51, 56, 62, 67, 69, 158
Lipid 51
Lyophilization 12-17

M

Macroporous 30, 80-82, 86, 90, 91, 155, 161
Measurement 32, 51, 59, 67, 68, 70, 71
Mechanism 21, 29, 43-45, 81, 83, 88, 90, 97, 104, 118, 126, 143, 150, 152, 167, 169, 170, 177, 182, 186
Membrane 1, 3, 6, 51, 55, 62, 68, 71, 80-93, 95, 166, 183
Memory 66, 86, 96
Metal oxide 26, 27, 30, 31, 35, 41-44, 48, 115, 202
Methacrylate 59, 127, 128, 154
Microparticle 4, 72, 158, 161
Microstructure 1, 7, 26, 28-30, 35, 42, 55
Modification of protein 13
Molecular imprinting 7, 12, 22, 23, 26-28, 30-32, 34-36, 41, 64, 65, 73, 81, 86, 95, 108, 112, 118, 122, 141, 142, 149, 164, 170, 179, 180, 182, 184, 187, 191, 196, 198
Molecular recognition 12, 13, 16, 17, 22, 23, 43, 80, 85, 86, 92, 93, 97, 99, 108, 110, 114, 164, 182
Molecular sieve 100

Molecularly imprinted polymer (MIP) 1-3, 6, 7, 23, 50, 64-76, 85-88, 90-92, 95-103, 107-110, 112-115, 117, 122, 123, 125-136, 140-146, 149-151, 153-161, 164, 170, 172, 173, 175-177, 179, 180, 182-186, 188, 189, 191-199, 200-204
Monolithic polymer 110, 154, 155, 157, 158, 160, 161

N

Nanoparticle 2, 3, 6, 87, 110, 118, 161

O

Oligomeric 53
Optical 51, 62, 64, 67, 69, 70, 72, 75, 95, 114, 185
Organic solvent 14, 16, 17, 19, 64, 66, 83, 96, 107, 108, 140, 143-145, 155, 179, 185
Organic-inorganic composite material 82
Oxidation catalysis 35, 45

P

Particles 1-5, 7, 30, 32, 43, 52, 57, 62, 83-85, 87, 91, 92, 98, 110-114, 116, 146, 154-156, 158-161, 183, 185, 188, 189
Patents 64, 192, 193, 196, 199-204
pH 16, 66, 75, 96, 102-107, 113, 144-146, 150-152, 160
Phase inversion 6, 82, 86, 90, 91
Photoinitiator 6, 87
Polyaddition 52
Polycondensation 6, 52
Polymer morphology 52
Polymer supported reagents 133
Polymerization 4, 31, 52, 56, 59, 65-67, 69, 83, 85-88, 90, 98, 106, 108, 110, 111, 114, 116, 118, 129, 149, 150, 153-155, 157-160, 175, 188, 189, 202
Polymers 1, 2, 4-7, 12, 23, 26, 27, 30, 31, 36, 41, 50-54, 56-58, 60, 62, 64-74, 82, 83, 85-91, 95-101, 104, 105, 107, 108, 110, 112-117, 122, 123, 126-136, 140, 141, 143, 144, 146, 149, 150, 153-161, 164, 170-173, 175-179, 182-186, 188, 189, 191, 195, 199-204

Polystyrene 56, 67, 86, 89
Polyurethane 52, 54, 57, 59, 68, 70, 71
Potentiometric 51, 69, 71, 105
Precipitation polymerization 4, 110, 111, 154, 189
Protecting groups 134, 135
Protein modification 18
Proteins 4, 7, 12-19, 21-23, 50, 59-61, 64, 65, 84, 91, 122, 123, 144, 145, 150, 166, 167, 169, 170, 187, 188
Proximity scintillation 2, 72, 185, 186

Q

Quartz crystal microbalance (QCM) 6, 51, 54-56, 58, 59, 61, 68, 69, 75, 114, 115

R

Radical polymerization 52, 98
Reaction 19, 22, 26-30, 32, 34-36, 41, 42, 45, 48, 50, 52, 57, 59, 72, 75, 80, 82-84, 86, 87, 92, 101, 116, 122-126, 128, 131-134, 136, 137, 153-155, 186, 188
Receptor 1, 3-5, 12, 16, 21, 64-67, 70-73, 75, 85, 91-93, 100, 101, 118, 122, 150, 159, 166-177, 179, 180, 182-184, 186, 192, 203

S

Screening 66, 75, 85, 95, 100, 107, 161, 164-166, 169, 170, 176, 177, 179, 180, 184, 186, 195, 202
Selectivity 12, 18, 20-23, 26, 28, 31, 32, 34-36, 41, 42, 44, 45, 47, 48, 50, 51, 55, 62, 68, 70, 71, 80, 81, 83-85, 87-92, 95-97, 99-101, 104-106, 110, 112, 114, 115, 117, 122, 134, 140-144, 149, 152, 155, 157-159, 170, 172, 173, 175, 177, 183, 192, 193, 195, 197
Self-organization 50, 54, 59
Sensitivity 47, 48, 51, 54, 56, 66, 68, 69, 71, 114, 115, 194
Sensors 1, 26, 27, 31, 35, 36, 41, 47, 48, 50-52, 54-62, 64-76, 81, 87, 92, 93, 110, 114, 117, 118, 164, 185, 186, 192, 194, 200, 203
Separation 2, 22, 26, 28, 31, 43, 80-85, 87, 88-93, 95, 97, 99, 100, 105, 110, 112, 114-118, 133, 140-143, 145, 146, 149-153, 155, 157-161, 171, 173, 175, 177, 188, 189, 192-195, 197, 201, 204

Shape selectivity 28, 32, 34-36, 41, 42, 44, 45, 47, 48
Signal 51, 54, 55, 58, 64, 65, 72, 114, 166, 185
Silica 2, 3, 5-7, 12, 13, 26-36, 41-45, 47, 48, 56, 57, 86, 112-114, 128, 152-154, 161, 194
Silica overlayer 35, 36, 41, 42, 48
Solvent 2, 4-7, 12-14, 16-19, 21, 64-67, 72, 73, 82-84, 89, 96, 98, 107, 108, 112, 115, 140-146, 150, 152-155, 157, 175, 179, 185-189, 194
Spin-coating 52
Stability 22, 32, 35, 36, 41, 50-52, 56, 64-67, 69, 82-86, 95, 146, 149, 154, 164, 179, 185, 188, 189
Superporous polymers 158
Supramolecular 52, 62, 80, 82, 85, 202
Surface 2-7, 12, 16, 19, 22, 23, 26-28, 30-32, 34-36, 41-45, 47, 48, 50-62, 67-69, 71, 81, 86-88, 91, 96, 102, 110, 112-116, 127, 128, 140, 141, 143-146, 152-154, 157, 166, 188, 195, 201, 202
Surface acoustic wave (SAW) 51, 56, 69
Surfactant 2-4, 29, 57, 202
Suspension polymerization 202
Swelling 2, 4, 5, 7, 81, 86, 88, 90, 110, 145
Synthetic receptor 64, 100, 179

T

Template molecule 2, 4, 7, 17, 26, 27, 30, 32, 35, 42, 44, 45, 47, 48, 69, 71, 107, 141, 146, 160, 170, 180, 185, 188, 201, 203
Transducer 50-52, 54-56, 60, 64-67, 75, 114, 203
Transesterification 16, 34, 126, 128
Transition state analog (TSA) 16-18, 122-133, 136, 186, 201
Transport 71, 80-82, 85, 87, 88, 90-93, 115, 152

U

UV-irradiation 60

V

Van-der-Waals 53
Vapor 28, 30, 35, 41, 42, 44, 47
Virus 50, 59, 62, 202
Volatile 17, 45
Voltammetry 30, 69

Y

Yeast 52-58, 68

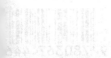

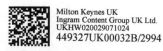